New Frontiers in Offender Treatment

Elizabeth L. Jeglic • Cynthia Calkins
Editors

New Frontiers in Offender Treatment

The Translation of Evidence-Based Practices to Correctional Settings

Springer

Editors
Elizabeth L. Jeglic
Department of Psychology
John Jay College of Criminal Justice
City University of New York
New York, NY, USA

Cynthia Calkins
Department of Psychology
John Jay College of Criminal Justice
City University of New York
New York, NY, USA

ISBN 978-3-030-01029-4 ISBN 978-3-030-01030-0 (eBook)
https://doi.org/10.1007/978-3-030-01030-0

Library of Congress Control Number: 2018962404

This Springer imprint is published by the registered company Springer Nature Switzerland AG
The registered company address is: Gewerbestrasse 11, 6330 Cham, Switzerland

This book is dedicated to the scholars, researchers and clinicians on the frontiers of offender treatment.

Acknowledgement

We would like to thank Kseniya Katsman for her incredible dedication and assistance in the publication of this book.

Contents

Chapter 1
Introduction: The Role of Evidence-Based Interventions in Forensic Settings

Elizabeth L. Jeglic and Cynthia Calkins

1.1 Introduction

In 2016, there were 2.2 million people being held in American prisons and jails representing a rate of 860 incarcerated individuals per 100,000 adults (Gramlich, 2018). While incarceration rates in the USA have been steadily declining since 2008, the USA has the highest per capita rate of incarceration in the world (Walmsley, 2016). Even though the purpose of imprisonment in the USA has always vacillated between punishment and the "rehabilitative ideal," scholars have agreed that with the introduction of policies such as mandatory sentences for drug crimes, three strikes laws, and the development of supermax prisons, the pendulum has swung largely toward the use of prison and jails as a means of punishment (Phelps, 2011). Rehabilitation these days is often just an ancillary goal.

But it wasn't always this way. Between the 1950s and 1970s, incarceration in the USA was mainly premised on the principles of rehabilitation. It was believed that those who were incarcerated could receive treatment and rehabilitative programs to "cure" them of their criminal behavior. During this time programs for education, training, and treatment were being developed. Further, new prisons were being designed and built to support this rehabilitative milieu (Garland, 2001). Education for inmates was a priority, and by 1968 11 state prison systems provided university-level programming with 13 other states planning to follow (Morris, 1968). In addition, the application of psychological theory to delinquent behavior was growing within corrections. Consequently, individual and group therapy programs, that were based primarily on psychoanalytic principles (which was the dominant psychological theory of the time), were being widely implemented in the criminal justice system in an effort to treat criminal behavior (Hollin, 2004).

E. L. Jeglic (✉) · C. Calkins
Department of Psychology, John Jay College of Criminal Justice, City University of New York, New York, NY, USA
e-mail: ejeglic@jjay.cuny.edu; ccalkins@jjay.cuny.edu

E. L. Jeglic, C. Calkins (eds.), *New Frontiers in Offender Treatment*,
https://doi.org/10.1007/978-3-030-01030-0_1

However, growing social unrest in the 1960s coupled with the rising rates of serious youth delinquency began the shift of public opinion away from rehabilitation. By the 1970s many Americans viewed rehabilitation as a means of coddling those who had committed crimes against society (Phelps, 2011). It was within this backdrop that in 1974 Robert Martinson published his seminal paper *What Works? Questions and Answers about Prison Reform* in which he presented the findings of a review of 231 studies of offender treatment programs published between 1945 and 1967. The review, which he conducted along with Douglas Lipton and Judith Wilks, was commissioned by New York State Governor's Commission on Criminal Offenders. Despite serious limitations to the methodology and quality of many of the treatments that were reviewed, Martinson (1974) concluded that "...with few and isolated exceptions the rehabilitative efforts that have been reported so far have had no appreciable effect on recidivism" (p. 25). While the media immediately caught on to the "nothing works" proclamation, little attention was paid to what Martinson (1974) said later on in his paper. More critical of the methods used to draw his conclusion, he clarified, "It is possible that some of our treatment programs are working to some extent, but that our research is so bad that it is incapable of telling" (p. 49). When the complete findings of the study were then published in 1975, it turned out that between 40 and 60% reported some degree of effectiveness (Lipton, Martinson, & Wilks, 1975).

The "nothing works" decree ushered in public support for "get tough on crime" and "war on drugs" policies in the 1980s, resulting in increased rates of incarceration, coupled with decreased funding for rehabilitative efforts which were now deemed to be ineffective (Phelps, 2011). It wasn't until Andrews, Bonta, and Hoge (1990) conducted a review with some meta-analytic calculations of the correctional treatment literature in 1990, as you will read about in Chap. 2, and concluded that "some service programs are working with at least some offenders under some circumstances" (p. 372) that rehabilitation once again became a focus of correctional interventions. They found that it was clear that some treatment approaches were better than others and thus began the era of evidence-based interventions for offenders. The Risk-Need-Responsivity (RNR) Model, first conceptualized in 1990 by Andrews, Bonta, and Hoge, has been the cornerstone of this more tailored treatment approach. Abandoning the one-size-fits-all model, the RNR approach grew out of this increasing awareness that treatment need and offender risk level should match the type of treatment offered. This required treatment providers to pay closer attention to individual characteristics so as to target programs to their specific needs. As described in Chap. 3, the development of the Good Lives Model in 2002 ushered in a new way that we have begun to think about offender treatment (Ward, 2002). Instead of the focus simply being on what offenders should avoid—in other words what they should not do—strengths-based approaches like GLM help clients work toward the goal of developing a meaningful and productive life, a goal incongruent with harm to others.

1.2 Evidence-Based Interventions

While still a relatively new concept in corrections, research examining the effectiveness of psychotherapy began in the general psychotherapy literature in the 1950s. In 1952, Hans Eysenck published the first review of 19 psychotherapy studies demonstrating treatment effects on over 7000 patients diagnosed as "neurotic" who were treated using primarily psychodynamic or eclectic interventions (Eysenck 1952). Similar to Martinson's conclusions about correctional interventions, Eysenck concluded that the studies of psychotherapy "fail to prove that psychotherapy, Freudian or otherwise, facilitates the recovery of neurotic patients. They show that roughly two-thirds of a group of neurotic patients will recover or improve to a marked extent within about two years of the onset of their illness, whether they are treated by means of psychotherapy or not." (p. 322). However, rather than dissuade further attempts to help patients, Eysenck's conclusions spurred many researchers into action to develop better interventions and evaluate them using more methodologically rigorous designs. In the next two decades, several additional reviews of the treatment outcome literature were published. These newer reviews produced more favorable outcomes, thus providing support for the effectiveness of psychotherapy in the reduction of symptoms of psychopathology and an increase in quality of life (Bergin, 1971; Emrick, 1975; Luborsky, Singer, & Luborsky, 1975). The first meta-analysis of psychotherapy outcome research was conducted in 1977 by Smith and Glass who analyzed the data from 375 studies of approximately 25,000 subjects, finding a large effect size ($d = 0.68$) for those receiving therapy as opposed to no treatment controls. The authors reported that in the studies they assessed, the average psychotherapy client was 75% better off than those who were not receiving treatment (Smith & Glass, 1977).

While the number of meta-analyses showing treatment effects continued to grow, the field of evidence practice in psychotherapy was revolutionized in 1993 when the Task Force on Promotion and Dissemination of Psychological Procedures was created by Division 12 (Clinical Psychology) of the American Psychological Association in order to determine how to disseminate information about the efficacy of psychological interventions to clinicians. This task force was established based upon a movement in the United Kingdom called evidence-based medicine (Sackett, Richardson, Rosenberg, & Haynes, 1997) which was created in response to the need to circulate current research findings to medical professionals working in the field. There were four main canons of the evidence-based medicine movement: (1) patient care would be improved with up-to-date empirical knowledge; (2) busy clinicians struggle to stay abreast with new research that is relevant to their work; (3) clinicians who do not stay well-informed of the current research will perform worse the longer they are from their initial training; and (4) clinicians need to be given easily available access to current treatment research along with directions on how these interventions should be applied with their clients (Sackett et al., 1997).

As part of the work on the task force, members were required to develop operational definitions of empirically supported treatments (ESTs) (initially referred to as empirically validated treatments). Guidelines for the defining ESTs were published by Chambless and Hollon (1998), and the task force produced a list of well-established treatments and probably efficacious treatments. While the EST movement was not without controversy, it resulted in a culture of scientific accountability and the development of further ESTs. Today there are over 80 different research-supported treatments for 17 diverse types of disorders.

In recent years, there has been a movement away from developing specific ESTs—but rather current psychotherapy researchers are focusing more on common factors and processes to create evidence-based practice (EBP; Hayes & Hofman, 2017). Evidence-based practices typically refer to those practices that are anchored in scientific knowledge. As such, evidence-based practices are more than just clinical impression or good therapeutic intention. Instead, they are practices grounded in data and methods which allow researchers to draw conclusions about whether a treatment works.

1.3 Evidence-Based Intervention within Corrections

There remains, however, a disjoint between the state of the art in the general research-based psychotherapy literature and what is being practiced in the world of corrections with forensic clients. In his Vollmer Award Address to the American Society of Criminology in 2004, Edward Latessa highlighted the challenges of bringing evidence-based practice to corrections. While he emphasized the personal and organizational impediments of changing policies and procedures at the administrative level, he also highlighted the failure of researchers and scholars to adequately disseminate what we know to those working in the field. Latessa (2004) argued that in order to get the evidence-based message out there, academics needed to go into the field and make their research more understandable and user-friendly. In addition, Latessa argued for integrating measures of program integrity and fidelity into the treatment design and providing better education, training, and supervision to future forensic clinicians.

Latessa's (2004) call to action was an impetus for developing this book. We invited expert researchers, scholars, and clinicians to discuss the exciting and cutting-edge work that they are doing and how they are translating what we know from the general psychology ligature and applying and adapting it for use with those in the criminal justice system. We view this book as a forum for them to share their work and disseminate what they know. Thus, the overarching goal of this book is to bridge this divide and demonstrate how these new and promising interventions can be used with those involved in the criminal justice system. This volume will highlight how these interventions can be used beyond targeting factors that have traditionally been thought to reduce recidivism, such as criminal thinking styles, anger, and aggression, and encompass issues related to a more holistic sense of well-being which more recent research suggests can promote desistance (Ronel & Segev, 2014).

This edited volume will be divided into three parts. In the first part, we will review current models of offender treatment including the Risk-Need-Responsivity (RNR) Model (Chap. 2), the Good Lives Model and Strengths-Based Approaches (Chap. 3), and Cognitive Behavioral Models (Chap. 4). These models will be described, and findings from treatment outcome studies integrating these models will be presented. Additionally, their role in the development of evidence-based practice with offending populations will be explained. These chapters will highlight how these models will provide the foundation for future correctional programming and how these models serve as the underpinning for new and innovative applications for use with forensic clients.

The second part of the book builds on what is known about psychotherapy process issues and how these can impact treatment outcome. One of the biggest criticisms of programs developed for criminal justice-involved clients is the lack of attention to responsivity issues, which as you will learn account for the largest proportion of change in treatment (Webb, DeRubeis, & Barber, 2010). While many of these clinical issues have been well-studied in the general psychology literature, they have been all but neglected when addressing treatment issues with clients involved in the criminal justice system. In Chap. 5, leading researchers will present research on the therapeutic alliance, how it is formed, and its importance when conducting treatment with those who have offended. Chap. 6 addresses the role of the therapist in treatment. Whereas most of the text will be dedicated to the "how" of offender treatment, this chapter focuses on the "who." While having an effective treatment is important, the treatment is only as good as the individual delivering it; thus, this chapter will review characteristics of effective therapists and therapist-related factors that may affect treatment outcome with criminal justice-involved clients, such as burnout, countertransference, and vicarious traumatization. Part II will conclude with a discussion of diversity as it applies to treatment within corrections (Chap. 7). We know from the general therapy literature that addressing issues related to diversity pertaining to issues such as race, ethnicity, gender, sexual orientation, and religion, among others all impact treatment outcome. However, there is a dearth of research on how diversity impacts treatment engagement and outcome among those who are involved in the criminal justice system. In this section we will review what is known about these clinical factors, including recent research examining these issues in forensic treatment research and avenues for future investigation and clinical training and supervision.

In the third and final part, we will present current adaptations of research-based interventions to criminal justice-involved populations. Numerous effective interventions have been identified within the evidence-based therapy movement. This section will present the work of those leading the charge in bringing these evidence-based interventions to the criminal justice system. Each chapter will present what is known about the treatment and its efficacy within the general psychotherapy research, and then the authors will present how these interventions are being adapted for use with forensically involved clients. Interventions that will be reviewed include Dialectical Behavior Therapy (Chap. 8), Trauma-Informed Care (Chap. 9), Mindfulness (Chap. 10), Motivational Interviewing (Chap. 11), Assertive Community Treatment (Chap. 12), and Multisystemic Treatment (Chap. 13). The final two chapters highlight emerging practices that are being applied to populations in the criminal justice system that have been traditionally more difficult to treat—those who perpetrate intimate partner violence (Chap. 14) and individuals with psychopathy (Chap. 15). The chapters in Part III will show how these evidence-based practices can be tailored to meet the needs of those involved in the criminal justice system. Many of these interventions have been shown to be effective in increasing motivation, treatment completion, and self-management—factors that are associated with better treatment outcome (Olver, Stockdale, & Wormith, 2011; Taxmans, Walters, Sloas, Lerch, & Rodriguez, 2015).

Psychological treatment within the criminal justice system remains a relatively new and understudied endeavor. Its history and existence are tied into the politics of rehabilitation and punishment and thus have not been without controversy. However, in this book we seek to show you that many of the same principles that have been well-researched and established in the general psychology literature can be adapted and applied to clients involved in the criminal justice system. We will conclude by integrating what we know and providing recommendations for research, teaching, and implementation of evidence-based practice with correctional populations.

References

Andrews, D. A., Bonta, J., & Hoge, R. D. (1990). Classification for effective rehabilitation: Rediscovering psychology. *Criminal Justice and Behavior, 17*(1), 19–52. https://doi.org/10.1177/0093854890017001004

Bergin, A. E. (1971). The evaluation of therapeutic outcomes. In A. E. Bergin & S. L. Garfield (Eds.), *Handbook of psychotherapy and behavior change* (pp. 217–270). New York, NY: John Wiley & Sons, Inc.

Chambless, D. L., & Hollon, S. D. (1998). Defining empirically supported therapies. *Journal of Consulting and Clinical Psychology, 66*(1), 7–18. https://doi.org/10.1037/0022-006X.66.1.7

Emrick, C. D. (1975). A review of psychologically oriented treatment of alcoholism. II. The relative effectiveness of different treatment approaches and the effectiveness of treatment versus no treatment. *Journal of Studies on Alcohol and Drugs, 36*(1), 88–108. https://doi.org/10.15288/jsa.1975.36.88

Eysenck, H. J. (1952). The effects of psychotherapy: An evaluation. *Journal of Consulting Psychology, 16*(5), 319–324. https://doi.org/10.1037/h0063633

Garland, D. (2001). *The culture of control: Crime and social order in contemporary society*. Chicago, IL: University of Chicago Press.

Gramlich, J. (2018, May 2). American's incarceration rate is at a two-decade low. Pew Research Center. Retrieved from http://www.pewresearch.org/fact-tank/2018/05/02/americas-incarceration-rate-is-at-a-two-decade-low/

Hayes, S. C., & Hofman, S. G. (2017). The third wave of cognitive behavioral therapy and the rise of process-based care. *World Psychiatry, 16*(3), 245–246. https://doi.org/10.1002/wps.20442

Hollin, C. R. (2004). To treat or not to treat? An historical perspective. In C. R. Hollin (Ed.), *The essential handbook of offender assessment and treatment* (pp. 1–16). Chichester, UK: John Wiley & Sons Ltd.

Latessa, E. D. (2004). The challenge of change: Correctional programs and evidence-based practices. *Criminology & Public Policy, 3*(4), 547–560. https://doi.org/10.1111/j.1745-9133.2004.tb00061.x

Lipton, D., Martinson, R., & Wilks, J. (1975). *The effectiveness of correctional treatment: A survey of treatment evaluation studies*. Westport, CT: Praeger Publishers.

Luborsky, L., Singer, B., & Luborsky, L. (1975). Comparative studies of psychotherapies: Is it true that "everyone has won and all must have prizes"? *Archives of General Psychiatry, 32*(8), 995–1008. https://doi.org/10.1001/archpsyc.1975.01760260059004

Martinson, R. (1974). What works? Questions and answers about prison reform. *The Public Interest, 35*, 22–54.

Morris, R. R. (1968). State programs in college education for inmates of correctional institutions. *American Journal of Corrections, 30*(2), 27–38.

Olver, M. E., Stockdale, K. C., & Wormith, J. S. (2011). A meta-analysis of predictors of offender treatment attrition and its relationship to recidivism. *Journal of Consulting and Clinical Psychology, 79*(1), 6–21. https://doi.org/10.1037/a0022200

Phelps, M. S. (2011). Rehabilitation in the punitive era: The gap between rhetoric and reality in U.S. prison programs. *Law and Society Review, 45*(1), 33–68. https://doi.org/10.1111/j.1540-5893.2011.00427.x

Ronel, N., & Segev, D. (2014). Positive criminology in practice. *International Journal of Offender Therapy and Comparative Criminology, 58*(11), 1389–1407. https://doi.org/10.1177/0306624X13491933

Sackett, D. L., Richardson, W. S., Rosenberg, W., & Haynes, R. B. (1997). *Evidence-based medicine*. New York, NY: Churchill Livingstone.

Smith, M. L., & Glass, G. V. (1977). Meta-analysis of psychotherapy outcome studies. *American Psychologist, 32*(9), 752–760. https://doi.org/10.1037/0003-066X.32.9.752

Taxmans, F. S., Walters, S. T., Sloas, L. B., Lerch, J., & Rodriguez, M. (2015). Motivation tools to improve probationer treatment outcomes. *Contemporary Clinical Trials, 43*, 120–128. https://doi.org/10.1016/j.cct.2015.05.016

Walmsley, R. (2016). *World prison population list* (11th ed.). London, UK: International Prison Publications.

Ward, T. (2002). Good lives and the rehabilitation of offenders: Promises and problems. *Aggression and Violent Behavior, 7*(5), 513–528. https://doi.org/10.1016/S1359-1789(01)00076-3

Webb, C. A., DeRubeis, R. J., & Barber, J. P. (2010). Therapists' adherence/competence and treatment outcome: A meta-analytic review. *Journal of Consulting and Clinical Psychology, 78*(2), 200–211. https://doi.org/10.1037/a0018912

Part I
Current Models of Correctional Treatment

Chapter 2
The Historical Roots, Current Status, and Future Applications of the Risk-Need-Responsivity Model (RNR)

J. Stephen Wormith and Alexandra M. Zidenberg

2.1 Introduction

The risk-need-responsivity (RNR) model is arguably the most dominant paradigm of offender programming and treatment in the field of corrections today. It is practiced by clinicians and frontline workers, not only in their intervention but in their offender assessments as well. It guides correctional policy makers and senior correctional officials. It is applicable to all demographics within the offender population, including age, race, gender, and ethnicity. Its reach has been pervasive and worldwide. It had been the subject of countless research studies and many meta-analyses, some of which contributed to its development and others to its ongoing validation. In her insightful review, Polaschek (2012) asserted that "the RNR model has made an original substantive contribution to the development of criminal justice assessment, intervention, research, programme accreditation, and programme integrity" (p. 8, emphasis in original). Yet its acceptance and adoption have not been universal. As it has grown, so too has the debate, most of which has been constructive, among academics, administrators, and practitioners.

This chapter traces the theoretical and empirical development of RNR from its historical beginning, through a number of updates and elaborations. It describes the core features of RNR, as well as the lesser known, but some would say, equally important principles that contribute to RNR being a fulsome and comprehensive model for the conceptualization, assessment, and intervention of offenders. It then reviews the implications of RNR for offender assessment and intervention practices and the extent to which RNR has impacted correctional practices since the turn of the century. Research pertaining to the development and validation of the RNR

J. S. Wormith (✉) · A. M. Zidenberg
Department of Psychology, University of Saskatchewan, Saskatoon, SK, Canada
e-mail: s.wormith@usask.ca; alexandra.zidenberg@usask.ca

E. L. Jeglic, C. Calkins (eds.), *New Frontiers in Offender Treatment*,
https://doi.org/10.1007/978-3-030-01030-0_2

model is described with particular attention to relevant meta-analyses, in part due to the very large number of individual studies that have been conducted and in part due to the capacity of meta-analyses to summarize such a substantial research literature in a fair and unbiased manner. The chapter describes some of the debate about offenders and their treatment that the RNR model has generated and some of the misunderstandings about the full RNR model. The chapter ends with an examination of the future, new directions that RNR may take us, and the kinds of research that will assist us on this important journey.

2.2 The Fundamental Principles of RNR

2.2.1 Historical Background

The story of RNR begins with the early research of Donald Andrews, a psychology professor at Carleton University in Ottawa, Canada (Wormith, 2011), which he continued with his collaborator James Bonta, from Public Safety Canada, with whom he published six editions of The *Psychology of Criminal Conduct* (Andrews & Bonta, 1994; Bonta & Andrews, 2017). The rehabilitation movement, popularized in the 1960s, had fallen into serious disrepute in the 1970s, lead in large part by Robert Martinson's (1974) scathing review of the rehabilitative ideal. Unconvinced, Andrews along with others including Paul Gendreau, Robert Ross, Herbert Quay, Ted Palmer, and Donald Gottfredson mounted a pro-rehabilitative campaign conducting and citing empirical studies that demonstrated, in varying degrees, a positive outcome of specific kinds of programming for juvenile and adult offenders (Ross & Gendreau, 1980).

What differentiated their work from the countless examples of "nothing works" with offenders was the focus of intervention that characterized these studies. Specifically, they tended to address characteristics and behavioral habits of offenders that were directly related to their offending behavior. The original and most central core of the RNR model is the concept of "criminogenic need," those dynamic aspects of the offender that contributed directly to their criminal behavior but were "dynamic" in that they were subject to change. A second apparent aspect of these successful interventions was that they tended to be behavioral in nature, reminiscent of the behavioral modification movement, as opposed to the popular, psychodynamic-driven therapeutic approach of that era and "nondirective" therapy that characterized the failure of the 1960s treatment tradition with offenders. These successful interventions also included an emerging treatment modality, cognitive-behavioral treatment that was empirically demonstrating success with a wide variety of behavioral and mental health problems. Finally, another theme was emerging with respect to successful offender intervention. Specifically, it was noted that the services offered to individuals whose contact with the law had been minimal and who did not display a plethora of serious criminogenic needs did not have an impact on what already was a low rate of recidivism. In other words, treating the compliant and willing volunteer offender was proving to be a waste of time, money, and resources, not to mention adding fuel for the nothing works doctrine.

Frustrated with failure to change the course of the nothing works debate, Andrews set to put his reading of the offender treatment research to the empirical test and did so with two important publications. The first paper (Andrews, Bonta, & Hoge, 1990) resembled a systematic review of the research on offender classification and early efforts at offender risk assessment, with some meta-analytic calculations included to illustrate what was professed in the paper, the principles of RNR and their first clearly presented definitions. First, their review provided convincing evidence for the predictive validity of six offender classification instruments that included both (static) risk and (dynamic) need factors among adult and juvenile offenders. It described 12 studies in which more service corresponded to better outcome for high-risk offenders, but no change or even poorer outcome for low-risk offenders. This leads to the development of the risk principle.

Second, it provided two illustrations of "dynamic predictive validity," whereby changes in risk (i.e., increases and decreases) from intake to some point later in time corresponded to differences in offender rates of recidivism (i.e., higher or lower than the no change offenders). It also described two studies, where changes in some attributes (antisocial attitudes, antisocial associates, antisocial personality trouble at school/home, and drug abuse) were related to commensurate differences in recidivism, whereas other offender characteristics (anxiety, low self-esteem, and empathy) were not. These latter two findings helped to solidify the need principle. Third, relying on two "box score" reviews by Hollett (1984) and Ross and Fabiano (1985), 85% of 27 studies that examined structured programs or focused on cognitive change had a positive influence on recidivism, while only 26% of the 46 unstructured, noncognitive programs had a positive impact on offender outcome. These findings lead to the principle of general responsivity.

Finally, they presented results from eight studies in which a particular kind of intervention was successful for some types of offenders, but not for others. For example, the performance of highly anxious offenders may deteriorate in highly confrontational modes of group intervention, but low-anxious offenders may profit from such a milieu (Andrews, 1980). Similarly, highly mature offenders may exhibit positive attitudinal change when exposed to highly interpersonally skilled staff, while low-maturity offenders are more likely to fail without clear rules to prevent acting out (Grant, 1965). Other client-by-type of intervention/therapist interactions identified the offender's self-control, antisocial personality, motivation, and sensation seeking as relevant characteristics to consider when planning an offender intervention. The authors also added a final caveat to these principles, one that acknowledged that criminal justice professionals may be required to look beyond these principles in making recommendations and decisions about the best means of offering the most effective services to the individual offender.

The second paper was a more fulsome true meta-analysis of concepts advanced in the first paper. Although not the first, his meta-analysis of 80 youth and adult offender treatment studies (Andrews et al., 1990) provided an optimistic and empirically defensible statement about the prospects of offender rehabilitation, although they came with a catch: treatment had to meet some important criteria in order to affect the recidivism rates of the treated offenders. However, our best interventions, when applied to our most selectively chosen offenders were capable of reducing the recidivism by up to 50%, while "inappropriate" treatment interventions that failed to follow these principles had a slightly deleterious effect on offender outcome. Collectively, these papers lead to a new mantra in corrections, namely, "what works for whom?" In other words, we must be smarter in our delivery services to offenders, both at the group and individual level.

2.2.2 Formalization of the RNR Principles

Derived from and initially coined in the two previously described papers, the principles of RNR have been popularized in three simple questions: whom to treat, what to treat, and how to treat them. More formally, they are described as follows. The risk principle states that interventions should be directed at moderate- and high-risk offenders. These interventions refer to programs, therapies, and services that are designed to reduce the likelihood of offender recidivism and not those that are offered for other humanitarian, ethical, and human rights-related reasons. Historically, there was a tendency in corrections to concentrate its resources on the most amenable, cooperative, and motivated offenders and its clinicians to focus their attention on the most receptive clientele, reminiscent of the YAVIS (young, attractive, verbal, intelligent, successful) syndrome in general community practice. These services are a poor and inefficient use of scarce financial and human resources in spite of the service providers' sense that they are having a positive impact on client outcome because of the ease with which their services are offered and the appreciativeness with which they are received.

Some versions of the risk principle cite that *only* high-risk offenders should be considered for recipients of rehabilitative interventions. Such a policy may be necessitated by a scarcity of resources to provide treatment. Another spin-off of the risk principle is that the delivery of services should vary in intensity with the highest-risk offenders receiving the greatest intensity of service, followed by moderate-risk offenders being referred to a moderate degree of intervention. Regardless of the version adapted by a correctional agency, the definition of high, moderate, and low risk, in both theoretical and operational terms, is essential. Clearly, a prerequisite of exercising the risk principle is the administration of an accurate offender risk assessment, which is reviewed below in more detail.

The need principle states that interventions should focus on those characteristics of the offender that contributed to his or her coming into conflict with the law and are likely to continue to do so if they do not change. Therefore, these characteristics must be dynamic, that is to say they must be capable of change, either naturally, for example, through maturation or spontaneous changes in the external environment or through some kind of direct intervention offered in the form of various kinds of programming, therapy, or service. Andrews and Bonta (1994) began calling these characteristics "criminogenic needs" for two reasons: one, to implicate their causal nature in contributing to criminal behavior, and two, to differentiate them with the many other legitimate human needs that offenders experience that are unrelated to the potential for further criminal behavior. The identification of legitimate criminogenic needs has proven more complicated than one might expect and has generated some considerable debate as to what offender attributes merit inclusion on this list. Implicit in the need principle is that fact that the characteristic must be a criminogenic need for the specific offender under consideration and not simply in a generic sense. In other words, referring an offender to substance abuse programming who has never abused alcohol or drugs, simply because substance abuse is a criminogenic need for many, perhaps most, offenders is not adhering to the need principle.

In their effort to identify the general and most common criminogenic needs, Andrews and Bonta (2003) identified what they referred to as the Central Eight risk/need domains for adult and youth offenders. Criminal history is a static risk domain, leaving the remaining criminogenic need domains. They are as follows: education and employment (typically for youth and adults, respectively), leisure/recreation, family (youth) and marital (adults), companions, procriminal attitudes, alcohol and drug problems, and antisocial pattern (a combination of the previous seven domains). It is also important to note what is not included in the Central Eight. This includes any demographic features of the offender (age, race, ethnicity, or gender), socioeconomic status (SES; although problems with education and employment are likely correlates of low SES), and personality characteristics such as anxiety, self-esteem, and well-being. However, the need principle allows for the identification of specific criminogenic needs that are not common, but may pertain very clearly to a particular offender, such as a person who suffers from schizophrenia and experiences violent command hallucinations, is particularly controlling or intimidating in interpersonal relationships, or harbors particularly racist or sexist attitudes. It follows that a thorough and detailed assessment of an offender's criminogenic needs is required if one plans to offer intervention that adheres to the need principle.

There are two components to the responsivity principle. The general responsivity principle states that the nature of the intervention should be based on a behavioral or cognitive-behavioral paradigm. By behavioral, they were referring to interventions that focused on overt behavior of clients and used the principles of reinforcement to change behavior, either individually as in behavior modification interventions or collectively in programs such as token economies. By cognitive-behavioral, they were referring to treatment approaches that focused on the thinking patterns of offenders and treated them as though they were explicit, identifiable, and changeable behaviors (Lipsey, Chapman, & Landenberger, 2001). As a "general" type of responsivity, this principle is meant to convey the undeniable finding that these sorts of interventions are routinely superior to other forms of intervention such as client-centered and psychodynamic therapy and therapeutic communities. Hence, it is quite straight forward and offered as a general "rule of thumb" to program administrators, clinicians, and other service providers.

The specific responsivity rule states that the treatment planner and service provider should attend to the personal characteristics of the offender that may impinge on his or her receptivity to intervention efforts. This may impact the nature of the intervention offered, the person offering it, and the style in which it is offered. Specific responsivity factors include the demographic characteristics of the offender (age, race, ethnicity, and gender), personality characteristics, (such as anxiety, psychopathy), mental health status, intellect and cognitive functioning, and motivation. This principle is founded on various type of treatment-by-type of offender and type of service provider-by-type of client interactions, in which a particular mode of intervention or characteristic of the therapist works well with one type of offender and does not, or is even harmful, with another type of offender. Together, the two prongs of responsivity ensure that the offender will absorb the maximum amount of the rehabilitative intervention that is offered.

Implicit in the principle of specific responsivity is the fact that "one size does not fit all." Rather, the style and mode of delivery of a particular intervention should be adapted to each and every individual offender. Underlying the specific responsivity principle is the very reliable finding of psychological intervention generally that positive outcome varies with the nature of the therapeutic relation between service provider and client (Horvath, Del Re, Flückiger, & Symonds, 2011). Quite likely, the ubiquity of the alliance–outcome connection in interventions generally has elevated the principle of specific responsivity from its former status as the "forgotten R" (Kennedy, 1999) during the first decade of RNR to more recently (Cohen & Whetzel, 2014). Once again, adherence to the specific responsivity principle requires a thorough and accurate assessment of the client, not just in terms of risk, but personality and interpersonal style as well. Finally, it should be noted that an offender attribute may simultaneously be both a responsivity factor and a criminogenic need. Examples include motivation, psychopathy, and some mental disorders.

2.3 RNR as a Comprehensive Model for Offender Assessment, Treatment, and Management

Not long after its initial articulation, the RNR model, as it came to be known, expanded substantially in its content and scope to offer a much more comprehensive framework for offender intervention (Andrews, 2001; Andrews & Bonta, 1994, 2010a; Bonta & Andrews, 2007, 2017). However, these additional principles have either been lost or never really integrated into the RNR model by many correctional administrators, clinicians, and other frontline practitioners. It appears that the strong, clearly articulated empirical support for the first four principles, the fact that they were promoted first, and the zeal with which agencies have rushed to implement the original tenets have led to their omission. It would appear that a large part of the criticism about the RNR model may be related to a general failure to appreciate and integrate these additional principles.

Although the number and specific description of these principles have varied over time, their themes and statements have remained consistent. In addition to the core RNR principles, they may be grouped as four types of principles (Andrews, 2011; Andrews & Bonta, 1995, 2010a; Bonta & Andrews, 2007, 2017). They are important to review for two reasons: one, most critiques of RNR appear to have been oblivious to them; two, more importantly, they have not been included or accommodated in many programs and services offered by otherwise RNR supportive agencies, which is likely to have limited the extent of their rehabilitative impact and generated even more criticism about such things as one-size-fits-all and excessively manualized interventions.

2.3.1 Overarching Principles

Four overarching principles set the stage for intervention at a political, policy, and agency level. Unlike the RNR principles that are theoretically based and empirically supported, these statements are fundamentally value-based (Andrews, 2011). First, respect for the person frames intervention and the agency and practitioners who provide it, as an ethical, legal, just, moral, humane, and decent activity. One's personal views of the offender or enthusiasm to have an impact on client outcome do not trump the rights and integrity of the offender.

Second, intervention should be theoretically based; according to Andrews and Bonta (1995) and Bonta and Andrews (2017), it should be founded on a solid psychological theory of human behavior at the individual level, as opposed to theories based on aggregated crime rates. They were particularly partial to what they coined a "general personality and cognitive social learning theory," which combines personal (disposition and attitude) and interpersonal (social) characteristics of the individual with environmental circumstances, learning opportunities, and their consequences and allows clinicians and frontline workers to better appreciate or understand how offenders have adopted an antisocial, criminal lifestyle (Bonta & Andrews, 2017).

Third, strategies that are meant to prevent or reduce criminal behavior should come through the delivery of human services and not through the sanction of the court and its reliance on deterrence. Punishment and incapacitation, by themselves, are not likely to be effective in the face of the kinds of unaddressed criminogenic needs that are described above.

Fourth, human services that are based on RNR should be widely disseminated and practiced throughout the criminal justice system and beyond, including programs found in mental health, social services, education, family services, and addictions. Stated simply, crime prevention is not the sole responsibility of the criminal justice system, and there is no reason to believe that RNR-compatible services in these related contexts will be less effective—they can be offered in a just, fair, and humane manner. In fact, the evidence is mounting in their favor (Campbell et al., 2015; Prendergast, 2009; Prendergast, Pearson, Podus, Hamilton, & Greenwell, 2013; Somers, Currie, Moniruzzaman, Eiboff, & Patterson, 2012).

2.3.2 Principles of Structured Assessment

As forewarned above, the core principles of RNR have implications for offender assessment. Consequently, four principles speak to the importance of structured offender assessment. First, the core concepts of risk, need, and responsivity must not only be assessed, but they should be assessed using a structured and validated instrument. Ideally, the validity evidence should pertain to the particular context of the assessment at hand, meaning the outcome that is being predicted, the demographic characteristics (age, race, ethnicity, and gender), and the justice context (custody, parole, sentencing, bail, probation) of the offender being assessed in the jurisdiction (state/province, country) in which he or she is being processed. This is best achieved by the development of local norms by the criminal justice agency responsible for the offender and his or her assessment. These assessments should not be based on traditional clinical (subjective) judgment, described as first-generation offender risk assessment (Andrews, Bonta, & Wormith, 2006; Bonta, 1996).

Second, in addition to the assessment of static risk factors and criminogenic needs, the assessment should also consider offender strengths and protective factors. Consideration of strengths serves three purposes. Although the evidence for their incremental predictive validity is sparse (e.g., Desmarais, Nicholls, Wilson, & Brink, 2012; Lodewijks, de Ruiter, & Doreleijers, 2010; Vincent, Chapman, & Cook, 2011), they may mitigate documented risks and needs. Further, they play an important role in the intervention process when the service provider integrates them into the interventions that are designed to challenge the offender's criminogenic needs. Lastly, the acknowledgment of strengths creates a more positive milieu for intervention and can enhance the working alliance between service provider and offender, a theme that has been advocated by proponents of the Good Lives Model (GLM) for many years (Ward, Gannon, & Birgden, 2007; Ward & Stewart, 2003b). Sadly, this principle has succeeded the responsivity principle as the most overlooked concept in the RNR model, as many proponents of the RNR model have focused exclusively on risk and needs. (Wormith & Truswell, in press).

Third, the assessment of the offender should have breadth beyond the traditional risk and need factors. It should include the assessment of noncriminogenic needs of the offender for at least three reasons. In compliance with the first overarching principle of fair, ethical, and humane treatment, the offender deserves to be assessed for outstanding needs that deserve service because they are related to basic human rights for all. Noncriminogenic needs, such as health or mental health problems, may serve as a barrier to any efforts to address criminogenic needs. Also, assisting offenders with noncriminogenic needs may facilitate the alliance between service provider and the offender or may enhance the motivation of the offender to participate in the intervention and address his or her criminogenic needs. This principle has also been widely ignored, and sometimes actively discouraged, by many supporters of the RNR model.

Fourth, professional discretion is allowed in the assessment of the offender. This principle, also known as the "override principle," was included in the initial declaration of RNR (Andrews, Bonta, & Hoge, 1990) but is also largely ignored. It allowed for deviation from the prescribed results of a structured offender assessment, but if and only if there were clearly articulated specific reasons for doing so. This concept harkens back to Meehl's (1957) "broken leg" analogy, a scenario whereby some extra-objective assessment information negates the prognostication about a particular behavior, for example, the likelihood that an offender would go out this evening and commit a burglary with his or her leg in a cast. This principle can work in either direction. An example need not be as dramatic as a broken leg. For example, a functional analysis of an offender may reveal that emotional distress, which is not generally criminogenic (Gendreau, Little, & Goggin, 1996), may be criminogenic for a particular offender (Andrews, 2011). This principle acknowledges the professional's capacity to accommodate unique client information that is out of the ordinary and makes clinical sense to consider in the assessment of the offender. However, effort to demonstrate the incremental predictive validity of the override principle has not been encouraging (Wormith, Hogg, & Guzzo, 2012). Andrews, Bonta, and Hoge's (1990) suggestion that "systematic monitoring and follow-up of the consequences of these overrides will surely be one source of new insights" (p. 44) is as true now has it was then.

2.3.3 Principles of Service Delivery

There are three principles focused on the delivery of programs and services to offenders. First, as an elaboration of the risk principle, the concept of dosage gets specific about the intensity of intervention and clarifies the point that intervention is not an all-or-none proposition. As demonstrated by Bourgon and Armstrong (2005) and Sperber, Latessa, and Makarios (2013a, 2013b), the most intensive interventions, typically measured in duration or number of sessions, are appropriate for the highest-risk offenders, while moderate-intensity interventions are sufficient for moderate-risk offenders. A corollary to this principle is the importance of minimizing dropout from intervention programs by high-risk offenders.

The other two principles focused on the skills of the service provider while working with offenders. Related to the importance of the service provider-offender relationship introduced previously, relationship skills of the service provider contribute to a positive outcome by the offender. They include presenting a respectful, caring, and collaborative disposition when interacting with clients. The service provider is enthusiastic and values the personal autonomy of the client. These skills are particularly characteristic of motivational interviewing (MI), particularly in the early stages (Miller, 1983). MI has become a mainstream model of intervention with reticent clients in many different contexts, particularly substance abuse, which is a criminogenic need for many offenders. Moreover, in their meta-analysis of 72 MI studies, Hettema, Steele, and Miller (2005) found that MI treatment effects were significantly larger for minorities samples ($d = 0.79$) that for nonminority, white samples ($d = 0.26$). This is encouraging for practitioners in the criminal justice system where minorities are routinely vastly overrepresented in the offender population (Nellis, 2016).

A second important staff practice is the use of structuring skills in one's work with offenders either individually or in group. They include the use of prosocial modeling in the spirit of social learning theory (Bandura, 1977), the appropriate use of reinforcement, articulated disapproval of antisocial statements and behavior, the effective use of authority, skill building, the practice of cognitive restructuring with the client, problem solving, client advocacy, and use of MI, particularly the more advanced stages. These staff skill principles have also been enshrined in the core correctional practice (CPP) movement that has been popular in many correctional jurisdictions for the past two decades (Dowden & Andrews, 2004).

2.3.4 *Organizational Principles*

Finally, four organizational principles are offered for correctional agencies to consider when designing their service delivery model. First, RNR services that are offered in the community are more effective than those offered in custodial settings (Andrews, Zinger, et al., 1990). This is understandable when one considers the cultural milieu of prison, where the prosocial milieu of a treatment program, perhaps a few hours per week, or even per day, are up against the pervasive contingencies that are in operation around the clock among an entrenched prison culture. However, this does not mean that institutional services should be abandoned. Empirical evidence supports that ongoing use of RNR-based interventions in custody (e.g., Andrews, Zinger, et al., 1990; Usher & Stewart, 2014). We simply needed to be mindful that their impact is not likely to be as impactful as services in the community and, where possible (e.g., for parolees), look to post-incarceration opportunities for RNR-based interventions.

Second, continuity of service should not be overlooked. It is insufficient to enroll an offender in a program or begin to provide an intervention and assume that the task is done. Ongoing monitoring of the service to ensure it stays on task and of the offender to chart progress or deterioration as part of the offender's case management is essential to determine if the plan is working as expected and the continuity of the service or services are being maintained or if modifications are required.

Third, at a higher, more administrative level, agency management is another important principle. Managers should consider relationship and structuring skills in their hiring and training of staff. A hierarchical model of staff supervision should ensure staff adherence to the core principles of RNR. This requires the use of organizational mechanisms to monitor, evaluate, and ensure the quality of offender assessment and intervention as per all of the previous principles. Correctional managers also have a responsivity to create a culture that supports effective practice that involves researchers and outside experts in the design, delivery, and evaluation of services (Andrews, 2011).

Finally, the correctional agency, be it institutional- or community-based, should have strong linkages with other community agencies, including nongovernmental organizations and non-justice-related programs. These linkages will assist the offender's case worker to fulfill other principles, such as client advocacy, continuity of service, and supplementing institutional-based RNR-based interventions with community support. Slowly, these extended principles are being acknowledged, and their value to RNR is being touted (Herzog-Evans, 2017; McNeill, 2012; Polaschek, 2012), although not by all as seen below.

2.4 Research and Meta-Analyses on RNR

The RNR principles have been the subject of empirical research since Andrews, Zinger, et al. (1990) conducted a meta-analysis examining what works in correctional treatment. Since this initial meta-analysis establishing the RNR principles, there has been an abundance of individual studies examining the principles individually and in conjunction with each other. Due of the volume of individual studies and the value of meta-analyses to systematically summarize findings in a standardized fashion, this summary of RNR-related research focuses on meta-analyses conducted since 2000; representing almost 20 years of meta-analyses evaluating the RNR model.

2.4.1 RNR-Informed Intervention

As seen in Table 2.1, there have been at least 14 meta-analyses (6 between 2000 and 2009 and 8 between 2010 and 2018) examining the effectiveness of RNR-informed interventions. The majority of studies examined offenders or subgroups of offenders (i.e., young offenders, Aboriginal/indigenous offenders, ethnically diverse offenders, sexual offenders, and mentally disordered offenders), and one meta-analysis examined the impact of RNR-informed intervention on drug abusers in a criminal and drug abuse context. Generally, the principles of RNR are well supported with the exception of the principle of risk which had mixed findings in the earlier studies. Specifically, the risk principle was not supported in four of the earlier meta-analyses (Dowden & Andrews, 2000; Dowden & Andrews, 2004; Dowden, Antonowicz, & Andrews, 2003; Hanson, Bourgon, Helmus, & Hodgson, 2009a, 2009b). On the other hand, six meta-analyses, five of which were after 2010, found support for the risk principle (Andrews & Dowden, 2006; Bonta, Blais, & Wilson, 2014; Gutierrez, Wilson, Rugge, & Bonta, 2013; James, Stams, Asscher, De Roo, & van der Laan, 2013; Koehler, Lösel, Akoensi, & Humphreys, 2013; Wilson & Hoge, 2013), and

Table 2.1 Meta-analyses of offender treatment programs and their findings with respect to RNR

Author	Offender type	Principle examined	Risk	Need	Responsivity	Outcome
2000–2009						
Andrews and Dowden (2005)	Not specified	Risk, need, responsivity	Not tested directly	Not tested directly	Not tested directly	When programs were clinically appropriate (adhered to RNR), mean effect sizes were greater for programs that incorporated elements of program integrity. No matter the integrity conditions, the mean effect size was always greater with more appropriate treatment
Andrews and Dowden (2006)	Not specified	Risk	Supported	Not tested	Not tested	Results show solid support for the risk principle (limited to clinically and psychologically appropriate treatment). Risk sample received most support in women and younger offenders
Dowden and Andrews (2000)	Not specified	Risk, need, responsivity	Not supported	Supported	General responsivity: Supported	Adherence to need and responsivity also had significant effect sizes, but risk did not
Dowden and Andrews (2004)	No specified	Risk, need, responsivity	Not supported	Supported	General responsivity: Supported	Mean effect sizes were higher (with the exception of noncriminogenic needs category) under conditions of adherence to CCP
Dowden et al. (2003)	Not specified	Risk, need, responsivity	Not supported	Supported	General responsivity: Supported	Need and general responsivity made significant contributions to program effectiveness—Programs that didn't target needs along with relapse prevention or failed to use CB/social learning strategies did not reduce recidivism. Risk was not a significant moderating variable
Hanson et al. (2009a, 2009b)	Sexual offenders	Risk, need, responsivity	Not supported	Supported	General responsivity: Supported	Treated group had lower rates of sexual and general recidivism. Adherence to need and responsivity principle made for more effective treatment. Adherence to the risk principle had no significant effect

Author	Offender type	Principle examined	Risk	Need	Responsivity	Outcome
2010–2018						
Bonta et al. (2014)	Mentally disordered offenders	Risk-need/the central eight	Supported	Supported	Not tested	Primary status of the big four may be more important for the prediction of violent recidivism compared to general recidivism for mentally disordered offenders. Drug abuse was a significantly better predictor of general recidivism, and alcohol abuse was a better predictor of violent recidivism
Gutierrez et al. (2013)	Aboriginal offenders	Risk-need/the central eight	Supported	Supported	Not tested	All of the central eight predicted general recidivism, and seven (not recreation/leisure) predicted violent recidivism. Criminal history, procriminal associates, and antisocial personality pattern were the best predictors of general recidivism
Gutierrez et al. (2018)	Indigenous offenders	Responsivity	Not tested	Not tested	Specific responsivity: Supported	Culturally relevant programs outperformed generic programs for indigenous offenders, consistent with the principle of specific responsivity. It is speculated that culturally relevant programing may work because it targets the risk/needs of indigenous offenders, but this was not tested directly
James et al. (2013)	Juveniles and young adult offenders	Risk, need, responsivity	Supported	Supported	Specific responsivity: Supported	Aftercare programs are suitable for youth who are at a high risk of recidivism. Aftercare interventions focused on the individual offender were more effective than those that focused on the social system; consistent with the needs and responsivity principles

(continued)

Table 2.1 (continued)

Author	Offender type	Principle examined	Risk	Need	Responsivity	Outcome
Koehler et al. (2013)	Young offenders	Risk, need, responsivity	Supported	Supported	Specific responsivity: Supported	Program in adherence with the RNR principles revealed the strongest mean effect (a reduction of 16% against a baseline of 50%)
Prendergast et al. (2013)	Drug abusers	Risk, need, responsivity	Partially supported	Partially supported	General responsivity: Partially supported	Standardized coefficients for crime outcomes for risk, 0.27; for need, 0.17; for responsivity, 0.33; and for appropriate service (a combination of risk, need, and responsivity), 0.46. Standardized coefficients for drug outcomes for risk, 0.06; for needs, 0.05; and for responsivity, 0.05
Usher and Stewart (2014)	Ethnically diverse offenders	Risk, need, responsivity	Not tested directly	Not tested directly	General responsivity: Supported	The four ethnic groups (Caucasian, aboriginal, black, other) demonstrated significant treatment gains from participating in CBT-based programing
Wilson and Hoge (2013)	Youth offenders	Risk, need, responsivity	Supported	Not tested	Supported	Programs that offered treatment targeting medium- to high-risk offenders were more effective in reducing recidivism. Only two studies adhered to the needs principle, so it was not possible to test the needs principle. Programs that adhered to the responsivity principle were more effective at reducing recidivism than those that did not

one study found support for the risk principle when applied to criminal outcomes but not drug outcomes (Prendergast et al., 2013).

When tested, the needs principle was supported in every meta-analysis. Two studies examined the Central Eight specifically, finding that they were generally supported (Bonta et al., 2014; Gutierrez et al., 2013). Gutierrez et al. (2013) found that the Big Four were not distinct from the other risk factors in the prediction of general recidivism but three (criminal history, procriminal attitudes and cognitions, and antisocial personality pattern) of the Big Four were supported in the prediction of violent recidivism (the exception was criminal companions). Additionally, education/employment, family/marital, and substance abuse—three of the moderate four—were found to be supported in the prediction of violent recidivism. For the responsivity principle, both general responsivity (Dowden et al., 2003; Dowden & Andrews, 2000; Dowden & Andrews, 2004; Hanson et al., 2009a, 2009b; Prendergast et al., 2013; Usher & Stewart, 2014; Wilson & Hoge, 2013) and specific responsivity, which however were only examined in two of the more recent meta-analyses (Gutierrez, Chadwick, & Wanamaker, 2018; James et al., 2013; Koehler et al., 2013), were supported for criminal outcomes. It is also encouraging to find that the more recent meta-analyses have been conducted by a wider range of researchers.

2.5 Criticisms, Oversights, and Debates about RNR

Two hallmarks of a good theory are that they have a practical application and impact (Lewin, 1964) and that they stimulate intellectual discourse. RNR has done both. The empirical research, which is summarized above, verifies the first component, while the ongoing dialogue and debate about RNR, which continues today, illustrate the second component. To begin this section, we submit that the discussion, although sometimes sounding adversarial, has benefited the RNR model and assisted both organizations and individual practitioners in its use. Indeed, the model continues to grow and develop as it becomes even more comprehensive and applicable to a wider range of offenders and contexts.

Many of the criticisms come from a failure to realize that the full RNR model consists not of 3 or 4, but 18 principles (Andrews, 2001) as discussed previously. Admittedly, these principles came after the original, and oft-cited, articulation of RNR by Andrews, Bonta, and colleagues in 1990. However, they have been widely touted now for the last 20 years (Andrews, 2001; Andrews & Bonta, 1998, 2003, 2006, 2010a, 2010b; Andrews, Bonta, & Wormith, 2011; Bonta & Andrews, 2007, 2017; Polaschek, 2012; Wormith, Gendreau, & Bonta, 2012). Examples of critiques of the core RNR principles include Taxman's (2014) call for a second generation of RNR and a spirited debate over the benefits of RNR (Andrews & Bonta, 2010a; Andrews, Bonta, & Wormith, 2011; Ogloff & Davis, 2004; Wormith, Gendreau, & Bonta, 2012) versus the Good Lives Model (Gannon & Ward, 2014; Ward & Brown, 2004; Ward, Melser, & Yates, 2007; Ward & Stewart, 2003a, 2003b; Ward, Yates, &

Willis, 2012) and Abracen and Looman's (2016b) application of the core RNR to the assessment and treatment of sexual offenders.

2.5.1 Strengths, Resilience, and Protective Factors

Perhaps the most prevalent criticism of RNR is its alleged exclusive focus on offender risk and neglect or any positive attributes that the offender might possess or that might be stimulated through intervention. This is a misunderstanding (or oversight) about RNR which has occurred for at least three reasons: one, the originators' perceived need to focus on risk/needs, which was driven in large part by their effort to overcome the traditional models of psychiatric and psychological assessment of offenders that were in vogue at the time; two, a failure to conduct the necessary research to enshrine strengths empirically and conceptually into the RNR model; and three, the variety of terms (strengths, protective factors, resilience, stabilizers) and definitions that were proposed to characterize positive attributes of offenders. Not surprising then, early practitioners of RNR would be unlikely to include strengths as part of their client assessments or incorporate them into their intervention. The first shortcoming can be readily addressed in the promotion and training of RNR. The second shortcoming is a longer-term proposition requiring careful, longitudinal research and clarification about the terms, their operational definitions, and hypothesizing as to how they interact with risk and needs and affect intervention. This is set out in the third reason that RNR has not demonstrably integrated strengths into its model either theoretically or empirically.

Numerous terms have been used to identify and describe those personal attributes and situational contexts that correlate positively with leading a prosocial lifestyle and negatively with an antisocial, criminal lifestyle. Interest in these aspects of offenders comes from various sources, including developmental psychology and its identification of the resilient child; the long tradition of research on desistence from criminal and antisocial behavior, which had its beginnings in Europe in the 1980s (e.g., Cusson & Pinsonneault, 1986); and, most generally, the positive psychology movement (Seligman & Csikszentmihalyi, 2000; Seligman, Steen, Park, & Peterson, 2005).

Resilience, according to Masten (2001), "refers to a class of phenomena characterized by good outcomes in spite of serious threats to adaptation or development … Individuals are not considered resilient if there has never been a significant threat" (p. 227). However, in the field of offender risk prediction protective factors are often characterized simply as "factors that diminish risk of violent recidivism" (Vogel, de, de Ruiter, Bouman, & de Vries Robbé, 2009, p. 13) or as "characteristics of an offender, his environment or situation that protect an individual from relapsing into violent behavior" (de Vries Robbé, de Vogel, & de Spa, 2011, p. 178). At the same time, the term *protective factor* has also been used extensively in conjunction with a model describing an interaction effect, while the term *promotive* factor (Sameroff, Bartko, Baldwin, Baldwin, & Seifer, 1998) has been used to describe the positive end of a characteristic that ranges from risk to strength (p. 112). Others have found main effects for both risk and promotive factors, as opposed to an interaction, and have suggested what has been referred to as a "compensatory" model, whereby risk factors and promotive factors may counterbalance each other (Van der Laan, Veenstra, Bogaerts, Verhulst, & Ormel, 2010). Specifically, Ttofi, Farrington, Piquero, and DeLisi (2016) described two kinds of protective factors. They defined a direct protective or promotive factor as one that predicts a low probability of offending, a risk-based protective factor as one that predicts a low probability of offending among a risk category, and an interactive protective (or buffering protective) factor as one that predicts a low probability of offending among a risk category but not among a non-risk category (p. 1). After examining a series of longitudinal studies, Ttofi et al. (2016) concluded that most protective factors from diverse studies in different geographic and sociopolitical contexts are in concordance with the broader literature on resilience, implying that protective factors may be equated with resilience or at least contribute to it.

Polaschek (2016) focused on risk and protective factors that are particularly dynamic, in part because of their implications for social policy and offender intervention. However, dynamic protective factors are no less complicated by various definitions and models. There are often obvious conceptual overlaps between dynamic protective and dynamic risk factors or criminogenic needs (e.g., emotional volatility vs. emotional regulation skills; absence of stable marital relationship vs. stable marital relationship). Statistical claims may be made that when dynamic protective factors contribute uniquely to risk prediction, they represent a unique class of variables. However, usually protective factor instruments and scales (e.g., the SAPROF; de Vogel, de Ruiter, Bouman, & de Vries Robbé, 2012; and the DRAOR; Serin, 2007; Serin, Mailloux, & Wilson, 2012) also correlate significantly with dynamic, need-based instruments and scales (e.g., de Vries Robbé et al., 2011; de Vries Robbé & de Vogel, 2013; Yesberg & Polaschek, 2015). Together, these two points suggest that when found to be incrementally predictive over the initial list of risk factors in regressions, their unique contribution might still be partially or entirely explained as the contribution of risk factors not in the original list, but now being called "protective factors."

With great interest among clinicians and researchers in resilience, strengths, and protective factors, their varied definitions notwithstanding, it is not surprising to find disenchantment with the original RNR principles. In our view, the nature and role of strengths are adequately described above in the extended RNR principles (Wormith & Truswell, in press). Yet much more research is required to document their contribution to offender risk assessment and service delivery.

2.5.2 The Failure of Knowledge Translation in the Application of RNR–Based Assessment and Intervention

Much of the criticism of RNR pertains to its application by correctional agencies and not to the model itself (McNeill, 2012). A number of examples have been described by Polaschek (2012). Programs have been focused solely on risk reduction and its impact on public good. They have ignored the goals and aspiration of offenders, failed to engage offenders and build a therapeutic alliance. They have targeted criminogenic needs exclusively, ignoring noncriminogenic needs whose successful resolution would have facilitated subsequent work on criminogenic needs. They have worked on skill development while ignoring offenders' motivation and social opportunities to acquire such skills (McNeill, 2009, 2012; McNeill & Whyte, 2007).

It is now clearly apparent that the enthusiasm with which many correctional agencies and their senior administrators have embraced RNR has caused some of the criticism and disillusionment that has been expressed with the model. It is also understandable. Claimed adherence to evidence-based practice has become a popular mantra in the field of corrections, and RNR-based intervention is arguably its most empirically established model of intervention as documented in the preceding section. In their zeal to implement RNR, particularly in large organizations, agencies trained and dispersed their service providers to deliver very specific programs in a very specific manner. This manualized fashion of program delivery by quasi-professional staff has led to justifiable criticisms about the "cookie cutter" approach that is used all too commonly in the delivery of RNR interventions (Ward, Melser, & Yates, 2007). Correctly, these interventions focus on content, specifically generalized criminogenic needs, but do so at the expense of relationship building, client motivation, and specific responsivity (Porporino, 2010; Raynor & Robinson, 2009). This is both regretful and ironic.

The precepts of RNR were founded upon a psychology of individual differences (Andrews, Bonta, & Hoge, 1990), and the specific responsivity principle was meant to individualize service delivery in a manner that would maximize the impact of the intervention by promoting client engagement and facilitating learning (Bourgon & Bonta, 2014). We now appreciate that its initial articulation was too vague (Polaschek, 2012) and its promotion was too muted (Cohen & Whetzel, 2014). Consequently, specific responsivity became oversimplified, misinterpreted, and overshadowed by general responsivity (McNeill, 2012; Robinson & Crow, 2009).

The failure of RNR to be implemented as prescribed in the field has also been noted and documented empirically at the level of the individual client with both adult and young offenders in Canada (Bonta, Rugge, Scott, Bourgon, & Yessine, 2008). Following the administration of a validated risk/needs assessment instrument to the offenders, probation officers' efforts in magnitude and focus bore little resemblance to the risk level and criminogenic needs of the offenders, with the exception of family and marital problems. Viglione, Rudes, and Taxman (2015) found similar results in the USA. Miller and Maloney (2013) have traced this kind of shortcoming to practitioners, who fail to make decisions based on their tools, and to agencies, that fail to monitor staff and project their lack of confidence in their RNR-based tools. However, we remain hopeful that these "wakeup calls" have been heard and are increasingly being accommodated by correctional agencies, at least by those that claim to adhere to the RNR model in their assessment, intervention, and case management process.

Responding to this shortfall, Bourgon and Bonta (2014) have suggested a way forward, one in which the following recommendations can be derived. One, do not focus only on client characteristics, but the mode of service delivery by which an optimal learning environment might be created for the offender client. This remains an under-researched endeavor. Two, examine whether such an environment has been created. This may be achieved, not by examining recidivism rates, but in two ways. The first is by monitoring behavioral indicators of responsive engagement, such as attrition, attendance, program participation, homework, and client-reported feedback. The second is by assessing the acquisition of specific knowledge and skills, which can vary from writing an employment resume to practicing self-regulation of anger, to practicing a cultural activity. Three, engage in motivational interviewing and its closely aligned correctional counterpart, core correctional practice, to produce a collaborative therapeutic environment. Four, develop a research agenda for responsivity, particularly specific responsivity, which is much more complex than general responsivity, but has been the subject of far less research. This may be done by breaking through the black box of treatment (Bonta et al., 2008) to determine how engagement can be enhanced and learning can be optimized, not by focusing on distal outcomes, such as recidivism, or on client only characteristics to the neglect of therapist characteristics and actions. We are encouraged by studies that have investigated these details pertaining to post-assessment intervention and supervision, particularly with young (juvenile) offenders, where empirical evidence of RNR adherence, although still some distance from perfection, is encouraging (e.g., Luong & Wormith, 2011; Nelson & Vincent, 2018; Peterson-Badali, Skilling, & Haqanee, 2015).

Thus, the translation of knowledge to practical application is a legitimate concern. Promoters of the model bear some responsibility to see the model implemented in a manner in which it was intended. This is easier said than done. RNR is not a copyrighted product that can be licensed, monitored, and sanctioned, like some of the assessment instruments that it might call into use. Rather, it is an open access set of principles. Therefore, its oversight is left to multiple stakeholders. This includes the agencies that have adopted RNR to monitor their programs critically, the practitioners to self-monitor their adherence to program manuals and the full array RNR principles, the independent observers who are offered the opportunity to examine programs by means of agency-created accreditation panels, and the general academic and research community through their critical analysis of public documents and accounts of agency-offered RNR services.

2.5.3 Responsivity

Polaschek (2012) is critical about the vagueness of the responsivity principle, noting that general responsivity has been overemphasized to the detriment of specific responsivity which is potentially rife with many nuanced clinical phenomena that impact client outcome. We agree only in that general responsivity, by virtue of being a general principle, is more easily understood, researched, and applied in the field, as evidenced in Table 2.1. But in the original enunciation of core RNR principles, specific responsivity gets more than its share of attention. In fact, Andrews, Bonta, and Hoge (1990) cited nine specific hypotheses pertaining to candidates for specific responsivity issues. Admittedly, only three of them were supported empirically at the time; hence the others were identified as hypotheses.

Moreover, in their Fifth Edition of *The Psychology of Criminal Conduct*, Andrews and Bonta (2010a) acknowledged "we have not developed the concept of specific responsivity to any serious degree" (p. 507), although they did add motivation and strengths to their nine candidates, no doubt in response to the criticisms of RNR to that time. Although RNR now considers issues of motivation to be a specific responsivity factor, it has been criticized for not yet integrating a theory of motivation. However, RNR advocates often embrace motivational interviewing in the context of core correctional practice (CCP), which consists of a set of empirically supported, RNR-based guidelines for practitioners to use in their work with offenders. Consequently, the link between RNR and motivation is implicit. Deci and Ryan's (1985, 2002) self-determination theory (SDT), with its distinction between intrinsic and external motivation, have clear implications for offender rehabilitation and the steps that one may logically follow as pointed out by advocates of the GLM (Ward & Fortune, 2013). If there is a failing, it is partly a failure of researchers and clinicians to collaborate in examining these and the many other specific responsivity issues that one might come across. Others have also been concerned about the definition and operationalization of responsivity, modified the name, and worked it into their own reformulation of RNR. Some of these modifications are reviewed below (e.g., Herzog-Evans, 2016; Taxman, 2014).

2.6 Variations and Enhancements of RNR

Taxman and colleagues (Crites & Taxman, 2013; Taxman, 2014; Taxman, Thanner, & Weisburd, 2006) have proposed a number of modifications and additions to the RNR model, culminating in a proposed second generation of RNR (Taxman, 2014). Some of the modifications, we believe, can equally be accommodated by principles in the expanded version of RNR described previously, while others focus on some of the necessary details that are likely required to maximize the impact of the RNR model on the offender population. With a particular focus on responsivity, their work calls for what amounts to a comprehensive, clinical evaluation of the offender client that acknowledges the individual differences that are unique to each individual offender and directs the service provider and agency to attend to each individual in the delivery of RNR services accordingly. This imposes important responsibilities on the correctional agency, what they describe as "systemic responsivity" and what we believe is subsumed under the RNR organizational principles listed previously. Regardless, all can agree that the agency must be prepared to offer a wide variety of services in varied ways and doses to a heterogeneous clientele and must do so with the commitment of managers within the agency. As Rudes, Kras, Meyer, and Magnuson (2017) revealed in their detailed analysis of organizational culture in three probation agencies in the USA, it is not sufficient simply to declare, "yes, we are doing evidence-based practice," and that would include RNR, when they do so begrudgingly, in a minimalist or distorted fashion, because of its draw on staff resources and the pressure this puts on other requirements of the office.

Similarly, Taxman's version of RNR offers a more complex appreciation of patterns of criminogenic needs and responsivity characteristics. This allows for the opportunity to look for patterns of these factors that may be found with some regularity and accommodated in any agencies offerings of intervention accordingly. Five examples include substance abuse, criminal cognitions, substance abuse with some other criminogenic needs, social and interpersonal skills, and life skills (Taxman, 2014). Its proponents also prefer to talk about "tailoring" instead of specific responsivity. This more clinical term is perhaps a better description of the process underlying specific responsivity and implies that the uniqueness of the individual offender requires a client-specific intervention. It also tends to set the process apart from general responsivity.

Their extension of RNR also introduces the concepts of stabilizers and destabilizers, as another dimension to the offender's risk-need profile. Stabilizers are very similar to strengths, but also imply the interaction definition of strengths, that they are not simply the opposite of risk/need, but directly serve to neutralize or minimize the impact of existing risk and needs as suggested by Andrews and Bonta (1994), Andrews (2011), and Bonta and Andrews (2007), while destabilizers exacerbate them. Even when they may be environmentally based, rather than personally based, we see no reason why destabilizers cannot be also construed as risks and needs since any combination of risks and needs can interact with each other making the overall risk of the client greater than the simple sum of said risk and needs. Again, this is the very principle that underlies the concept of antisocial pattern, one of the Central Eight domains.

The RNR Simulation Tool, developed by the Center for Advancing Correctional Excellence, is a creative and handy mechanism based on Taxman's integrated version or RNR (Caudy & Taxman, n.d.). It consists of three online portals. One is used to assess the offender and assign him or her to one of the five offender groups mentioned above based on their risk and needs. The second assesses the agency's programs in terms of their adherence to the RNR practices and corresponding core correctional practices. The third assesses the agency's overall capacity to provide the necessary RNR-based interventions, given the nature of its offender population, and makes recommendations where the analysis detects shortfalls. Hopefully, this easy access query mechanism will improve the translation of RNR to field practice, make programs and services truly evidence-based, and, in so doing, improve their impact on offenders.

Following a thorough and balanced inspection of the competing perspectives on RNR, including GLM and desistence theory, Herzog-Evans (2017) has called for a truce among competing models and their proponents. In their stead, she has also proposed an "integrative theory" that realigns theoretical perspective of offender behavior and change and sets a course for her integrative theory to guide future offender assessment and intervention. To begin, she has suggested that a host of non-programmatic factors, namely, "staff characteristics; offender characteristics; the interaction of staff and client characteristics; size of caseload, frequency of contact, individualized/flexible programming and explicitness of intervention strategies; and setting" (p. 110) be considered a part of responsivity in its two forms. Intrinsic responsivity includes demographic and psychological characteristics, as per specific responsivity, but also includes personal goals and priorities, and type and level of agency and autonomy as per SDT. Extrinsic responsivity refers to institutional characteristics and is reminiscent of Taxman's (2014) systemic responsivity. They would replace general and specific responsivity.

In this framework, Herzog-Evans (2017) also called not only for an extrinsic responsive correctional system but an extrinsic responsive legal system, one in which laws sustain rehabilitation by tailoring obligations to criminogenic need, accommodating the time required to address such needs, and supporting client agency. However, all of these concepts and their applicability to offender rehabilitation require more empirical research, which is perhaps the reason they were not included as core components of the original RNR framework. Finally, Herzog-Evans (2017) provided what we would describe as a series of guidelines for applying the core RNR principles that were derived from a number of research, clinical, and legal traditions including mental health, motivation theory (SDT), MI, psychometrics, the law, justice, therapeutic jurisprudence, human rights, CCP, GLM, attachment theory, feminism, and CBT. As such, it offers an excellent road map for applying the complete model of RNR to offenders.

Hanson et al.' (2009a, 2009b) meta-analysis supported the applicability of the three core RNR principles to the treatment of sexual offenders. However, citing additional factors related to the recidivism of sexual offenders, such as prior trauma and mental health problems (Douglas, Guy, & Hart, 2009), but noting the lack of empirical support for GLM, Looman and Abracen (2013) have called for a more *integrated* version of RNR. Their RNR-I considers how high-risk behaviors interact with each other to exacerbate risk and interfere with desired outcomes, somewhat reminiscent of the Central Eight's pattern of antisocial behavior. It also integrates trauma, mental health, and insecure attachment, but not vague and unsubstantiated notions of "inner peace," into their model of sexual offender treatment (Abracen & Looman, 2016b).

With respect to offending more generally, Herzog-Evans (2016, 2017) has also advocated for the following: a more integrative theory of RNR, one that moves general responsivity to a principle of treatment, changes specific responsivity to "intrinsic responsivity," and adds mental health, as per Abracen and Looman (2016a); other factors, such as intelligence, personality, ethnicity, and gender that RNR considers specific responsivity; and personal goals and agency, as proposed by GLM. Similar to Taxman's (2014) systemic responsivity, she also proposed "extrinsic responsivity," which, as noted previously, is not unlike the organizational principles in the expanded version of RNR. Finally, her version brings a legal perspective by means of therapeutic jurisprudence (Wexler & Winick, 1996) to the model, which is reminiscent, but not identical to the extended RNR and its call for a just and humane delivery of sentence and service and is prescient of Rogan's (2017) appeal to international human rights in the application of risk and needs. In sum, Herzog-Evans puts an array of factors from law/jurisprudence, mental health, demography, GLM, and clinical and organizational psychology under a single umbrella. Her appeal to make RNR more integrative is helpful and important in that it reminds one to consider the full 18 principles of RNR, but is nonspecific as to how they might all interact.

2.7 The Future of RNR-Based Assessment and Intervention

Risk-need assessment tools are getting increasingly complex with their use of sophisticated decision trees and other algorithms in their effort to become more precise in their prediction of offenders' antisocial behavior, including recidivism (e.g., Correctional Offender Management Profiling for Alternative Sanctions; COMPAS; Brennan, Dieterich, & Ehret, 2009). Although not without difficulty (Wormith, 2017), there is no reason to believe that these more advanced procedures cannot supersede our current or theoretically sound, but simplistic, practice of assigning offender to the most appropriate course of intervention. The array of possible static risks, dynamic criminogenic needs, strengths, noncriminogenic needs, and responsivity factors that constitute a single offender's profile is mind-boggling.

Borrowing from Taxman's (2014) attention to patterns of risk, need, and responsivity characteristics, consider an agency's high-risk offenders who score high on two of the Central Eight risk/need domains. That alone generates 56 possible combinations or offender risk-need profiles. To illustrate further, consider whether (a) they do or do not have at least one strength on another domain; (b) they do or do not have a noncriminogenic need (say, general mental health needs); (c) they have any of three specific responsivity factors that are demographic in nature, let us say gender (males and female), race and ethnicity (White, Black, Asian, Latino, and indigenous), and age (young adult, middle-aged adult, and senior); or (d) they possess or do not possess one personality-related responsivity characteristic (say, psychopathy). The number of possible offender profiles balloons to 2160, and this is only for those offenders who are high risk on two of the Central Eight domains. It is time to merge RNR theory with sophisticated mathematical models to tailor individualized intervention and to cluster offender profiles into workable and feasible groupings that are both practical and effective.

The general responsivity principle and the service delivery-related principles of the expanded RNR model have been operationalized for use in the field in the name of "core correctional practice" (CCP; Dowden & Andrews, 2004). CCPs are techniques of influence that are designed for service providers, such as probation and parole offices, to use in their face-to-face work with their clientele. Although some staff come by these skills naturally, the techniques can also be trained. They include structuring skills, relationship-building skills, behavioral techniques, and cognitive techniques. "These CCPs have been validated on more than 700 individual adult and juvenile programs by correlating scores with offender recidivism" (Latessa, Smith, Schweitzer, & Labrecque, 2013, p. 12). Bonta et al. (2010) have developed a programmatic version of CCP in which the core practices are delivered in a group format. The Strategic Training Initiative in Community Supervision (STICS) has produced encouraging results in both in-program change and recidivism outcome (Bonta et al., 2011), in spite of what some might call its "prescriptive" format. More research and practice are required to evaluate and to fully understand this kind of strongly based RNR intervention.

To date, with few exceptions (e.g., Newcome & Cullen, 2017), RNR proponents have not yet integrated understanding about the biological, particularly the neuropsychological, basis of behavior into the model. The impact of insults to the brain (e.g., head injuries, anoxia, toxic exposure, and fetal alcohol spectrum disorder, FASD) has been well known for many years, as have their personality and behavioral repercussions (e.g., deficits in impulse control, problem solving, self-control, delay of gratification, empathy, intellect, executive functioning, and diagnoses of antisocial personality disorder and psychopathy). The implications of these consequences are obvious for the three core RNR principles. They contribute to offender risk, they generate criminogenic needs, some of which we submit are dynamic in spite of their biological bases, and they can generate specific responsivity traits that demand consideration in offenders' treatment and case management (Newcome & Cullen, 2017).

The mechanisms for change in risk and its consequences require more research and attention by correctional agencies and their staff. There is some research on the dynamic predictive validity of risk-need assessments (Andrews & Bonta, 2010a; Andrews & Wormith, 1984; Labrecque, Smith, Lovins, & Latessa, 2014; Raynor, 2007; Vose, Lowenkamp, Smith, & Cullen, 2009), but more is required (Cohen & VanBenschoten, 2014). This speaks to the need for independent reassessment of offenders on a common instrument. In particular, linking the complete chain (risk-need assessment, followed by assessment-driven intervention, followed by risk-need reassessment, followed by offender (intermediate) gain on various dimensions including positive, prosocial indicators, followed by ultimate outcome, including measures of recidivism) is essential to verify the RNR model without reservation.

In sum, the many implications of the full RNR model for correctional agencies are clear. In addition to adhering to the core RNR principles, the overarching principles, the principles of structured assessment, the principles of service delivery, and the organizational principles offer numerous directions for offender assessment and intervention. In order to implement the full RNR model, or any of its integrative variations, responsibility and effort are required from organizational management, researchers, and field-level practitioners. However, many questions asked about RNR more than a decade ago, particularly those pertaining to therapeutic alliance, motivation, responsivity, organizational context, and ethics of intervention (McGuire, 2004), still remain.

References

Abracen, J., & Looman, J. (2016a). The risk–need–responsivity model: An expansion and revision with an emphasis on groups of high-risk, high-need offenders. In D. B. Boer, A. R. Beech, & T. Ward (Eds.), *The Wiley handbook on the assessment, treatment and theories of sexual offending* (pp. 399–420). West Sussex, UK: John Wiley & Sons, Ltd.

Abracen, J., & Looman, J. (2016b). *Treatment of high-risk sexual offenders: An integrated approach*. West Sussex, UK: John Wiley & Sons, Ltd.

Andrews, D. A. (1980). Some experimental investigations of the principles of differential association through the deliberate manipulation of the structure of service systems. *American Sociological Review, 45*(3), 448–462. https://doi.org/10.2307/2095177

Andrews, D. A. (2001). Principles of effective correctional programs. In L. L. Motiuk & R. C. Serin (Eds.), *Compendium 2000 on effective correctional treatment* (pp. 9–17). Ottawa, ON: Research Branch: Correctional Service of Canada.

Andrews, D. A. (2011). The risk-need-responsivity (RNR) model of correctional assessment and treatment. In J. A. Dvoskin, J. L. Skeem, R. W. Novaco, & K. S. Douglas (Eds.), *Using social science to reduce violent offending* (pp. 127–156). New York, NY: Oxford University Press.

Andrews, D. A., & Bonta, J. (1994). *The psychology of criminal conduct*. Cincinnati, OH: Anderson.

Andrews, D. A., & Bonta, J. (1995). *Level of supervision-revised (LSI-R): An offender assessment system. User's guide*. Toronto, ON: Multi-Health Systems.

Andrews, D. A., & Bonta, J. (1998). *The psychology of criminal conduct* (2nd ed.). Cincinnati, OH: Anderson.

Andrews, D. A., & Bonta, J. (2003). *The psychology of criminal conduct* (3rd ed.). Cincinnati, OH: Anderson.

Andrews, D. A., & Bonta, J. (2006). *The psychology of criminal conduct* (4th ed.). Newark, NJ: LexisNexis.

Andrews, D. A., & Bonta, J. (2010a). *The psychology of criminal conduct* (5th ed.). New Providence, NJ: LexisNexis.

Andrews, D. A., & Bonta, J. (2010b). Rehabilitating criminal justice policy and practice. *Psychology, Public Policy, and Law, 16*(1), 39–55. https://doi.org/10.1037/a0018362

Andrews, D. A., Bonta, J., & Hoge, R. D. (1990). Classification for effective rehabilitation: Rediscovering psychology. *Criminal Justice and Behavior, 17*(1), 19–52. https://doi.org/10.1177/0093854890017001004

Andrews, D. A., Bonta, J., & Wormith, J. S. (2006). The recent past and near future of risk and/or need assessment. *Crime and Delinquency, 52*(1), 7–27. https://doi.org/10.1177/0011128705281756

Andrews, D. A., Bonta, J., & Wormith, J. S. (2011). The risk-need-responsivity (RNR) model: Does adding the good lives model contribute to effective crime prevention? *Criminal Justice and Behavior, 38*(7), 735–755. https://doi.org/10.1177/0093854811406356

Andrews, D. A., & Dowden, C. (2005). Managing correctional treatment for reduced recidivism: A meta-analytic review of program integrity. *Legal and Criminological Psychology, 10*(2), 173–187. https://doi.org/10.1348/135532505X36723

Andrews, D. A., & Dowden, C. (2006). Risk principle of case classification in correctional treatment: A meta-analytic investigation. *International Journal of Offender Therapy and Comparative Criminology, 50*(1), 88–100. https://doi.org/10.1177/0306624X05282556

Andrews, D. A., & Wormith, J. S. (1984). *Criminal sentiments and criminal behavior. Programs branch user report*. Ottawa, ON: Solicitor General Canada.

Andrews, D. A., Zinger, I., Hoge, R. D., Bonta, J., Gendreau, P., & Cullen, F. T. (1990). Does correctional treatment work? A clinically relevant and psychologically informed meta-analysis. *Criminology, 28*(3), 369–404. https://doi.org/10.1111/j.1745-9125.1990.tb01330.x

Bandura, A. (1977). *Social learning theory*. Englewood Cliffs, NJ: Prentice-Hall.

Bonta, J. (1996). Risk-needs assessment and treatment. In A. T. Harland (Ed.), *Choosing correctional options that work: Defining the demand and evaluating the supply* (pp. 18–32). Thousand Oaks, CA: Sage Publications, Inc.

Bonta, J., & Andrews, D. A. (2007). *Risk-need-responsivity model for offender assessment and rehabilitation. (report no. 2007–06)*. Ottawa, Canada: Department of Public Safety and Emergency Preparedness Canada.

Bonta, J., & Andrews, D. A. (2017). *The psychology of criminal conduct* (6th ed.). New York, NY: Routledge.

Bonta, J., Blais, J., & Wilson, H. A. (2014). A theoretically informed meta-analysis of the risk for general and violent recidivism for mentally disordered offenders. *Aggression and Violent Behavior, 19*(3), 278–287. https://doi.org/10.1016/j.avb.2014.04.014

Bonta, J., Bourgon, G., Rugge, T., Scott, T.-L., Yessine, A. K., Gutierrez, L., & Li, J. (2010). *The strategic training initiative in community supervision: Risk-need-responsivity in the real world*. Ottawa, ON: Public Safety Canada.

Bonta, J., Bourgon, G., Rugge, T., Scott, T.-L., Yessine, A. K., Gutierrez, L., & Li, J. (2011). An experimental demonstration of training probation officers in evidence-based community supervision. *Criminal Justice and Behavior, 38*(11), 1127–1148. https://doi.org/10.1177/0093854811420678

Bonta, J., Rugge, T., Scott, T.-L., Bourgon, G., & Yessine, A. (2008). Exploring the black box of community supervision. *Journal of Offender Rehabilitation, 47*(3), 248–270. https://doi.org/10.1080/10509670802134085

Bourgon, G., & Armstrong, B. (2005). Transferring the principles of effective treatment into a "real world" prison setting. *Criminal Justice and Behavior, 32*(1), 3–25. https://doi.org/10.1177/0093854804270618

Bourgon, G., & Bonta, J. (2014). Reconsidering the responsivity principle: A way to move forward. *Federal Probation Journal, 78*(2), 3–10.

Brennan, T., Dieterich, W., & Ehret, B. (2009). Evaluating the predictive validity of the COMPAS risk and needs assessment system. *Criminal Justice and Behavior, 36*(1), 21–40. https://doi.org/10.1177/0093854808326545

Campbell, M. A., Canales, D. D., Wei, R., Totten, A. E., Macaulay, W. A. C., & Wershler, J. L. (2015). Multidimensional evaluation of a mental health court: Adherence to the risk-needs-responsivity model. *Law and Human Behaviour, 39*(5), 489–502. https://doi.org/10.1037/lhb0000135

Caudy, M. S., & Taxman, F. S. (n.d.). *The RNR simulation tool: Putting RNR to work to improve client outcomes*. Fairfax, VA: Center for Advancing Correctional Excellence (ACE!), George Mason University.

Cohen, T. H., & VanBenschoten, S. W. (2014). Does the risk of recidivism for supervised offenders improve over time? Examining changes in the dynamic risk characteristics for offenders under federal supervision. *Federal Probation Journal, 89*(2), 41–56.

Cohen, T. H., & Whetzel, J. (2014). The neglected "R" – Responsivity and the federal offender. *Federal Probation Journal, 78*(2), 11–18.

Crites, E. L., & Taxman, F. S. (2013). The responsivity principle: Determining the appropriate program and dosage to match risk and needs. In F. S. Taxman & A. Pattavina (Eds.), *Simulation strategies to reduce recidivism: Risk need responsivity (RNR) modeling in the criminal justice system* (pp. 143–166). New York, NY: Springer.

Cusson, M., & Pinsonneault, P. (1986). The decision to give up crime. In D. B. Cornish & R. V. Clarke (Eds.), *The reasoning criminal: Rational choice perspectives on offending* (pp. 72–82). New York, NY: Springer-Verlag.

de Vogel, V., de Ruiter, C., Bouman, Y., & de Vries Robbé, M. (2012). *Structured assessment of protective factors for violence risk*. Utrecht: Van Der Hoeven Stichting.

de Vries Robbé, M., & de Vogel, V. (2013). Protective factors for violence risk: Bringing balance to risk assessment and management. In C. Logan & L. Johnstone (Eds.), *Managing clinical risk: A guide to effective practice* (pp. 293–310). Abingdon, UK: Routledge.

de Vries Robbé, M., de Vogel, V., & de Spa, E. (2011). Protective factors for violence risk in forensic psychiatric patients: A retrospective validation study of the SAPROF. *International Journal of Forensic Mental Health, 10*(3), 178–186. https://doi.org/10.1080/14999013.2011.600232

Deci, E. L., & Ryan, R. M. (1985). *Intrinsic motivation and self-determination in human behavior*. New York, NY: Plenum Press.

Deci, E. L., & Ryan, R. M. (Eds.). (2002). *Handbook of self-determination research*. Rochester, NY: University of Rochester Press.

Desmarais, S. L., Nicholls, T. L., Wilson, C. M., & Brink, J. (2012). Using dynamic risk and protective factors to predict inpatient aggression: Reliability and validity of START assessments. *Psychological Assessment, 24*(3), 685–700. https://doi.org/10.1037/a0026668

Douglas, K. S., Guy, L. S., & Hart, S. D. (2009). Psychosis as a risk factor for violence to others: A meta-analysis. *Psychological Bulletin, 135*(5), 679–706. https://doi.org/10.1037/a0016311

Dowden, C., & Andrews, D. A. (2000). Effective correctional treatment and violent reoffending: A meta-analysis. *Canadian Journal of Criminology, 42*(4), 449–467.

Dowden, C., & Andrews, D. A. (2004). The importance of staff practice in delivering correctional treatment: A meta-analytic review of core correctional practice. *International Journal of Offender Therapy and Comparative Criminology, 48*(2), 203–214. https://doi.org/10.1177/0306624X03257765

Dowden, C., Antonowicz, D., & Andrews, D. A. (2003). The effectiveness of relapse prevention with offenders: A meta-analysis. *International Journal of Offender Therapy and Comparative Criminology, 47*(5), 516–528. https://doi.org/10.1177/0306624X03253018

Gannon, T. A., & Ward, T. (2014). Where has all the psychology gone? A critical review of evidence-based psychological practice in correctional settings. *Aggression and Violent Behavior, 19*(4), 435–446. https://doi.org/10.1016/j.avb.2014.06.006

Gendreau, P., Little, T., & Goggin, C. (1996). A meta-analysis of the predictors of adult recidivism: What works. *Criminology, 34*(4), 575–608. https://doi.org/10.1111/j.1745-9125.1996.tb01220.x

Grant, J. D. (1965). Delinquency treatment in an institutional setting. In H. C. Quay (Ed.), *Juvenile delinquency: Research and theory* (pp. 29–57). Princeton, NJ: Van Nostrand.

Gutierrez, L., Chadwick, N., & Wanamaker, K. A. (2018). Culturally relevant programming versus the status quo: A meta-analytic review of the effectiveness of treatment of indigenous offenders. *Canadian Journal of Criminology and Criminal Justice, 60*(3), 321–353. https://doi.org/10.3138/cjccj.2017-0020.r2

Gutierrez, L., Wilson, H. A., Rugge, T., & Bonta, J. (2013). The prediction of recidivism with aboriginal offenders: A theoretically informed meta-analysis. *Canadian Journal of Criminology and Criminal Justice, 55*(1), 55–99. https://doi.org/10.3138/cjccj.2011.E.51

Hanson, R. K., Bourgon, G., Helmus, L., & Hodgson, S. (2009a). *A meta-analysis of the effectiveness of treatment for sexual offenders: Risk, need and responsivity*. Ottawa, ON: Public Safety Canada.

Hanson, R. K., Bourgon, G., Helmus, L., & Hodgson, S. (2009b). The principles of effective correctional treatment also apply to sexual offenders: A meta-analysis. *Criminal Justice and Behavior, 36*(9), 865–891. https://doi.org/10.1177/0093854809338545

Herzog-Evans, M. (2016). Law as an extrinsic responsivity factor: What is just is what works! *European Journal of Probation, 8*(3), 146–169. https://doi.org/10.1177/2066220316678750

Herzog-Evans, M. (2017). The risk-need-responsivity model: Evidence diversity and integrative theory. In P. Ugwudike, P. Raynor, & J. Annison (Eds.), *Evidence-based skills in criminal justice: International research on supporting rehabilitation and desistance* (pp. 99–124). Bristol, UK: Policy Press.

Hettema, J., Steele, J., & Miller, W. R. (2005). Motivational interviewing. *Annual Review of Clinical Psychology, 1*, 91–111. https://doi.org/10.1146/annurev.clinpsy.1.102803.143833

Hollett, J. (1984). *Effective elements of correctional programs. Unpublished comprehensive examination.* Ottawa, ON: Carleton University.

Horvath, A. O., Del Re, A. C., Flückiger, C., & Symonds, D. (2011). Alliance in individual psychotherapy. In J. C. Norcross (Ed.), *Psychotherapy relationships that work: Evidence-based responsiveness* (2nd ed., pp. 25–69). New York, NY: Oxford University Press.

James, C., Stams, G. J. J. M., Asscher, J. J., De Roo, A. K., & van der Laan, P. H. (2013). Aftercare programs for reducing recidivism among juvenile and young adult offenders: A meta-analytic review. *Clinical Psychology Review, 33*(2), 263–274. https://doi.org/10.1016/j.cpr.2012.10.013

Kennedy, S. (1999). Responsivity: The other classification principle. *Corrections Today, 61*(1), 48–51.

Koehler, J. A., Lösel, F., Akoensi, T. D., & Humphreys, D. K. (2013). A systematic review and meta-analysis on the effects of young offender treatment programs in Europe. *Journal of Experimental Criminology, 9*(1), 19–43. https://doi.org/10.1007/s11292-012-9159-7

Labrecque, R. M., Smith, P., Lovins, B. K., & Latessa, E. J. (2014). The importance of reassessment: How change in the LSI-R risk score can improve the prediction of recidivism. *Journal of Offender Rehabilitation, 53*(2), 116–128. https://doi.org/10.1080/10509674.2013.868389

Latessa, E. J., Smith, P., Schweitzer, M., & Labrecque, R. M. (2013). *Evaluation of the effective practices in community supervision model (EPICS) in Ohio.* Cincinnati, OH: University of Cincinnati.

Lewin, K. (1964). *Field theory in social science—Selected theoretical papers by Kurt Lewin.* New York, NY: Harper & Row.

Lipsey, M. W., Chapman, G. L., & Landenberger, N. A. (2001). Cognitive-behavioral programs for offenders. *The Annals of the American Academy of Political and Social Science, 578*(1), 144–157. https://doi.org/10.1177/000271620157800109

Lodewijks, H. P., de Ruiter, C., & Doreleijers, T. A. (2010). The impact of protective factors in desistance from violent reoffending: A study in three samples of adolescent offenders. *Journal of Interpersonal Violence, 25*(3), 568–587. https://doi.org/10.1177/0886260509334403

Looman, J., & Abracen, J. (2013). The risk need responsivity model of offender rehabilitation: Is there really a need for a paradigm shift. *International Journal of Behavioral Consultation and Therapy, 8*(3–4), 30–36. https://doi.org/10.1037/h0100980

Luong, D., & Wormith, J. S. (2011). Applying risk/need assessment to probation practice and its impact of the recidivism of young offenders. *Criminal Justice and Behavior, 38*(12), 1177–1199. https://doi.org/10.1177/0093854811421596

Martinson, R. (1974). What works? Questions and answers about prison reform. *The Public Interest, 35*, 22–54.

Masten, A. S. (2001). Ordinary magic: Resilience processes in development. *American Psychologist, 56*(3), 227–238. https://doi.org/10.1037/0003-066X.56.3.227

McGuire, J. (2004). Commentary: Promising answers and the next generation of questions. *Psychology Crime and Law, 10*(3), 335–345. https://doi.org/10.1080/10683160410001662816

McNeill, F. (2009). *Towards effective practice in offender supervision.* Glasgow, UK: The Scottish Centre for Crime & Justice Research.

McNeill, F. (2012). Four forms of 'offender' rehabilitation: Towards an interdisciplinary perspective. *Legal and Criminological Psychology, 17*(1), 18–36. https://doi.org/10.1111/j.2044-8333.2011.02039.x

McNeill, F., & Whyte, B. (2007). *Reducing reoffending: Social work and community justice in Scotland*. Cullompton, UK: Willan.

Meehl, P. E. (1957). When shall we use our heads instead of the formula? *Journal of Counseling Psychology, 4*(4), 268–273. https://doi.org/10.1037/h0047554

Miller, J., & Maloney, C. (2013). Practitioner compliance with risk/needs assessment tools: A theoretical and empirical assessment. *Criminal Justice and Behavior, 40*(7), 716–736. https://doi.org/10.1177/0093854812468883

Miller, W. R. (1983). Motivational interviewing with problem drinkers. *Behavioural and Cognitive Psychotherapy, 11*(2), 147–172. https://doi.org/10.1017/S0141347300006583

Nellis, A. (2016). *The color of justice: Racial and ethnic disparity in state prisons*. Washington, DC: The Sentencing Project.

Nelson, R. J., & Vincent, G. M. (2018). Matching service to criminogenic needs following comprehensive risk assessment implementation in juvenile probation. *Criminal Justice and Behavior, 45*(8), 1136–1153. https://doi.org/10.1177/0093854818780923

Newcome, J., & Cullen, F. T. (2017). The risk-need-responsivity model revisited: Using biosocial criminology to enhance offender rehabilitation. *Criminal Justice and Behavior, 44*(8), 1030–1049. https://doi.org/10.1177/0093854817715289

Ogloff, J. R. P., & Davis, M. R. (2004). Advances in offender assessment and rehabilitation: Contributions of the risk-need-responsivity approach. *Psychology Crime and Law, 10*(3), 229–242. https://doi.org/10.1080/10683160410001662735

Peterson-Badali, M., Skilling, T., & Haqanee, Z. (2015). Implementation of risk assessment in case management for youth in the justice system. *Criminal Justice and Behavior, 42*(3), 304–320. https://doi.org/10.1177/0093854814549595

Polaschek, D. L. L. (2012). An appraisal of the risk–need–responsivity (RNR) model of offender rehabilitation and its application in correctional treatment. *Legal and Criminological Psychology, 17*(1), 1–17. https://doi.org/10.1111/j.2044-8333.2011.02038.x

Polaschek, D. L. L. (2016). Desistance and dynamic risk factors belong together. *Psychology Crime and Law, 22*(1–2), 171–189. https://doi.org/10.1080/1068316X.2015.1114114

Porporino, F. J. (2010). Bringing sense and sensitivity to corrections: From programmes to 'fix' offenders to services to support desistence. In J. Brayford, F. Crowe, & J. Deering (Eds.), *What else works? Creative work with offenders* (pp. 61–86). Abingdon, UK: Willan Publishing.

Prendergast, M. L. (2009). Interventions to promote successful re-entry among drug-abusing parolees. *Addiction Science & Clinical Practice, 5*(1), 4–13. https://doi.org/10.1151/ascp09514

Prendergast, M. L., Pearson, F. S., Podus, D., Hamilton, Z. K., & Greenwell, L. (2013). The Andrews' principles of risk, needs, and responsivity as applied in drug treatment programs: Meta-analysis of crime and drug use outcomes. *Journal of Experimental Criminology, 9*(3), 275–300. https://doi.org/10.1007/s11292-013-9178-z

Raynor, P. (2007). Risk and need assessment in British probation: The contribution of the LSI-R. *Psychology Crime and Law, 13*(2), 125–138. https://doi.org/10.1080/10683160500337592

Raynor, P., & Robinson, G. (2009). *Rehabilitation, crime and justice*. Basingstoke, UK: Palgrave Macmillan.

Robinson, G., & Crow, I. (2009). *Offender rehabilitation: Theory, research and practice*. London, UK: Sage Publications Inc.

Rogan, M. (2017). Human rights, risk and need: The right to rehabilitation and the right to fairness. In F. S. Taxman (Ed.), *Handbook on risk and need assessment: Theory and practice* (pp. 447–464). New York, NY: Routledge.

Ross, R. R., & Fabiano, E. A. (1985). *Time to think: A cognitive model of delinquent prevention and offender rehabilitation*. Johnson City, NJ: Institute of Social Science and Arts.

Ross, R. R., & Gendreau, P. (Eds.). (1980). *Effective correctional treatment*. Toronto, ON: Butterworths.

Rudes, D. S., Kras, K. R., Meyer, K. S., & Magnuson, S. (2017). Implementation uptake: Organisational factors affecting evidence-based reform in community corrections in the United States. In P. Ugwudike, P. Raynor, & J. Annison (Eds.), *Evidence-based skills in criminal justice: International research on supporting rehabilitation and desistance* (pp. 79–96). Bristol, UK: Policy Press.
Sameroff, A. J., Bartko, W. T., Baldwin, A., Baldwin, C., & Seifer, R. (1998). Family and social influences on the development of child competence. In M. Lewis & C. Fairing (Eds.), *Families, risk, and competence* (pp. 161–186). Mahwah, NJ: Lawrence Erlbaum Associates, Inc.
Seligman, M. E. P., & Csikszentmihalyi, M. (2000). Positive psychology [special issue]. *American Psychologist, 55*(1), 5–14.
Seligman, M. E. P., Steen, T. A., Park, N., & Peterson, C. (2005). Positive psychology in progress: Empirical validation of interventions. *American Psychologist, 60*(5), 410–421. https://doi.org/10.1037/0003-066X.60.5.410
Serin, R. (2007). *The dynamic risk assessment scale for offender re-entry (DRAOR). Unpublished scale*. Ottawa, ON: Carleton University.
Serin, R. C., Mailloux, D. L., & Wilson, N. J. (2012). *The dynamic risk assessment for offender re-entry (DRAOR), New Zealand adaptation (unpublished user manual)*. Ottawa, ON: Carleton University.
Somers, J. M., Currie, L., Moniruzzaman, A., Eiboff, F., & Patterson, M. (2012). Drug treatment court of Vancouver: An empirical evaluation of recidivism. *International Journal of Drug Policy, 23*(5), 393–400. https://doi.org/10.1016/j.drugpo.2012.01.011
Sperber, K. G., Latessa, E. J., & Makarios, M. D. (2013a). Examining the interaction between level of risk and dosage of treatment. *Criminal Justice and Behavior, 40*(3), 338–348. https://doi.org/10.1177/0093854812467942
Sperber, K. G., Latessa, E. J., & Makarios, M. D. (2013b). Establishing a risk-dosage research agenda: Implications for policy and practice. *Justice Research and Policy, 15*(1), 123–141. https://doi.org/10.3818/JRP.15.1.2013.123
Taxman, F. S. (2014). Second generation of RNR: The importance of systemic responsivity in expanding core principles of responsivity. *Federal Probation Journal, 78*(2), 32–40.
Taxman, F. S., Thanner, M., & Weisburd, D. (2006). Risk, need, and responsivity (RNR): It all depends. *Crime & Delinquency, 52*(1), 28–51. https://doi.org/10.1177/0011128705281754
Ttofi, M. M., Farrington, D. P., Piquero, A. R., & DeLisi, M. (2016). Protective factors against offending and violence: Results from prospective longitudinal studies. *Journal of Criminal Justice, 45*, 1–3. https://doi.org/10.1016/j.jcrimjus.2016.02.001
Usher, A. M., & Stewart, L. A. (2014). Effectiveness of correctional programs with ethnically diverse offenders: A meta-analytic study. *International Journal of Offender Therapy and Comparative Criminology, 58*(2), 209–230. https://doi.org/10.1177/0306624X12469507
Van der Laan, A. M., Veenstra, R., Bogaerts, S., Verhulst, F. C., & Ormel, J. (2010). Serious, minor, and non-delinquents in early adolescence: The impact of cumulative risk and promotive factors. The TRAILS study. *Journal of Abnormal Child Psychiatry, 38*(3), 339–351. https://doi.org/10.1007/s10802-009-9368-3
Viglione, J., Rudes, D. S., & Taxman, F. S. (2015). Misalignment in supervision: Implementing risk/needs assessment instrument in probation. *Criminal Justice and Behavior, 42*(3), 263–285. https://doi.org/10.1177/0093854814548447
Vincent, G. M., Chapman, J., & Cook, N. E. (2011). Risk-needs assessment in juvenile justice: Predictive validity of the SAVRY, racial differences, and the contribution of needs factors. *Criminal Justice and Behavior, 38*(1), 42–62. https://doi.org/10.1177/0093854810386000
Vogel, d., de, V., de Ruiter, C., Bouman, Y., & de Vries Robbé, M. (2009). *SAPROF. Guidelines for the assessment of protective factors for violence risk*. Utrecht, The Netherlands: Forum Educatief.
Vose, B., Lowenkamp, C. T., Smith, P., & Cullen, F. T. (2009). Gender and the predictive validity of the LSI-R: A study of parolees and probationers. *Journal of Contemporary Criminal Justice, 25*(4), 459–471. https://doi.org/10.1177/1043986209344797

Ward, T., & Brown, M. (2004). The good lives model and conceptual issues in offender rehabilitation. *Psychology Crime and Law, 10*(3), 243–257. https://doi.org/10.1080/10683160410001662744

Ward, T., & Fortune, C.-A. (2013). The good lives model: Aligning risk reduction with promoting offenders' personal goals. *European Journal of Probation, 5*(2), 29–46. https://doi.org/10.1177/206622031300500203

Ward, T., Gannon, T. A., & Birgden, A. (2007). Human rights and the treatment of sex offenders. *Sexual Abuse: A Journal of Research and Treatment, 19*(3), 195–216. https://doi.org/10.1007/s11194-007-9053-4

Ward, T., Melser, J., & Yates, P. M. (2007). Reconstructing the risk–need–responsivity model: A theoretical elaboration and evaluation. *Aggression and Violent Behavior, 12*(2), 208–228. https://doi.org/10.1016/j.avb.2006.07.001

Ward, T., & Stewart, C. A. (2003a). Criminogenic needs and human needs: A theoretical model. *Psychological, Crime, and Law, 9*(2), 125–143. https://doi.org/10.1080/10683160310001162 47

Ward, T., & Stewart, C. A. (2003b). The treatment of sex offenders: Risk management and the good lives model. *Professional Psychology: Research and Practice, 34*(4), 353–360. https://doi.org/10.1037/0735-7028.34.4.353

Ward, T., Yates, P. M., & Willis, G. M. (2012). The good lives model and the risk need responsivity model: A critical response to Andrews, Bonta, and Wormith (2011). *Criminal Justice and Behavior, 39*(1), 94–110. https://doi.org/10.1177/0093854811426085

Wexler, D. B., & Winick, B. J. (Eds.). (1996). *Law in a therapeutic key: Developments in therapeutic jurisprudence*. Durham, NC: Carolina Academic Press.

Wilson, H. A., & Hoge, R. D. (2013). The effect of youth diversion programs on recidivism: A meta-analytic review. *Criminal Justice and Behaviour, 40*(5), 497–518. https://doi.org/10.1177/0093854812451089

Wormith, J. S. (2011). The legacy of D. A. Andrews in the field of criminal justice: How theory and research can change policy and practice. *International Journal of Forensic Mental Health, 10*(2), 78–82. https://doi.org/10.1080/14999013.2011.577138

Wormith, J. S. (2017). Automated offender risk assessment: The next generation or a black hole? *Criminology & Public Policy, 16*(1), 281–303. https://doi.org/10.1111/1745-9133.12277

Wormith, J. S., Gendreau, P., & Bonta, J. (2012). Deferring to clarity, parsimony, and evidence in reply to Ward, yates, and Willis (2011). *Criminal Justice and Behavior, 39*(1), 111–120. https://doi.org/10.1177/0093854811426087

Wormith, J. S., Hogg, S., & Guzzo, L. (2012). The predictive validity of a general risk/needs assessment inventory on sexual offender recidivism and an exploration of the professional override. *Criminal Justice and Behavior, 39*(12), 1511–1538. https://doi.org/10.1177/0093854812455741

Wormith, J. S., & Truswell, K. (in press). Strengths in the risk-needs-responsivity model of offender assessment and rehabilitation. In C. M. Langton & J. R. Worling (Eds.), *The Wiley handbook of offender desistance from aggression and crime: Theory, research, and evidence-based practice*. Hoboken, NJ: John Wiley & Sons, Inc.

Yesberg, J. A., & Polaschek, D. L. L. (2015). Assessing dynamic risk and protective factors in the community: Examining the validity of the dynamic risk assessment for offender re-entry. *Psychology, Crime & Law, 21*(1), 80–99. https://doi.org/10.1080/1068316X.2014.935775

Chapter 3
Protective Factors and the Good Lives Model: Combining Positive Approaches to Assessment and Treatment

Sophie R. Dickson, Gwenda M. Willis, and Danielle Mather

3.1 Introduction

In the year 2000, the *American Psychologist* devoted its millennial issue to the emerging field of positive psychology, tying together disparate research that looked at what makes life worth living (Seligman & Csikszentmihalyi, 2000). Positive psychology has been defined as "the scientific study of optimal functioning, focusing on aspects of the human condition that lead to happiness, fulfilment, and flourishing" (Linley & Harrington, 2005, p. 13). Since that time, the field has flourished, and a myriad of articles and books have been written on the promotion of mental health and well-being, which was a significant shift from the previous focus on pathology within the psychology profession (Seligman, Steen, Park, & Peterson, 2005). While in the criminal justice arena the focus of psychology has understandably been on risk management and minimizing harm to the community, positive factors associated with ceasing offending after an individual has come into contact with the criminal justice system have attracted increasing attention in recent years (e.g., Laws & Ward, 2011). A shift toward the inclusion of positive factors has a number of potential benefits including adding incremental predictive validity to recidivism risk assessments, improving risk management, and reducing the likelihood of stigmatization of persons who have offended (de Vries Robbé, Mann, Maruna, & Thornton, 2015). It has been argued that the promotion of an individual's well-being should sit alongside reducing their risk of engaging in further harmful behavior for treatment to be most effective (Ward & Stewart, 2003). The current chapter will discuss two examples of approaches within criminal justice psychology

S. R. Dickson
Psychological Services, New Zealand Department of Corrections, Wellington, New Zealand
e-mail: sophie.dickson@corrections.govt.nz

G. M. Willis (✉) · D. Mather
School of Psychology, The University of Auckland, Auckland, New Zealand
e-mail: g.willis@auckland.ac.nz; dmat217@aucklanduni.ac.nz

E. L. Jeglic, C. Calkins (eds.), *New Frontiers in Offender Treatment*,
https://doi.org/10.1007/978-3-030-01030-0_3

that have their roots in positive psychology: The emerging focus on "protective factors" within risk assessment and the Good Lives Model (GLM), which is a strengths-based theory of rehabilitation developed by Tony Ward and colleagues (e.g., Laws & Ward, 2011; Ward, Mann, & Gannon, 2007; Ward & Stewart, 2003). The chapter will describe both and explore how the two could work together to provide a positive psychological approach to both assessment and treatment of individuals within the criminal justice system.

3.2 Positive Approaches to Assessment

For many years, a major focus in the forensic psychology field was on identifying risk factors for reoffending. As defined in Andrews and Bonta's (2010) seminal text, risk factors are "characteristics of people and their circumstances that are associated with an increased chance of future criminal activity" (p. 20). Research has consistently identified a number of risk factors that predict reoffending, such as antisocial personality, antisocial associates, and substance use (e.g., Gendreau, Little, & Goggin, 1996). Actuarial tools that combine a number of risk factors enable practitioners to identify the relative risk level posed by individual clients in the criminal justice system. They provide a transparent and consistent method for estimating risk for recidivism, which outperforms unstructured professional judgment (the first approach to recidivism risk assessment). To illustrate, the Violence Risk Scale (Wong & Gordon, 2006) and a combination of the Static-99 and Stable-2007 (Hanson, Helmus, & Harris, 2015) predict violent and sexual recidivism with moderate predictive accuracy (AUCs of 0.73 and 0.74, respectively). By contrast, the predictive accuracy of unstructured professional judgment more closely approximates chance (estimated AUC of 0.56; Grove, Zald, Lebow, Snitz, & Nelson, 2000). Given their clear superiority to unstructured professional judgments about risk, risk assessment tools have become a major component of assessment within criminal justice psychology and are at the cornerstone of a number of decisions around sentencing, treatment, and release into the community.

Despite the empirical support for a variety of risk assessment tools, they are not without their limitations. Their emphasis on risk factors has led to the development of an approach that is deficits-focused, thus generating pessimism and negative views of the individual being assessed (Cording & Beggs Christofferson, 2017; de Vries Robbé & Willis, 2017). Risk assessments that examine solely risk factors fixate on unfavorable aspects of the individual and their environment, producing stigmatization of not only the individual who offended but also those around them (Kewley, 2016). It is not unreasonable to assume that an assessment focused on identifying the things that are "wrong" with an individual would not be particularly enjoyable or motivating for the client, or even for the assessor. In addition, current risk assessment tools can overestimate recidivism risk. For example, of individuals assessed in the "high" risk category on the Violence Risk Scale (VRS; Wong & Gordon, 2006), 51.5% went on to violently reoffend, meaning that almost half of those individuals assessed as "high risk" did not reoffend. By relying on risk factors alone, we are unable to differentiate the 48.5% of this group who did not go on to reoffend from those who did. Inaccurately identifying someone as high risk can have significant consequences including unnecessary interventions that come at a high cost to the taxpayer and seriously limit the individual's autonomy (Cording & Beggs Christofferson, 2017; de Vries Robbé & Willis, 2017). Therefore, it has become increasingly apparent that a less biased assessment of recidivism risk is needed, one that focuses not just on deficits or flaws but on positive aspects of the individual that may counteract risk factors.

Alongside criminal justice psychology's focus on risk assessment, researchers in the field of criminology have explored the phenomena of desistance from crime, or personal and environmental characteristics that disrupt the continuation of criminal behavior (e.g., Laub & Sampson, 2001; Maruna, 2001; Sampson & Laub, 1993). Recent scholarly work has integrated desistance research and criminal justice psychology research to inform new, positive approaches to assessment and treatment of individuals in the criminal justice system (e.g., de Vries Robbé, Mann, et al., 2015; Laws & Ward, 2011). One such development has been the introduction of new assessment tools designed to bring balance to predominantly risk-focused tools through the incorporation of protective factors, which we discuss next.

3.2.1 The Introduction of Protective Factors in Risk Assessment

The concept of "protective factors" has attracted steady scholarly attention in recent years. de Vries Robbé, Mann, et al. (2015) define protective factors as "a feature of a person that lowers the risk of reoffending" and noted that "the definition of a protective factor should encompass social, interpersonal, and environmental factors as well as psychological and behavioral features" (p. 18). The positive effect of protective factors is thought to weigh against the negative effect of risk factors (de Vries Robbé, de Vogel, & de Spa, 2011). In a similar vain to Andrews and Bonta's (2010) differentiation between static and dynamic risk factors, de Vries Robbé, de Vogel, Koster, and Bogaerts (2015) noted that protective factors could be static (e.g., secure attachment in childhood) or dynamic (e.g., good social skills) in nature. They emphasized that while many protective factors likely exist in the same domain as risk factors, they must exist in their own right: The absence of a risk factor does not imply the presence of a protective factor. While risk and protective factors can resemble opposing ends of the same continuum, they can also co-occur within an individual. For example, in the domain of social influences, both negative social influences (a risk factor) and prosocial social influences (a protective factor) can co-occur. Similarly, in the domain of sexual interests, an individual can demonstrate both deviant sexual interests (e.g., sexual interest in children, a risk factor for sexual reoffending) and prosocial sexual interests (interest in and arousal to adult consenting sex—a proposed protective factor against sexual reoffending; Willis,

Thornton, Kelley, & de Vries Robbé, 2017). Thus, single measures for a given domain may not capture the complexity of individual presentations (see also Klepfisz, Daffern, & Day, 2017). We contend that a balanced approach to risk assessment requires considering the psychological, social, and environmental variables related to criminal behavior for both their risk enhancing and risk mitigating or "protective" potential.

Compared to risk factor research, the literature exploring protective factors is still in its infancy. The earliest comprehensive investigation into protective factors was a doctoral thesis by de Vries Robbé (2014) assessing the psychometric properties of the Structured Assessment of Protective Factors for Violence Risk (SAPROF; de Vogel, de Ruiter, Bouman, & de Vries Robbé, 2012). The SAPROF authors considered protective factors that may exist on the opposite end of a continuum with risk factors (e.g., self-control versus impulsivity), as well as protective factors that may operate independently from risk factors to promote an enhanced sense of personal agency and desistance from crime (e.g., prosocial life goals). Ultimately, the SAPROF incorporated protective factors that were separated into three categories: *internal factors* such as intelligence, empathy, and self-control; *motivational factors* such as work, leisure activities, life goals, and medication; and *external factors* such as intimate relationships, professional care, and living circumstances.

Research examining the predictive validity of the SAPROF has produced promising results. For example, SAPROF scores have predicted violent incidents in forensic psychiatric patients during treatment (Abidin et al., 2013), as well as violent recidivism posttreatment (de Vries Robbé, de Vogel, & Douglas, 2013). When used alongside the Historical-Clinical-Risk Management-20 (HCR-20), the SAPROF has demonstrated added incremental predictive validity to the prediction of violent recidivism in some studies (e.g., de Vries Robbé et al., 2011) but not others (e.g., Abidin et al., 2013). A study of individuals convicted for sexual offending demonstrated that the SAPROF was also a significant predictor of new convictions of any (including sexual) violence over a follow-up period of 15 years. When controlling for scores on the HCR-20, the SAPROF remained a significant predictor of recidivism over that period (de Vries Robbé, de Vogel, et al., 2015). Thus, emerging empirical evidence suggests that protective factors can add value in our ability to predict recidivism, and their inclusion in risk assessment tools may reduce the likelihood that risk is overestimated. However, further research is needed to better understand the relative contribution of protective factors to recidivism risk assessments.

Notwithstanding the early stages of empirical research into the predictive validity of protective factors, they accommodate the addition of an individual's strengths into assessment. Importantly, the inclusion of protective factors can counteract the bias produced by risk assessment tools that concentrate solely on risk factors (de Vries Robbé & Willis, 2017). Not only might protective factors improve the accuracy of risk assessments, but they might also shift the focus of assessment from problems and negative aspects of an individual toward strengths and positive change, which is inherently more engaging. A positive approach is likely to strengthen the therapeutic alliance between client and therapist, which is an important and often overlooked variable related to treatment outcome (Marshall et al., 2003). Moreover, attending to protective factors may improve the receptiveness of communities to individuals who have offended, as an emphasis on an individual's capacities and capabilities could reduce stigmatization (Cording & Beggs Christofferson, 2017; Nee & Vernham, 2017). While reducing stigmatization might not be an immediate concern for therapists working with clients in the criminal justice system, to the extent that individuals who have offended are outed by communities, opportunities for safe (re)integration and long-term desistance from offending may be compromised (Willis, Levenson, & Ward, 2010).

The potential for protective factors to improve assessment practices in a meaningful and consistent way may rest on addressing salient definitional and conceptual issues surrounding the term "protective factor." Ward (2017) highlighted that it is common for researchers to lack a comprehensive conceptual understanding of protective factors which limits their ability to meaningfully incorporate protective factors into both risk assessment instruments and strengths-based interventions. There has been debate within the field regarding the definition of protective factors, and it remains unclear what exactly the term is referring to. Often, a number of terms are used interchangeably. These terms include "strengths," "promotive factor," "resilience," and "positive factors." However, these terms can all refer to different things and may not be describing the same processes (Ward, 2017). As highlighted by Ward, definitions and theoretical conceptualizations of protective factors should consider the different terms used in empirical research and explain how they relate to risk factors. Some researchers argue that protective factors are simply the absence or reversal of particular risk factors and do not exist as independent entities (Harris & Rice, 2015). Therefore, the relationship between the protective factor and offending can be interpreted through the corresponding risk factor (Cording & Beggs Christofferson, 2017). If true, the inclusion of protective factors that are the reversal of risk factors may be redundant when used in conjunction with tools that focus on risk factors. Considering the SAPROF (de Vogel, de Ruiter, Bouman, & de Vries Robbé, 2009), many items have a corresponding risk factor on the Historical-Clinical-Risk Management-20 version 3 (HCR-20^{V3}; Douglas, Hart, Webster, & Belfrage, 2013), which likely explains their similar levels of predictive validity. However, the SAPROF also includes protective factors that do not have a corresponding risk factor (e.g., medication and life goals) and has demonstrated incremental predictive validity for predictions of both sexual and violent reoffending when used with risk-based assessment instruments (e.g., de Vries Robbé et al., 2013; Kivisto, 2015). These findings challenge the suggestion that protective factors are simply the opposite of risk factors. Alternatively, as recently suggested by Helmus (2018), tools designed to measure protective factors may not be measuring constructs that are distinct from risk factors, "...but the possibility remains that they are measuring existing factors *better*" [emphasis in original] (p. 5). In other words, perhaps attending to protective factors allows for considering greater variance in functioning across risk-relevant domains than the variance captured by risk tools alone.

Related to definitional ambiguities, there is also debate regarding the causal nature of protective factors. Nee and Vernham (2017) negate the idea that protective factors are the opposite of risk factors and argue that they are not causes of reduced recidivism, but rather predictors of desistance. de Vries Robbé (2014) argues that protective factors have a causal influence on risk factors and criminal behavior. Durrant (2017) acknowledges that the causal processes are unclear and that there is a lack of research exploring why certain factors protect an individual from risk of offending. Much like risk factors, protective factors have been identified through studies that explore desistance from crime at a group or population level. As highlighted by Ward and Fortune (2016) regarding dynamic risk factors, it would be a mistake to assume that such factors therefore represent appropriate treatment targets at an individual level. Protective factors are merely predictive constructs that aid in our assessment of the likelihood of future offending. They may represent proxies or signals for underlying processes that can assist the individual to desist from crime, but they require further theoretical interpretation to inform individualized treatment. In other words, the empirical approach used to identify protective factors in large samples does little to explain causal processes of desistance at an individual level. When protective factors are transposed into treatment goals, treatment may miss the specific mechanism(s) responsible for counteracting risk factors and/or promoting desistance. For example, employment has been identified as a protective factor against reoffending and a predictor of desistance (e.g., de Vries Robbé, Mann, et al., 2015). But to state that there is a link between employment and non-offending does not identify the causal link between the two. Employment may protect the individual against offending in a variety of ways, such as providing an income for material needs (especially when the individual offended for material gain), providing structure to one's day and removing opportunities to offend, buffering an individual from peers who reinforce antisocial attitudes and offending, and increasing exposure to peers who model and reinforce prosocial attitudes and behavior. In other words, employment may protect against reoffending in different ways for different clients—and might offer little or no protection for other clients (e.g., if an individual's work brings them into contact with antisocial peers).

The simple identification of protective factors cannot replace a comprehensive theoretically informed case formulation that *explains* desistance from offending at the individual level. A theoretically informed case formulation will delineate causal mechanisms that protect an individual from future offending and inform an appropriate treatment approach. Explanations for the causal processes underlying protective factors are in their infancy and lack empirical testing. Later in this chapter, we draw on the theoretical resources of the Good Lives Model (GLM) to explore one possible mechanism through which protective factors might exert their effect. The GLM is an overarching theory or framework of rehabilitation and is described in the next section.

3.3 Positive Approaches to Treatment

Traditional treatment approaches, like traditional approaches to assessment, focus on risk factors. The dominant Risk Need Responsivity model (RNR; Andrews & Bonta, 2010) claims that reoffending is reduced through minimizing the presence of risk factors, which represent problems in the individual's life that need to be addressed (Ward & Brown, 2004). There have been a number of criticisms of risk-focused approaches to treatment, including difficulties motivating and engaging clients and associated high rates of treatment dropout (Ward & Stewart, 2003; Ware & Bright, 2008). Risk-focused treatment often relies heavily on treatment goals that are negative or avoidant in nature, such as avoiding antisocial peers or children (Ward & Brown, 2004). The distinction between positive, or "approach" goals, and avoidant goals is important, because research has demonstrated a variety of benefits to framing goals in a positive manner (Coats, Janoff-Bulman, & Alpert, 1996). Approach goals direct us to move toward a positive or desirable outcome (e.g., build a prosocial support network), whereas avoidance goals guide us to move away from a negative or undesirable outcome (e.g., avoid antisocial peers). Both of these goals may lead to the same outcome—a reduced likelihood of reoffending—but we achieve them in different ways, and they have different effects on us (Coats et al., 1996). Approach goals have been linked to a variety of positive outcomes and processes, such as increased effort, more persistence, improved performance, more intrinsic motivation, and more interest (Elliot, 1999; Elliot & Church, 1997). Avoidance goals have been linked to more negative outcomes and processes, such as low self-esteem, lower optimism, depression, low self-determination, anxiety, distraction, unwillingness to seek help, and poorer performance (Coats et al., 1996; Elliot, 1999; Gable, 2006). Treatment aimed at reducing risk is therefore likely to lead to poorer outcomes than treatment aimed at increasing strengths. The Good Lives Model provides a framework for correctional rehabilitation that promotes positive, approach-oriented treatment goals and is described next.

3.3.1 The Good Lives Model

The Good Lives Model (GLM; Ward, 2002; Ward & Stewart, 2003) was developed as a complementary approach to traditional risk-focused treatment to offset some of the issues with the deficits focus of RNR. The GLM is an overarching framework that guides rehabilitation in a way that is more person-centered and holistic compared to the traditional risk/deficit-focused approach. At its core, the GLM recognizes that all humans are naturally driven to seek similar underlying needs that once realized allow them to flourish. Referred to in the GLM as *primary human goods,* these needs are inherently valuable in their own right and include "life" (physical safety) and "relatedness" (relationships with others including intimate relationships, familial relationships, and friendships). Drawing from cross-disciplinary research, Ward and Stewart (2003) identified 10 classes of primary goods: life, relationships, community, agency, knowledge, excellence in work and play, inner peace, spirituality, happiness, and creativity. The pursuit of these goods in a prosocial manner promotes the well-being of an individual. Accordingly, the GLM promotes a dual focus in treatment on promoting prosocial attainment of primary human goods alongside reducing/managing reoffense risk. The GLM's focus on positive and prosocial aspirations reduces the stigma associated with a focus on deficits (Ward & Gannon, 2006).

According to the GLM, different individuals will prioritize different primary goods and achieve these goods through different means. The means by which an individual pursues primary goods are referred to as instrumental or *secondary goods* and are informed by the individual's capacities, resources, personal identity, and specific cultural context. In contrast to risk management approaches, the GLM seeks to decrease risk of recidivism by strengthening the competencies needed to accomplish primary goods in meaningful and prosocial ways. The GLM asserts that individuals turn to crime when they do not possess the personal and environmental characteristics needed to achieve their prioritized primary goods in socially acceptable ways (Ward, Göbbels, & Willis, 2014; Ward & Stewart, 2003). Crime is motivated by attempts to seek out one or more primary human goods, and criminal behavior can therefore be understood as a maladaptive strategy to attain a primary good or goods, or a maladaptive secondary good. For example, theft might be motivated by the primary good of life (e.g., to obtain food). In other cases, theft might be motivated by the primary goods of community (e.g., to strengthen connections to a gang), or autonomy. Sexual offending might be motivated by the primary good of relatedness (e.g., seeking sexual and emotional intimacy with a child), inner peace (e.g., sexual offending to relieve tension/stress), autonomy, or pleasure. Rehabilitation efforts consistent with the GLM focus on strengthening an individual's skills and resources to achieve primary goods in alternative, more adaptive ways, including addressing risk factors related to reoffending. For example, an individual who offended sexually in an attempt to attain inner peace would benefit from strengthening their emotional regulation skills to access inner peace in more adaptive ways. Naturally, the dynamic risk factor of using sex to cope with negative affect would be addressed as the individual identifies and strengthens alternative emotional regulation strategies. Ultimately, rehabilitation aims to assist clients seek out desired primary goods without causing harm (Ward & Stewart, 2003). Treatment is therefore tailored to the individual, based on their personal identity and conceptualization of a good life (i.e., including primary goods that are most valued to the individual and those implicated in offending).

A significant advantage of the GLM is that it has potential to simultaneously address risk management and increase treatment engagement (Ward & Maruna, 2007). While research evaluating the effectiveness of GLM-derived treatment programs is lacking, a few studies have documented beneficial effects. Harkins, Flak, Beech, and Woodhams (2012) developed a treatment program for individuals who had sexually offended that incorporated the GLM. They found that staff and client perceptions of the GLM program were more positive than perceptions of the standard (relapse prevention oriented) program, and a focus on meaningful goals enabled individuals to develop a more optimistic outlook for themselves and their future. However, there were no differences in rates of treatment attrition between the standard and GLM programs, and within treatment change to criminogenic needs was similar across programs. Follow-up data are thus needed to examine whether positive perceptions of the GLM program were associated with long-term behavior change and desistance from crime. In a multi-site study exploring the integration of the GLM in 13 North American sexual offending treatment programs, program directors were asked about what supported their efforts to integrate a GLM approach. Across programs, directors identified that buy-in from both clients and staff supported their adoption of the GLM (Willis, Ward, & Levenson, 2014). While the GLM has been most extensively researched in the adult male sex offending literature, the GLM offers a strengths-based framework for addressing criminal behavior in general and across different populations, including with youth (Fortune, 2018) and females (Sorbello, Eccleston, Ward, & Jones, 2002). Notwithstanding a lack of long-term outcome data, preliminary studies suggest that the GLM offers a more engaging approach compared to traditional risk/deficit-focused approaches.

3.4 Linking Positive Approaches to Assessment and Treatment

Overall, protective factors and the GLM provide more balanced approaches to the assessment and treatment of people in the criminal justice system. Rather than focusing on deficits, or things to avoid, they provide frameworks for systematically identifying strengths and building on them. Together, protective factors and the GLM offer a number of benefits over the predominant focus on criminogenic needs/dynamic risk factors: They hold promise for more accurate prediction of who will go on to commit further crimes, allowing for improved allocation of resources; they promote more individualized treatment planning; they are more engaging for clients and clinicians; and they reduce stigma by focusing on the client as a whole person who has strengths as well as deficits.

We believe that protective factors and the GLM are like good partners in marriage: They can support each other in mutually beneficial ways. First, the systematic assessment of protective factors bridges the gap between current risk assessment tools and treatment from a GLM framework by orienting the clinician to the client's strengths, rather than beginning treatment knowing primarily about the client's risk factors. Second, the GLM offers a framework through which to develop a deeper, theoretically driven understanding of how protective factors might operate to reduce the likelihood of future offending and promote desistance from crime.

GLM scholars advocate for a comprehensive assessment including identifying valued primary goods and goods implicated in offending, and strategies used (i.e., secondary goods) to access prioritized primary goods (e.g., Willis, Yates, Gannon, & Ward, 2013). However, owing partly to the lack of structured tools to assist with this exercise, the GLM is rarely integrated into assessment practices—even in treatment programs advocating a GLM approach (Willis et al., 2014). By contrast, clinicians have several tools at their perusal to assist in the identification of criminogenic needs (dynamic risk factors). Structured tools like the SAPROF orient the clinician to consider a client's existing strengths, which may help to elucidate existing prosocial instrumental or secondary goods that provide sources of primary human goods. More generally, a focus on existing strengths can facilitate an exploration of a client's life values and priorities (i.e., their conceptualization of a "good life"). To illustrate, items included in the SAPROF include life goals, work, and leisure activities. Enquiring about life goals might help the clinician to develop an understanding of what a good life means to the client and their prioritized primary goods. Enquiring about the extent to which prosocial, structured, and enjoyable work and leisure activities are present might help the clinician to identify prosocial sources of primary goods (i.e., secondary goods). Work and leisure activities may provide sources of any number of primary human goods, especially mastery (primary good = being good at work and play), relationships, and community. Certain work and leisure activities might additionally provide sources of pleasure, inner peace, life, agency, and creativity. Early opportunities to validate a client's personal goals and reinforce existing strengths (including prosocial ways of attaining primary goods) can help build rapport and prevent any disconnect between a deficits-focused assessment and strengths-based treatment.

In addition, structured approaches to assessing protective factors might improve our ability to detect within treatment change, especially in treatment programs utilizing strengths-based frameworks such as the GLM. Existing tools used to assess within treatment change focus on changes made across dynamic risk factors (e.g., Olver, Wong, Nicholaichuk, & Gordon, 2007; Wong & Gordon, 2006), which might not capture broader changes related to the prosocial pursuit of primary human goods and ultimately desistance from crime. Given the GLM's dual focus on preventing future offending and assisting clients live a fulfilling, meaningful life, an important implication for future research is developing outcome measures that align with these dual goals. While existing measures of protective factors were not derived from the GLM (or any theoretical model), they may detect treatment-related changes not captured by risk tools, such as the extent to which someone is working toward prosocial life goals. Thus, the assessment of protective factors alongside risk factors in pre-/posttreatment assessment might enhance our ability to detect within treatment changes in comparison to what is possible using risk tools alone. It is hoped that the burgeoning interest in assessing protective factors leads to the development of tools that are sensitive to underlying processes or mechanisms that protect the individual from future offending.

The GLM offers a theoretical lens from which to understand possible mechanisms underlying protective factors. More specifically, the GLM can help us understand *how* different protective factors might mitigate risk propensities or protect against reoffending, and in doing so provide explanatory/theoretical depth to the current empirical debate surrounding the nature of protective factors. To reiterate, protective factors as they are currently conceptualized in tools such as the SAPROF are predictive constructs useful in risk assessment, but without further theoretical interpretation such factors do not provide sufficient information to inform an individualized positive approach to treatment. The GLM provides a framework to bridge prediction and explanation—in other words, the GLM can help explain one of the ways in which protective factors may operate. For example, work and leisure activities might be protective if they provide the individual with sources of primary goods previously sought through offending. To illustrate, an individual with a history of bullying and long-standing social anxiety around peers may have felt less threatened around children and gravitated toward children to seek emotional and sexual intimacy (primary human good = relatedness). He may have described his offending against children in a romanticized fashion, explaining that he was "in relationships" with child victims. In this example, sexual offending can be conceptualized as a maladaptive attempt to seek out the legitimate human experience or primary human good of relatedness. Utilizing the GLM, treatment would focus on building up the individual's capacity to seek relatedness in an adaptive way—that is, to develop relationships with same-age peers—which would necessarily include addressing social anxiety. After effective treatment for social anxiety, work or leisure activities might be protective if they provide opportunities for prosocial, meaningful connections with adults. However, work or leisure activities that are solitary, or bring the individual into contact with children, would not provide prosocial sources of primary goods previously sought through offending and would not protect the individual from future offending. Thus, it is not the work or leisure activities per se that are protective, but how they operate to mitigate risk and/or promote desistance.

Researchers seeking to develop and refine tools to measure protective factors might benefit from consideration of the processes or mechanisms responsible for protection and identify measurable proxies for those mechanisms. In this chapter we have highlighted one such mechanism—that is, the prosocial attainment of valued primary goods or, as described by other scholars, the experience of prosocial reward (for further discussion of possible mechanisms underlying protective factors, see Thornton, Kelley, & Nelligan, 2017).

3.5 Concluding Comments

We believe that positive approaches to assessment and treatment with individuals who have offended brings much needed balance to a field that has been concerned primarily with risk and individual deficits. A focus on protective factors and strengths-based rehabilitation frameworks such as the GLM offers potential for better engaging individuals in therapeutic treatment programs and improving treatment outcomes. However, debate continues regarding whether these positive approaches offer unique contributions to assessment and treatment with individuals who have offended (e.g., Andrews, Bonta, & Wormith, 2011; Harris & Rice, 2015). We hope that this chapter inspires further research on strengths-based and positive approaches to assessment and treatment, so that their relative contributions to preventing future crime and improving the lives of persons who have offended are better understood.

References

Abidin, Z., Davoren, M., Naughton, L., Gibbons, O., Nulty, A., & Kennedy, H. G. (2013). Susceptibility (risk and protective) factors for in-patient violence and self-harm: Prospective study of structured professional judgement instruments START and SAPROF, DUNDRUM-3 and DUNDRUM-4 in forensic mental health services. *BMC Psychiatry, 13*(1), 197–215. https://doi.org/10.1186/1471-244X-13-197

Andrews, D. A., & Bonta, J. (2010). *The psychology of criminal conduct* (5th ed.). New York, NY: Routledge.

Andrews, D. A., Bonta, J., & Wormith, J. S. (2011). The risk-need-responsivity (RNR) model: Does adding the good lives model contribute to effective crime prevention? *Criminal Justice and Behavior, 38*(7), 735–755. https://doi.org/10.1177/0093854811406356

Coats, E. J., Janoff-Bulman, R., & Alpert, N. (1996). Approach versus avoidance goals: Differences in self-evaluation and well-being. *Personality and Social Psychology Bulletin, 22*(10), 1057–1067. https://doi.org/10.1177/01461672962210009

Cording, J. R., & Beggs Christofferson, S. M. (2017). Theoretical and practical issues for the measurement of protective factors. *Aggression and Violent Behavior, 32*, 45–54. https://doi.org/10.1016/j.avb.2016.12.007

de Vogel, V., de Ruiter, C., Bouman, Y. H. A., & de Vries Robbé, M. (2009). *SAPROF. Guideline for the assessment of protective factors for violence risk.* Utrecht, The Netherlands: Forum Educatief.

de Vogel, V., de Ruiter, C., Bouman, Y. H. A., & de Vries Robbé, M. (2012). *SAPROF. Guidelines for the assessment of protective factors for violence risk* (2nd ed.). Utrecht, The Netherlands: Van der Hoeven Stichting.

de Vries Robbé, M. (2014). Protective factors. Validation of the structured assessment of protective factors for violence risk in forensic psychiatry (Doctoral dissertation). Retrieved from http://www.saprof.com/content/2012/11/Research%2D%2Darticles

de Vries Robbé, M., de Vogel, V., & de Spa, E. (2011). Protective factors for violence risk in forensic psychiatric patients: A retrospective validation study of the SAPROF. *International Journal of Forensic Mental Health, 10*(3), 178–186. https://doi.org/10.1080/14999013.2011.600232

de Vries Robbé, M., de Vogel, V., & Douglas, K. S. (2013). Risk factors and protective factors: A two-sided dynamic approach to violence risk assessment. *The Journal of Forensic Psychiatry and Psychology, 24*(4), 440–457. https://doi.org/10.1080/14789949.2013.818162

de Vries Robbé, M., de Vogel, V., Koster, K., & Bogaerts, S. (2015). Assessing protective factors for sexually violent offending with the SAPROF. *Sexual Abuse, 27*(1), 51–70. https://doi.org/10.1177/1079063214550168

de Vries Robbé, M., Mann, R. E., Maruna, S., & Thornton, D. (2015). An exploration of protective factors supporting desistance from sexual offending. *Sexual Abuse, 27*(1), 16–33. https://doi.org/10.1177/1079063214547582

de Vries Robbé, M., & Willis, G. M. (2017). Assessment of protective factors in clinical practice. *Aggression and Violent Behavior, 32*, 55–63. https://doi.org/10.1016/j.avb.2016.12.006

Douglas, K. S., Hart, S. D., Webster, C. D., & Belfrage, H. (2013). *HCR-20V3: Assessing risk for violence – user guide.* Burnaby, BC: Mental Health, Law, and Policy Institute, Simon Fraser University.

Durrant, R. (2017). Why do protective factors protect? An evolutionary developmental perspective. *Aggression and Violent Behavior, 32*, 4–10. https://doi.org/10.1016/j.avb.2016.12.002

Elliot, A. J. (1999). Approach and avoidance motivation and achievement goals. *Educational Psychologist, 34*(3), 169–189. https://doi.org/10.1207/s15326985ep3403_3

Elliot, A. J., & Church, M. A. (1997). A hierarchical model of approach and avoidance achievement motivation. *Journal of Personality and Social Psychology, 72*(1), 218–232. https://doi.org/10.1037/0022-3514.72.1.218

Fortune, C.-A. (2018). The good lives model: A strength-based approach for youth offenders. *Aggression and Violent Behavior, 38*, 21–30. https://doi.org/10.1016/j.avb.2017.11.003

Gable, S. L. (2006). Approach and avoidance social motives and goals. *Journal of Personality, 74*(1), 175–222. https://doi.org/10.1111/j.1467-6494.2005.00373.x

Gendreau, P., Little, T., & Goggin, C. (1996). A meta-analysis of the predictors of adult offender recidivism: What works. *Criminology, 34*(4), 575–608. https://doi.org/10.1111/j.1745-9125.1996.tb01220.x

Grove, W. M., Zald, D. H., Lebow, B. S., Snitz, B. E., & Nelson, C. (2000). Clinical versus mechanical prediction: A meta-analysis. *Psychological Assessment, 12*(1), 19–30. https://doi.org/10.1037/1040-3590.12.1.19

Hanson, R. K., Helmus, L.-M., & Harris, A. J. R. (2015). Assessing the risk and needs of supervised sexual offenders: A prospective study using STABLE-2007, Static-99R, and Static-2002R. *Criminal Justice and Behavior, 42*(12), 1205–1224. https://doi.org/10.1177/0093854815602094

Harkins, L., Flak, V. E., Beech, A. R., & Woodhams, J. (2012). Evaluation of a community-based sex offender treatment program using a good lives model approach. *Sexual Abuse, 24*(6), 519–543. https://doi.org/10.1177/1079063211429469

Harris, G. T., & Rice, M. E. (2015). Progress in violence risk assessment and communication: Hypothesis versus evidence. *Behavioral Sciences and the Law, 33*(1), 128–145. https://doi.org/10.1002/bsl.2157

Helmus, L. M. (2018). Sex offender risk assessment: Where are we and where are we going? *Current Psychiatry Reports, 20*(6), 46–54. https://doi.org/10.1007/s11920-018-0909-8

Kewley, S. (2016). Strength based approaches and protective factors from a criminological perspective. *Aggression and Violent Behavior, 32*, 11–18. https://doi.org/10.1016/j.avb.2016.11.010

Kivisto, A. J. (2015). Violence risk assessment and management in outpatient clinical practice. *Journal of Clinical Psychology, 72*(4), 329–349. https://doi.org/10.1002/jclp.22243

Klepfisz, G., Daffern, M., & Day, A. (2017). Understanding protective factors for violent reoffending in adults. *Aggression and Violent Behavior, 32*, 80–87. https://doi.org/10.1016/j.avb.2016.12.001

Laub, J. H., & Sampson, R. J. (2001). Understanding desistance from crime. *Crime and Justice, 28*, 1–69. https://doi.org/10.1086/652208

Laws, D. R., & Ward, T. (2011). *Desistance from sex offending: Alternatives to throwing away the keys*. New York, NY: The Guilford Press.

Linley, P. A., & Harrington, S. (2005). Positive psychology and coaching psychology: Perspectives on integration. *The Coaching Psychologist, 1*(1), 13–14.

Marshall, W. L., Fernandez, Y. M., Serran, G. A., Mulloy, R., Thornton, D., Mann, R. E., & Anderson, D. (2003). Process variables in the treatment of sexual offenders: A review of the relevant literature. *Aggression and Violent Behavior, 8*(2), 205–234. https://doi.org/10.1016/S1359-1789(01)00065-9

Maruna, S. (2001). *Making good: How ex-convicts reform and rebuild their lives*. Washington, DC: American Psychological Association.

Nee, C., & Vernham, Z. (2017). Expertise and its contribution to the notion of protective factors in offender rehabilitation and desistance. *Aggression and Violent Behavior, 32*, 37–44. https://doi.org/10.1016/j.avb.2016.12.004

Olver, M. E., Wong, S. C., Nicholaichuk, T., & Gordon, A. (2007). The validity and reliability of the violence risk scale-sexual offender version: Assessing sex offender risk and evaluating therapeutic change. *Psychological Assessment, 19*(3), 318–329. https://doi.org/10.1037/1040-3590.19.3.318

Sampson, R. J., & Laub, J. H. (1993). *Crime in the making: Pathways and turning points through life*. Cambridge, MA: Harvard University Press.

Seligman, M. E. P., & Csikszentmihalyi, M. (2000). Special issue on happiness, excellence, and optimal human functioning [special issue]. *American Psychologist, 55*(1), 5–183.

Seligman, M. E. P., Steen, T. A., Park, N., & Peterson, C. (2005). Positive psychology progress: Empirical validation of interventions. *American Psychologist, 60*(5), 410–421. https://doi.org/10.1037/0003-066X.60.5.410

Sorbello, L., Eccleston, L., Ward, T., & Jones, R. (2002). Treatment needs of female offenders: A review. *Australian Psychologist, 37*(3), 198–205. https://doi.org/10.1080/0005006021000170 6876

Thornton, D., Kelley, S. M., & Nelligan, K. E. (2017). Protective factors and mental illness in men with a history of sexual offending. *Aggression and Violent Behavior, 32*, 29–36. https://doi.org/10.1016/j.avb.2016.12.003

Ward, T. (2002). Good lives and the rehabilitation of offenders: Promises and problems. *Aggression and Violent Behavior, 7*(5), 513–528. https://doi.org/10.1016/S1359-1789(01)00076-3

Ward, T. (2017). Prediction and agency: The role of protective factors in correctional rehabilitation and desistance. *Aggression and Violent Behavior, 32*, 19–28. https://doi.org/10.1016/j.avb.2016.11.012

Ward, T., & Brown, M. (2004). The good lives model and conceptual issues in offender rehabilitation. *Psychology, Crime & Law, 10*(3), 243–257. https://doi.org/10.1080/1068316041000166 2744

Ward, T., & Fortune, C. A. (2016). The role of dynamic risk factors in the explanation of offending. *Aggression and Violent Behavior, 29*, 79–88. https://doi.org/10.1016/j.avb.2016.06.007

Ward, T., & Gannon, T. A. (2006). Rehabilitation, etiology, and self-regulation: The comprehensive good lives model of treatment for sexual offenders. *Aggression and Violent Behavior, 11*(1), 77–94. https://doi.org/10.1016/j.avb.2005.06.001

Ward, T., Göbbels, S., & Willis, G. (2014). Good lives model. In G. Bruinsma & D. Weisburd (Eds.), *Encyclopedia of criminology and criminal justice* (pp. 1966–1976). New York, NY: Springer.

Ward, T., Mann, R. E., & Gannon, T. A. (2007). The good lives model of offender rehabilitation: Clinical implications. *Aggression and Violent Behavior, 12*(1), 87–107. https://doi.org/10.1016/j.avb.2006.03.004

Ward, T., & Maruna, S. (2007). *Rehabilitation: Beyond the risk paradigm*. New York, NY: Routledge.

Ward, T., & Stewart, C. A. (2003). The treatment of sex offenders: Risk management and good lives. *Professional Psychology: Research and Practice, 34*(4), 353–360. https://doi.org/10.1037/0735-7028.34.4.353

Ware, J., & Bright, D. A. (2008). Evolution of a treatment programme for sex offenders: Changes to the NSW custody-based intensive treatment (CUBIT). *Psychiatry, Psychology and Law, 15*(2), 340–349. https://doi.org/10.1080/13218710802014543

Willis, G. M., Levenson, J. S., & Ward, T. (2010). Desistance and attitudes towards sex offenders: Facilitation or hindrance? *Journal of Family Violence, 25*(6), 545–556. https://doi.org/10.1007/s10896-010-9314-8

Willis, G. M., Thornton, D. T., Kelley, S. M., & de Vries Robbé, M. (2017). The structured assessment of protective factors for violence risk - sexual offence version (SAPROF-SO). Pilot manual. Retrieved from http://www.saprof.com/

Willis, G. M., Ward, T., & Levenson, J. S. (2014). The Good Lives Model (GLM): An evaluation of GLM operationalization in North American treatment programs. *Sexual Abuse, 26*(1), 58–81. https://doi.org/10.1177/1079063213478202

Willis, G. M., Yates, P. M., Gannon, T. A., & Ward, T. (2013). How to integrate the good lives model into treatment programs for sexual offending: An introduction and overview. *Sexual Abuse, 25*(2), 123–142. https://doi.org/10.1177/1079063212452618

Wong, S. C. P., & Gordon, A. (2006). The validity and reliability of the violence risk scale: A treatment-friendly violence risk assessment tool. *Psychology, Public Policy, and Law, 12*(3), 279–309. https://doi.org/10.1037/1076-8971.12.3.279

Chapter 4
Cognitive Behavioral Therapy in Forensic Treatment

Damon Mitchell, Raymond Chip Tafrate, and Tom Hogan

4.1 Overview of Cognitive Behavioral Therapy (CBT)

Over the past six decades, the term CBT has come to encompass a plethora of models, interventions, and techniques for altering thinking and behavior, making it challenging to provide a distinct definition for this treatment approach. A review of the CBT literature and a perusal of the websites of well-known CBT training institutes reveals that a consensus definition of CBT does not currently exist. For example, the definitions below come from three leading CBT institutes that provide training in the United States and Australia:

- *Cognitive Behavior Therapy (CBT) is a time-sensitive, structured, present-oriented psychotherapy directed toward solving current problems and teaching clients skills to modify dysfunctional thinking and behavior* (Beck Institute for Cognitive Behavior Therapy, n.d.).
- *... an action-oriented psychotherapy that teaches individuals to identify, challenge, and replace their self-defeating beliefs with healthier ones that promote emotional well-being and goal achievement* (Albert Ellis Institute, n.d.).
- *Cognitive behaviour therapy is the term used for a school of therapies that share the underlying assumption that people are disturbed not by events in their lives but by their beliefs about those events. It is a logical and practical approach to help people with their emotional problems ...* (CBT Australia, n.d.).

D. Mitchell (✉) · R. C. Tafrate
Department of Criminology and Criminal Justice, Central Connecticut State University, New Britain, CT, USA
e-mail: mitchelldam@ccsu.edu; tafrater@ccsu.edu

T. Hogan
Institute for the Study of Crime and Justice, Central Connecticut State University, New Britain, CT, USA
e-mail: thogan@ccsu.edu

E. L. Jeglic, C. Calkins (eds.), *New Frontiers in Offender Treatment*,
https://doi.org/10.1007/978-3-030-01030-0_4

Some have characterized the CBT "package" as evolving from three distinct intellectual waves (DiGiuseppe, 2008; Leahy, 2008). The first wave includes traditional *behavioral principles* (e.g., positive and negative reinforcement, punishment, behavioral activation, exposure and response prevention) derived from the animal learning models of the early twentieth century (e.g., Thorndike, Watson, Pavlov, Watson, & Skinner). Behavioral interventions that developed from this wave focus on altering observable behaviors (as opposed to internal processes), which are largely viewed as a function of environmental influences such as reinforcement history and associative learning. The interventions emphasize the teaching, rehearsal, and acquisition of new behaviors that will become reinforced in the client's natural environment. Well-known interventions from this wave include contingency management, systematic desensitization, and assertiveness training.

The second wave traces its origin to the ancient Stoic Greek and Roman philosophers (e.g., Zeno, Seneca, Epictetus) and rests on the premise that disturbances in emotion and behavior can be modified by altering cognitive processes through testing one's thoughts through evidence and logic. These philosophical ideas were later formalized by Ellis (1957, 1962) and Beck (1963, 1967) into a set of intervention procedures. Ellis' model became known as *rational emotive behavior therapy* (REBT) and Beck's model *cognitive therapy*. A related intervention, known as *self-instructional training*, emphasizes verbal self-statements as a means of directing new behaviors, interrupting learned maladaptive patterns by replacing them with more adaptive internal self-instructions (Meichenbaum & Cameron, 1973). Currently, the generic term *cognitive restructuring* is frequently used to describe interventions that target thinking and self-talk.

The third wave incorporates elements of Buddhist philosophy and emphasizes mindful awareness and values-based actions (Hayes, 2008). The best-known intervention in this arena is *acceptance and commitment therapy* (ACT). The acronym ACT stands for *a*ccept thoughts and feelings, *c*hoose directions, and *t*ake action (Hayes & Smith, 2005). The focus is not on eliminating or changing client's upsetting thoughts and feelings but rather on learning to accept them and acting in ways that move the client in the direction they want to go. The identification of clients' personal values is used to establish anchor points to guide future behavioral choices, aiding in minimizing behaviors that will interfere with core values and developing behavioral activation plans likely to lead to a happier and more meaningful life (Amrod & Hayes, 2014).

4.1.1 Basic CBT Principles

Specific CBT interventions and programs contain elements from each historical wave, albeit with different emphasis and proportionality. Based on the three waves, some common hallmarks of the CBT approach can be derived.

1. *Address both behaviors and cognitions in treatment.* From a CBT perspective, people behave according to their thoughts and they think according to their behaviors. For example, consider a socially anxious person who avoids dating. If she were to change her thoughts from "I can't stand getting rejected. I'm terrible at dating" to "I have a lot to offer. Rejection is a normal, and I can deal with it," she would be more likely to explore online dating. Similarly, taking active steps to engage in romantic relationships (e.g., going on four dates per month) will challenge entrenched thinking patterns and foster new thoughts such as "Online dating is not so terrible. I'm having fun connecting with people, and I'm getting good at this." To have the greatest impact over the longer term, CBT practitioners focus on changing both thinking and behavior.
2. *Target cognitions that immediately precede emotional upset and self-defeating behavior.* In applying cognitive therapy, the first step is for practitioners to identify the cognitions (e.g., irrational logic or distortions) that actively drive the target behavior or emotional excess. The second step is to replace such patterns with more accurate and realistic thinking that will guide improved functioning. New thinking is actively rehearsed both in and out of sessions. The cognitions that become the focal point in treatment tend to differ according to the mental health disorder being addressed. For example, a tendency to overestimate danger is associated with worry; the belief "I'm special" is common in narcissism; the guiding idea that "I must never make mistakes" is often seen in compulsiveness. Different disorders can be understood as having their own set of typical unhealthy thinking patterns.

   The cognitions that become the focal point in treatment also tend to differ according to the specific CBT model of the practitioner. In Ellis' REBT model, the goal is to teach clients to think realistically about negative situations and to view them for what they usually are—Unpleasant, problematic inconveniences. In terms of relevant cognitive targets, *demandingness* (insisting that other people or the world confirm to one's own terms), *awfulizing* (exaggerating the consequences or level of hardship associated with difficult or challenging situations), *low frustration tolerance* (the tendency to underestimate one's ability to deal with discomfort or adversity), and *self or other ratings* (blaming or condemning other people or oneself "in total" for limited and specific things that they do) are viewed as the major culprits leading to disturbed functioning (DiGiuseppe, Doyle, Dryden, & Backx, 2013; O'Kelly, 2010).

   Beck's model of cognitive therapy takes into account several levels of cognitive processes. At the most basic level are *core beliefs* (or *schemas*), which tend to be global and overgeneralized conceptions about the self, other people, and the world. Core beliefs can be likened to a pair of eyeglasses; they are the lenses that color perceptions of the world and are formed in early childhood and often remain below the level of conscious awareness. It has been theorized that typical negative core beliefs for mental health clients fall into three categories: Helplessness, unlovability, and worthlessness (Beck, 2011).

   Core beliefs influence the next level of thinking, *intermediate beliefs* (*attitudes*, *rules*, and *assumptions*), which form the basis for how a person thinks, feels, and behaves across different situations. Such guiding rules of life may be maladaptive and potentially self-destructive. However, since intermediate beliefs have their origins in core beliefs, clients may not always consider such thinking patterns to be problematic. Practitioners are often astounded at the tenacity with which clients cling to their way of thinking in the face of negative consequences.

Lastly, emerging from intermediate beliefs are *automatic thoughts*. These are quick evaluative thoughts that spring up in response to different stimuli and form the stream of consciousness that people can learn to identify with minimal effort (Beck, 2011). Such thoughts are spontaneous, unrehearsed, and frequently articulated by clients. Since automatic thoughts directly affect how people feel and behave, they are often the first targets in cognitive therapy.

3. *Case formulation guides treatment*. Case formulation means developing an individualized treatment plan for each client and having a clear rationale for which thinking and behavior patterns will become the focal points across sessions. Before launching into active change techniques, practitioners spend time assessing and considering the cognitions and reinforcement contingencies that are most important in maintaining the client's maladaptive behaviors. In CBT, there is a continuity of focus across sessions on altering such relevant long-standing patterns.
4. *Sessions are structured and organized*. In addition to having an overall game plan for the course of treatment, practitioners approach sessions in an organized and structured manner, with an identified agenda, beginning, middle, and end. This means thinking ahead about the focus of a particular meeting and the strategy to be used in the session. Of course, not all sessions go according to plan. The ability to be flexible and adjust to new information and crises is often necessary.
5. *A skills-building orientation is adopted*. The emphasis in sessions is on improving clients' functioning (e.g., reducing emotional upset, lessening avoidance, and improving accurate and realistic thinking). Although listening to and understanding how clients' personal histories have influenced their present life circumstances is attended to in sessions, insight in and of itself will not be enough to bring about change. Rather, CBT practitioners emphasize a "here and now" focus, introducing new skills to alter clients' entrenched patterns of thinking and behavior.
6. *Treatment fosters psychological flexibility*. Inflexibility is viewed as a significant source of psychopathology (Hayes, Strosahl, & Wilson, 2012). One of the goals of CBT is to get clients to step back from their conditioned "dysfunctional autopilot reactions" in terms of thinking and behavior. Treatment fosters awareness of personal patterns, openness to new ways of facing life's problems, and the active pursuit of what clients value the most.
7. *Sessions are active and collaborative*. CBT is often described as "active-directive." Although practitioners frequently set the agenda for specific sessions, clients are not merely "along for the ride"; they are actively involved in participating in repeated practice of new thoughts and behaviors for improving their lives. CBT practitioners are creative in tailoring activities and assignments

to the unique context of clients' lives. In that sense, CBT is delivered in a collaborative spirit.

8. *Treatment incorporates homework.* Between sessions, assignments—or homework—are essential in CBT. Homework provides ongoing practice opportunities and is seen as a critical mechanism for transferring new thinking and behavioral skills to clients' day-to-day lives. Such assignments tend to be structured, concrete, and specific and have a real-world emphasis.

4.1.2 For What Types of Problems Is CBT Most Effective?

CBT has established itself as one of the most empirically supported intervention modalities for a wide variety of mental health disorders (Butler, Chapman, Forman, & Beck, 2006; Kazantzis et al., 2018). The bulk of this research has focused on the treatment of depression with meta-analyses published in the 1980s (Dobson, 1989), the 1990s (Gloaguen, Cottraux, Cucherat, & Blackburn, 1998; Hollon, Shelton, & Loosen, 1991), the 2000s (Cuijpers, van Straten, Andersson, & van Oppen, 2008; Wampold, Minami, Baskin, & Callen Tierney, 2002), and more recently (Johnsen & Friborg, 2015; Johnsen & Thimm, 2018). Impressive meta-analytic support also exists for the treatment of anxiety disorders (Carpenter et al., 2018; Gould, Otto, Pollack, & Yap, 1997; Hofmann & Smits, 2008; Norton & Price, 2007). A promising innovation is the emergence of CBT protocols that address whole classes of "emotional disorders" (Barlow et al., 2017; Newby, McKinnon, Kuyken, Gilbody, & Dalgleish, 2015).

The developmental progression of most CBT interventions, in terms of science, dissemination, and practice, typically follows a trajectory that begins with a focus on internalizing syndromes, such as depression and anxiety, and later extends to externalizing problems, such as substance misuse (Beck, Wright, Newman, & Liese, 2001; Bishop, 2001, 2014), anger dysregulation (Deffenbacher & McKay, 2000; Tafrate & Kassinove, in press), personality pathology (Beck, Davis, & Freeman, 2015), and criminal behavior (Tafrate & Mitchell, 2014; Tafrate, Mitchell, & Simourd, 2018).

Because the majority of CBT models are so strongly embedded within a mental health context, such interventions are typically oriented toward DSM diagnoses, session-by-session treatment manuals, and individualized therapy meetings. Although CBT has been shown to be effective with forensic clients (Hoffman, Asnaani, Vonk, Sawyer, & Fang, 2012; Landenberger & Lipsey, 2005; Lipsey, Chapman, & Landenberger, 2001; Lipsey & Cullen, 2007), significant adaptations of cognitive and behavioral principles to forensic environments are often required. In the remaining parts of this chapter, we describe (a) what is known about the effectiveness of CBT with offenders, (b) the most significant adaptations necessary to make CBT effective in forensic contexts, and (c) the integration of CBT into probation work.

4.2 The Effectiveness of CBT in Forensic Treatment

In Martinson's (1974) influential review of the forensic treatment literature *What works? Questions and answers about prison reform*, he noted that "with few and isolated exceptions, the rehabilitation efforts that have been reported so far have had no appreciable effect on recidivism" (p. 25). This conclusion, along with the title of the review, led to the use of the phrase "nothing works" as a characterization of forensic treatment efforts and was accompanied by a turn toward more punitive strategies such as incarceration, intensive supervision, and boot camps to reduce reoffending (Cullen & Gendreau, 2001). The long shadow cast on the field of correctional psychology by the "nothing works" perspective was evidenced in the choice of the title (*Does correctional treatment work*?) for a subsequent forensic treatment meta-analysis that reached far more optimistic conclusions (Andrews et al., 1990) and in the adoption of the phrase "what works" to refer to the developing literature on evidence-based practices in forensic treatment (Cullen & Gendreau, 2001; Smith, Gendreau, & Swartz, 2009).

Three key findings from the Andrews et al. (1990) meta-analysis are particularly relevant to this chapter: (1) punitive strategies of incarceration/community supervision with no treatment were associated with an *increase* rather than a decrease in reoffending, (2) treatment that targeted criminal risk factors for reoffending was found to be associated with significant reductions in reoffending, and (3) treatments that used a CBT modality had larger effects on recidivism than other treatment modalities. These three findings have been supported in subsequent reviews and meta-analyses (Aos, Miller, & Drake, 2006; Koehler, Lösel, Akoensi, & Humphreys, 2013; Lipsey & Cullen, 2007), and CBT has, in turn, emerged as the recommended treatment modality for offenders in the leading implementation and practice guidelines for correctional psychology (Bonta & Andrews, 2017; Dowden & Andrews, 2004; National Institute of Corrections & Crime and Justice Institute, 2004; Taxman, Sherpardson, & Byrne, 2004). CBT-based programs and models have been developed for antisocial conduct in general (Tafrate et al., 2018) as well as for specific offense types including drug (Bishop, 2014; Wanberg & Milkman, 2014), sex (Marshall & O'Brien, 2014; Wheeler & Covell, 2014), and violent offenses (Eckhardt, Crane, & Sprunger, 2014; Ronan, Maurelli, & Holman, 2014). Research on the effectiveness of CBT in forensic treatment is briefly reviewed below with an emphasis on the recidivism as the primary outcome variable.

4.2.1 CBT for Antisocial Conduct

The majority of the individual studies that comprise meta-analyses on the impact of CBT on general recidivism have used either Moral Reconation Therapy (MRT) or Reasoning and Rehabilitation (R&R), two popular manualized group treatment programs. MRT focuses on improving client deficits in moral reasoning (Little &

Robinson, 1986). R&R focuses on improving problem-solving and coping skills (Ross, Fabiano, & Ross, 1986). Other manualized programs that are included in some of the meta-analyses, such as Thinking for a Change, the Cognitive Interventions Program, and Aggression Replacement Training, have somewhat different emphases but all of the above programs' aim to help offenders become more aware of the thought processes that facilitate their antisocial conduct. These programs are "general" in that they do not target specific types of offenses (e.g., sex, intimate partner violence, drug use).

The first published meta-analysis specifically devoted to the impact of CBT on general recidivism involved just 14 studies, some with adult and some with juvenile offenders (Lipsey et al., 2001), which were selected because of their relatively strong methodological qualities. Although there was variation in the degree of treatment effectiveness from study to study, all of them found treatment to be associated with lower recidivism compared to incarceration or community supervision with no treatment. On average, the recidivism rate was reduced by a third for offenders in CBT treatment programs, with some studies reducing reoffending by as much as two thirds.

Subsequent reviews have yielded similar findings. One meta-analysis of 58 studies found that, on average, participation in a manualized CBT treatment program was associated with a 25% reduction in the recidivism rate compared to control conditions, and when the CBT programs were delivered with high-quality implementation practices, recidivism rates declined by an average of 50% compared to control conditions (Lipsey, Landenberger, & Wilson, 2007). A second meta-analysis of 20 studies found that MRT reduced recidivism by 16% over control conditions, while R&R reduced recidivism by 8% over control conditions (Wilson, Bouffard, & MacKenzie, 2005).

One additional finding, relevant to clinical practice, that emerges from the meta-analytic literature is that programs being tested as part of research and demonstration projects yield larger effect sizes than programs evaluated in the course of routine practice (Lipsey et al., 2001, 2007; Wilson et al., 2005). As research and demonstration projects are marked by greater adherence to a program's model, and often include intensive training to the treatment providers and greater diligence in adhering to program fidelity, the implication for practice is that attention to quality implementation is an important factor for success. By the same token, the ineffectiveness of a given treatment program in an outcome study may be related more to the poor manner of its implementation than to the underlying model or curriculum that the program relies upon.

4.2.2 Specialized CBT Programs: Sex, Drugs, and Violence

Offenders Who Committed Sexual Crimes

CBT is currently the dominant modality in the field of sex offender treatment. While the specific components of programs vary, in general CBT sex offender treatment programs include modules on (1) altering thinking patterns that facilitate or justify sex offending, (2) improving relationship skills and empathy, and (3) preventing "relapse" by identifying and coping with triggers for the sex offense cycle (Jeglic, Hanson, & Calkins, 2016; McGrath, Cumming, Burchard, Zeoli, & Ellerby, 2009). The two largest sex offender treatment meta-analyses, which included both CBT and alternative treatments, found lower rates of reoffending in participants who attended treatment compared to control groups: Lösel and Schmucker's (2005) meta-analysis of 69 studies found a 37% reduction in reoffending for treatment compared to control, while Hanson et al. (2002) meta-analysis of 43 studies found a 27% reduction in reoffending. Both meta-analyses found that CBT or purely behavioral treatments were associated with larger reductions in reoffending than other types of psychotherapy. However, sex offender treatment meta-analytic evaluations have been hindered by the limited methodological rigor (such as a lack of randomized designs, frequent use of nonequivalent control groups) of many individual studies (Hanson, Bourgon, Helmus, & Hodgson, 2009; Schmucker & Lösel, 2015). Studies that compare treated clients to nonequivalent comparison groups produce exaggerated and likely unreliable treatment effects.

Meta-analyses that restrict themselves to studies with a more rigorous methodological caliber produce more conservative findings: Schmucker and Lösel's (2015) meta-analysis of 29 higher-quality studies found that sex offender treatment was associated with a 10.1% rate of reoffending in the treatment groups and compared to a rate of 13.7% in control conditions, a small percentage-wise difference that translates into a 26% reduction in reoffending. Compared to alternative treatments, CBT produced somewhat stronger effects than insight or therapeutic communities but was less effective than multisystemic therapy (MST), a family therapy for juvenile offenders who committed sexual crimes.

Drug Offenders

CBT is not the dominant modality in the crowded field of offender substance abuse treatment, where approaches include drug courts, therapeutic communities, motivational enhancement groups, boot camps, and a variety of pharmacological agents (McMurran, 2007). However, like its application to sex offender treatment, CBT for substance abuse treatment typically has a relapse prevention orientation. Offenders are taught to identify their high-risk situations for substance use and to develop strategies for coping with, or avoiding, those situations. Purely behavioral approaches include contingency management programs, in which offenders are offered a reward (such as money or gift cards) for rendering clean urine toxicology tests. Meta-analyses of substance abuse treatment that are not restricted to offender samples have found CBT to have a small but significant effect size on subsequent substance use: For example, Magill and Ray (2009) found that 58% of clients in CBT programs had better outcomes than those in comparison treatments, while Dutra et al. (2008) found that CBT was effective in reducing substance use but that contingency management programs produced larger reductions.

When the first meta-analysis specifically devoted to substance abuse treatment for offenders was published, the data on CBT interventions were only mentioned as a promising approach because of the dearth of studies (Pearson & Lipton, 1999). Subsequent reviews, while few in number, have been more encouraging and produced findings consistent with the substance abuse treatment literature on non-offenders. One review of studies employing relatively higher-quality methodologies found CBT, therapeutic communities, and drug courts to produce significant reductions in reoffending and substance use compared to no treatment conditions (Bahr, Masters, & Taylor, 2012), while another review of a small number of programs in the United Kingdom and Canada also found that CBT was associated with reduced reoffending and subsequent use compared to no treatment (McMurran, 2007). While the existing literature indicates CBT can reduce both substance use and offending, there is insufficient data at present to indicate that it is more effective than other available treatments.

Violent Offenders

The offender treatment literature around violence includes programs specifically designed to treat intimate partner violence (IPV) and those intended to treat violent behavior that also occurs outside of intimate relationships. The theoretical and empirical literature concerning the treatment of IPV is in a state of flux (Gardner, Moore, Birkley, & Eckhardt, 2016). For nearly two decades, the dominant IPV treatment model (often referred to as the Duluth model) rested on the assumption that IPV is rooted in patriarchal socialization patterns that produced men's sexist attitudes and toward women. The Duluth model, which was not based in CBT, could not address IPV perpetrated by women, nor did it integrate treatment related to the empirical risk factors associated with IPV (Gardner et al., 2016). A lack of empirical support for the theoretical underpinnings and effectiveness of the Duluth model (Arias, Arce, & Vilariño, 2013; Langhinrichsen-Rohling, McCullars, & Misra, 2012) has led to a call for the integration of new CBT-based models into court-mandated IPV programming (see Chap. 14 of this volume and Gardner et al., 2016). With the development of CBT-based IPV therapies that incorporate mindfulness- and acceptance-based principles (Gardner & Moore, 2014), risk-based factors (Eckhardt et al., 2014), and problem-solving skills (Ronan et al., 2014), IPV treatment may be transformed in another generation.

CBT has also been applied to violent behavior that is not limited to intimate partner relationships. The existing research, while limited, has been promising. A systematic review of 11 studies using a variety of treatment approaches found that the impact of treatment of general and violent recidivism was inconsistent across studies. Two of 11 studies demonstrated a statistically significant impact on general recidivism, and 2 of 8 demonstrated a statistically significant impact on violent recidivism (Jolliffe & Farrington, 2007). However, examination of the impact of treatment components on recidivism indicated that programs that involved anger control skills, cognitive skills, or role plays produced statistically significant reductions in general and violent recidivism, suggesting a possible benefit of CBT-oriented violence treatment programs over other modalities. More recently, a meta-analysis of 14 studies found that CBT-based anger treatment was associated with a 23% reduced rate of general recidivism and a 28% reduced rate of violent recidivism for treatment over control groups (Henwood, Chou, & Browne, 2015). As in the other areas of forensic treatment, reviewers noted a need for more studies using rigorous designs such as random assignment to groups and measures of program fidelity to control for variations in implementation quality (Henwood et al., 2015; Jolliffe & Farrington, 2007).

4.3 Practical Considerations in Adapting CBT to Forensic Populations

4.3.1 Taking a Risk Versus a Symptom-Focused Approach

CBT interventions seek to change thinking and behavior patterns. As applied to mental health problems, this has traditionally meant that the techniques are applied with a symptom-focused approach. For example, because low energy and cessation of social activities are symptoms commonly found in depression, combating these symptoms with exercise and scheduled activities might be part of the behavioral component of a CBT treatment plan. Similarly, because thinking patterns around worthlessness and hopelessness are commonly found in depression, the monitoring and examination of the accuracy of these types of thoughts might be part of the cognitive component of a treatment plan.

In contrast, applying CBT to a forensic treatment context requires a shift from targeting the client's symptoms of psychological distress to their functioning in the major risk domains associated with continued offending. The need for a focus on risk of recidivism rather than symptoms of psychological distress means that practitioners need to be familiar with the nature of those risk domains (which are commonly referred to as the Central Eight; Bonta & Andrews, 2017), assess their client's functioning in those domains, and formulate and implement interventions in those domains. This, in turn, requires some familiarity with the theoretical and empirical work on the risk-need-responsivity (RNR) model of forensic assessment and treatment. This risk-based approach to forensic rehabilitation has been increasingly influential in correctional psychology and probation/parole supervision.

Because RNR is reviewed elsewhere in this text, we will limit discussion of this model to the implications for integrating the Central Eight risk domains into CBT case formulation (see Chap. 2 for a detailed review of RNR as well as a Bonta & Andrews, 2017).

Risk-Focused Assessment and Case Formulation

A useful way of understanding the connection between CBT and RNR in forensic treatment is that CBT provides a structure and a set of techniques for how treatment is implemented while RNR informs the content of that treatment, guiding the practitioner to areas in the client's life where those techniques can be applied. Table 4.1 provides a list of the Central Eight along with a brief description of core

Table 4.1 The Central Eight risk domains: assessment and case formulation considerations

Risk domain	Key assessment/case formulation considerations
History of antisocial/criminal behavior	What is the extent and nature of the client's involvement with criminal activities, including those detected by the justice system as well as those that are undetected? How is the client looking at those situations before, during, and after they occur? What is the person's history of community supervision and incarceration? What kinds of correctional programs have been helpful in the past?
Antisocial personality characteristics	What signs of antisocial personality disorder, dissocial personality disorder, and/or psychopathy seem to be present? To what extent is the client aware that these symptoms are part of a pattern that are having a negative impact on his or her life?
Antisocial attitudes/ criminogenic thinking	What are the immediate thoughts and long-standing thinking patterns that facilitate the client's antisocial behavior? What does the client tell him/herself before he/she makes criminal/antisocial decisions?
Antisocial companions	What is the degree to which the client associates with, and/or seeks approval from, antisocial friends? What kind of impact do antisocial friends have the client's own antisocial behavior? To what extent are prosocial friends in the client's life?
Family/marital dysfunction	To what extent do the client's family and/or marital bonds that lack nurturance and ignore, reinforce, or model antisocial behavior? What prosocial influences are in the client's family network?
Poor performance/ satisfaction with school/work	What is the client's current status with respect to work or school? What is their performance and attitude? What kinds of interpersonal or behavioral problems exist in this domain? How does the client's school/work life relate to criminal/antisocial behavior?
Unproductive use of leisure/ recreational pursuits	How does the client spend his or her free time? What organized activities does the person engage in or used to engage in? What kinds of risky activities are present? How does he/she handle boredom? What's the connection between leisure time and criminal/antisocial behavior?
Substance abuse	What is the client's quantity/frequency of use? What negative consequences have they experienced due to use? What's the connection between use and criminal/antisocial behavior?

assessment/case formulation concerns in each of the areas (see Tafrate et al., 2018 for practical guidelines for forensic assessment and case formulation). Practitioners accustomed to working with traditional mental health clients will already be familiar with assessment and formulation of several of the Central Eight (e.g., substance use, prior criminal behavior, dysfunctional family relationships) as part of standard intake and assessment procedures, while others (e.g., criminal companions, unproductive use of leisure time, criminal thinking) are less unfamiliar.

Although the Central Eight are commonly referred to as risk *factors*, for CBT assessment and case formulation purposes, they are better conceptualized as risk *domains*. The term risk factor implies a single characteristic about a person that is linked with a negative outcome (e.g., high cholesterol is a risk factor for heart disease), whereas each of the Central Eight encompasses the client's history, thinking, and behavior in a broad life area. For example, when it comes to assessing the work/school risk domain, it is not enough to simply learn if the client is unemployed (if they are an adult) or enrolled in school (if they are juvenile). Assessing the work domain may include learning (1) *why* an unemployed client is not working, (2) their stability in maintaining employment over the years, (3) interpersonal problems with peers and supervisors, (4) behavioral problems at work, (5) training/skills/certifications they have obtained, (6) overall attitudes toward employment, (7) level of enjoyment in working, (8) degree of congruence between the types of positions they are qualified for versus and the positions that they apply for, (9) plans and aspirations for employment in the future, and (10) how their difficulties in employment contribute to their offense history. For a juvenile client, the assessment process will seek to answer a parallel set of information about education.

A distinction needs to be made between case *formulation* and *risk assessment* in forensic CBT. Forensic case formulation is about identifying those treatment targets most likely to reduce future criminal behavior for an individual client. The topic of criminal risk assessment is a specialty area with its own unique terminology and practices. A specific feature of risk assessment is the prediction of outcomes (e.g., reoffending) through using probability estimates derived from validated risk instruments. Our case formulation guidelines are not recommended for making statistical estimates regarding probabilities of future criminal behavior. For more information about risk assessment, see Singh, Kroner, Wormith, Desmarais, and Hamilton (2018).

One of the benefits of a risk-based approach to forensic treatment is the optimistic and preventative framework within which it places treatment. As noted earlier, there has been a long-standing pessimism about the ability of forensic treatment to reduce reoffending. Yet the Central Eight are largely dynamic and changeable, rather than static, aspects of human functioning. A client's employment status, attitude toward employment, and performance at work can change. In fact, the client's history of criminal behavior is the only truly static risk domain and will therefore always, in a statistical sense, contribute to an increased likelihood of reoffending. The term often used to describe the seven dynamic risk areas is *criminogenic needs* (Bonta & Andrews, 2017). The implication of the dynamic nature of seven of the eight risk domains for treatment is that clients whose criminogenic needs worsen will be at increased risk for recidivism, while clients who make positive changes in these areas will decrease that likelihood. Therefore, improving a client's deficits in these areas has a preventative function.

Ideally the assessment of each risk domain should provide enough information, so that the practitioner can develop a case formulation—an understanding of what makes the domain a risk (or a strength) and a plan for improving this area if it is a source of concern. How a given risk factor translates into antisocial behavior can differ from client to client. For example, two clients may have numerous criminal companions, but they may significantly differ in *how* their companions contribute to their risk of recidivism. For one client, friends may present opportunities for impulsive criminal activities the client may not have sought out or initiated on his own. For the other client, the desire to obtain approval and respect from friends may lead him to initiate criminal behavior that he believes will be met with their approval.

Case formulation also entails understanding how a client's functioning in one risk domain is impacting their behavior in others. Tables, figures, and other visual representations of the risk domains (or criminogenic needs) may convey the impression that these are discrete factors operating in isolation from each other. In fact, criminal risk domains are connected in ways that can be complex, reinforce destructive patterns, and interfere with the development of the newer prosocial thinking and behavior patterns introduced in treatment. For example, consider the case below:

> Mike is a 29-year-old male on probation for the theft of computers from an officer-trailer on a construction site. His assessment reveals significant problems in four criminal risk domains: companions, substance abuse, employment, and leisure. Mike's primary social circle consists of a small group of close friends that are unemployed, smoke a lot of marijuana, and do not express much interest in conventional employment or a prosocial lifestyle. Mike is currently unemployed with limited job skills. He recently failed a pre-employment drug screen. He has never remained in the same job for more than 6 months, and he is supported by his mother with whom he still lives. Mike spends his excessive free time with his close friends or aimlessly hanging around his neighborhood and smoking marijuana. He smokes marijuana most days and drinks to intoxication on weekends, when he has the money. For Mike, these four risk domains are not unrelated: his marijuana smoking makes it impossible for him to pass pre-employment drug screens, which contribute to his excessive free time, which provides him opportunities to spend time with the companions that encourage his drug use and unstructured lifestyle in a self-perpetuating destructive cycle.

Importantly, the interconnectedness of criminal risk domains also means that positive changes in one domain can ripple into improvements in other risk domains and reinforce new prosocial patterns. For example, if Mike stopped smoking marijuana (even temporarily), he might be able to pass a drug screen and obtain full-time employment. Being at work would restrict his time with his friends (further reducing his opportunities to smoke marijuana) and expose him to co-workers and potentially new friends and acquaintances who have more prosocial lifestyles. Over time, reinforcement for his impulsive and unstable lifestyle habits might diminish as newer prosocial thinking, pursuits, and friends are rewarded. The implication of the synergistic quality of criminal risk domains for case formulation is that not every relevant domain for a client has to be addressed all at once in treatment. Practitioners can prioritize criminal risk domains and begin with the one that they believe has the greatest likelihood of producing more wide-ranging effects.

The Role of Mental Health Symptoms

Noticeably absent from the Central Eight are common mental health problems, such as depression, anxiety, and low self-esteem. Also absent are more severe and chronic conditions, such as schizophrenia and bipolar disorder. While there may be a common belief among mental health and criminal justice practitioners that mental disorders and criminality are strongly linked, the empirical literature indicates that the link is indirect and quite limited. Offenders with a mental disorder are not more likely to reoffend than those without a mental disorder (Bonta, Law, & Hanson, 1998; Phillips et al., 2005). Even in offenders with a severe mental disorder, such as schizophrenia or bipolar disorder, symptoms are rarely linked to their instant offense (Skeem, Kennealy, Monahan, Peterson, & Appelbaum, 2016). Furthermore, providing mental health treatment to offenders with a mental disorder reduces their symptoms but does not reduce their rate of reoffending (Bonta, Blais, & Wilson, 2014; Morgan et al., 2012). In fact, among offenders with a mental disorder, the best predictors of reoffending appear to be the Central Eight (Bonta et al., 1998; Phillips et al., 2005), and reductions in reoffending are found when treatment targets their relevant criminal risk domains (Morgan et al., 2012). Thus, reducing recidivism in offenders with mental disorders requires a focus on the same risk domains (e.g., criminogenic needs) as those without such disorders.

It would be incorrect, however, to assume that mental health problems are unimportant or should be not be addressed in forensic treatment. The mistake would be to assume that addressing mental health symptoms will improve the client's antisocial behavior. Addressing mental health problems will help the client feel better and can help them focus, attend, and participate fully in the interventions that target their criminal risk domains.

To provide a practical example, if Mike was also significantly depressed and had low self-esteem, a CBT program that only targeted his depressed mood and low self-esteem would help him feel better but would not reduce his likelihood to reoffend. It may, in fact, increase his antisocial conduct if he has more energy and focus to put in the wrong direction. On the other hand, effectively addressing his criminal risk domains will be difficult if he is too depressed to engage in the interventions designed to improve his employability, substance use, and choices about who he spends his time with and how he spends that time. In Mike's case, addressing the depression and self-esteem might be necessary so he can work on improving the relevant criminal risk areas of his life. In that sense, mental health treatment is considered as an adjunct, not a replacement, for addressing criminal risk domains.

Engagement and Motivation

Unfortunately, the fact that practitioners can identify risk areas that, if addressed, will lower a client's risk of further justice involvement does not automatically mean that client will want to make changes in any or all of those areas. As a contrast, consider the client who seeks CBT for depression. They are in distress, experiencing low mood, rumination, insomnia, and low energy. The client is seeking help because they want these symptoms to go away. Their motivation to change is intrinsic and likely to be quite high.

Now consider the case of Mike. Even after a fourth arrest for larceny, Mike was not in distress regarding his behavior. In fact, his behavior was more distressing to others than to himself. His initial motivation to change was purely extrinsic (forced upon him by the court) and quite low. The fact that offenders are rarely seeking help voluntarily and are mandated means that they often present with a lack of interest, and sometimes hostility, toward intervention programs. This puts both practitioners and clients in a difficult circumstance. Practitioners will have to work harder to develop a therapeutic alliance (see Chap. 5) and improve the client's readiness to change. The latter is particularly important given the results of a forensic treatment meta-analysis which found that mandated programs were significantly less effective than voluntary treatment in both institutional and community settings (Parhar, Wormith, Derkzen, & Beauregard, 2008). For treatment to be effective, practitioners must find a way to generate their mandated clients' interest in treatment to be more akin to that of their voluntary counterparts. In essence, practitioners will need to create an atmosphere in which clients who start treatment by saying they are "forced to be here" come to find that they "want to make changes anyway."

One increasingly common practice in forensic treatment settings is for practitioners to integrate motivational interviewing (MI) (see Chap. 11), or adaptations of MI, into their interventions (Tafrate, Mitchell, & Novaco, 2014). MI (Miller & Rollnick, 2013) has immediate practical advantages in the early stages of treatment of moving forensic clients toward greater engagement and collaboration and moving practitioners away from confrontation, advice-giving, and practical steps for which the client is not yet ready. Instead of practitioners telling the client what to do, clients and practitioners collaboratively discuss reasons *why* change would be important as well as *how* the client might go about it. The main objective in using MI is to elicit and explore clients' own motivations for making changes in their criminal risk domains (Tafrate, Hogan, & Mitchell, in press; Tafrate & Luther, 2014).

4.3.2 Cognitive Components of Treatment

Across a wide variety of mental disorders and behavior problems, the cognitive restructuring process may include one or all of the following components: (1) assessing the distorted or irrational automatic thoughts and/or intermediate beliefs associated with the symptoms or problem area, (2) having the client monitor the occurrence of their cognitive processes between sessions, (3) guiding the client through examination of the (in)accuracy of specific destructive automatic thoughts or intermediate beliefs, and (4) helping the client develop newer, more accurate and healthier thoughts and beliefs (Beck, 2011; Leahy, Holland, & McGinn, 2012). These same components are also relevant to cognitive restructuring with justice-involved clients. The primary difference is in the nature of thoughts and thinking patterns that are targeted for change.

For practitioners familiar with anxiety and depressive disorders, it is useful to think of the automatic thoughts and intermediate beliefs that facilitate criminal and self-destructive behavior as a mirror image of those found in clients suffering from anxiety and depression (Kroner & Morgan, 2014; Mitchell, Tafrate, & Freeman, 2015; Seeler, Freeman, DiGuiseppe, & Mitchell, 2014; Walters, 2014). For example, it was noted earlier that the thinking of clients suffering from anxiety is marked by exaggerations of potential threats and dangers (e.g., "I know my boss is going to fire me if I'm late, and then I'll never find another job ever again."). Offenders, on the other hand, may underestimate danger, challenges, or difficulties in favor of overly optimistic and self-serving predictions (e.g., "It's no big deal if I'm late for work. My boss won't mind at all, and nothing much happens in the first hour of my shift anyway."). Similarly, while the clients suffering from depression may blame and judge themselves harshly when they make a mistake (e.g., "It's my fault for being late. I'm such a failure and a screw up. No wonder my boss hates me."), offenders may seek to blame situations or others for their problems and exaggerate their positive qualities (e.g., "It's not my fault I'm late—people drive too slowly on the highway. My boss is lucky I showed up to begin with.").

A variety of terms have appeared in the literature to describe the kinds of thoughts that produce criminal behavior including criminal thinking, antisocial attitudes, and criminogenic thoughts. We use the term *criminogenic thoughts* to refer to those automatic and spontaneous thoughts that facilitate criminal and antisocial behavior and the term *criminogenic thinking patterns* to refer to the intermediate beliefs and assumptions that produce those thoughts (a review of schemas related to forensic treatment is beyond the scope of this chapter, but the interested reader is referred to Keulen-de Vos, Bernstein, & Arntz, 2014). A literature identifying and measuring different criminogenic thinking patterns has developed along with seven assessment instruments for adult offenders: the Psychological Inventory of Criminal Thinking Styles (PICTS; Walters, 1995), Criminal Sentiments Scale-Modified (CSS-M; Simourd, 1997), Measure of Criminal Attitudes and Associates (MCAA; Mills, Kroner, & Forth, 2002), Texas Christian University Criminal Thinking Scales (TCU CTS; Knight, Garner, Simpson, Morey, & Flynn, 2006), Measure of Offender Thinking Styles (MOTS; Mandracchia, Morgan, Garos, & Garland, 2007), Criminogenic Thinking Profile (CTP; Mitchell & Tafrate, 2012), and Criminal Cognitions Scale (Tangney et al., 2012).

Each criminogenic thinking instrument measures multiple thinking patterns (ranging from 3 to 8). The total number of thinking patterns measured across all the instruments adds up to 32; however, taking into account overlapping content reduces the number of distinct thinking patterns to a clinically practical 13. These instruments are free for practitioners and researchers and can be easily administered and scored in clinical settings. As recommended by Kroner and Morgan (2014), administering more than one instrument will provide a useful range of potentially relevant thinking targets for treatment. A description of the 13 key patterns along with sample thoughts connected with them is presented in Table 4.2 (for a listing and description of criminogenic thinking patterns, see also Mitchell et al., 2015; Tafrate et al., 2018).

A prominent criminogenic thinking patterns may impact a client in multiple risk domains as well as in other areas of his or her daily life, because the client brings the thinking pattern with them from one situation to the next. For example, Mike was high in two criminogenic thinking patterns: (a) *exploiting systems, situations, and/relationships for personal benefit* and (b) *excitement and thrill seeking and difficulty with "down time."* His tendency to exploit contributed to his theft of some

Table 4.2 Criminogenic thinking patterns and criminogenic thoughts

Description of criminogenic thsinking pattern	Sample criminogenic thought from pattern
Disregard for others; Lack of empathy/remorse	"I don't have time to care about anyone else. My life's about me and only me. Only the strong survive"
Avoiding intimacy and vulnerability	"Why should I open up to you? You're just going to leave anyway"
Grandiose beliefs about self and/or that special treatment is deserved	"I'm super smart, your program couldn't possibly teach me anything I don't already know"
Identifying with and valuing the opinions and expectations of antisocial companions	"I can only relate to people who are on the streets like me rippin' and runnin'"
Hostility toward criminal justice professionals	"Parole officers just want to keep you in the system so they can collect a paycheck"
Seeking dominance and control over others	"I need to be in charge of others. I don't take orders from anyone"
Justifying and minimizing, antisocial behaviors	"The store has insurance. What I stole isn't going to put them out of business"
Underestimating negative consequences	"I can time my drug use so that it'll be out of my system when my probation officer tests me. I won't get violated"
Avoiding problems by procrastination and avoidance	"I don't need to render clean urines or worry about how my behavior looks for the judge. I trust that everything will work out ok by itself"
Easily giving up or acting out in the face of adversity	"When life gets hard, I just get high and give up"
Exploiting systems, situations, and/or relationships for personal benefit	"I have a friend that just hustled a disability, so I'm just going to look into that. Maybe I can score something like"
Hostility toward laws and authority	"That's the way I am. If someone tells me to do something, I'm going to do the opposite"
Excitement and thrill seeking and difficulty with "down time"	"I like the excitement of selling drugs, always having to look over my shoulder, making my own hours"

electronic equipment that he believed was not being closely monitored and presented "an opportunity to make some quick money off a situation." His tendency to exploit was also apparent in his personal life. He lived with, and off of, his mother and relied on her for basic needs (e.g., laundry, cooking, and cleaning). His thinking pattern is reflected in statements such as, "Why shouldn't she do it for me? She has nothing else to do. It's not a problem." In the past, he had a similar parasitic relationship with girlfriends. His tendency toward excitement was reflected in past arrests for shoplifting, "Just wanted to see if I could get away with it" and reckless driving for "drag racing." His excitement seeking also contributed to his poor school and work history. He had found school and work boring, "I can't work a 9 to 5 trapped in a room, I need action." While criminogenic thinking patterns have the potential to facilitate poor decision-making in many areas of a client's life, improvements in a thinking pattern can lead to positive changes and reduced risk in multiple areas of a client's life, making criminogenic thinking an important component of treatment.

While treatment for anxiety and depression often involves helping clients connect their distorted intermediate beliefs and automatic thoughts with their dysfunctional emotional reactions, the focus in CBT with offenders is on helping them connect their criminogenic thinking patterns and thoughts with the choices they make in their criminal risk domains (Kroner & Morgan, 2014; Mitchell et al., 2015; Walters, 2014). For a client like Mike, this process may start by raising his awareness of a specific thinking pattern (such as excitement seeking) on his life by having him review different times when the thinking pattern emerged and led to poor decisions in different life areas. Once made aware of the pattern, Mike may be asked to monitor the pattern through homework assignments in which he notes occasions during the week when the pattern emerges. The homework then becomes fodder for treatment sessions in which those occasions are discussed, the thinking examined, and Mike being coached on the development of healthier thinking in those risky situations (Tafrate et al., 2018). Hopefully, over time and with practice, the newer and more prosocial thoughts developed through treatment become more typical of Mike's thinking, his criminogenic thoughts become weaker and less common, and better choices are made.

4.3.3 Behavioral Components of Treatment

Behavioral interventions are also oriented around criminal risk domains with emphasis given to behavioral *movement* and deliberate *actions* justice-involved clients can take to improve their overall lifestyles (e.g., ongoing routines, risky relationships, and destructive habits). Similar to cognitive restructuring, behavioral interventions are not single-session endeavors, require a continued focus across sessions, and emphasize the development of concrete skills over time. Below, we will briefly highlight a few examples relevant for forensic clientele. For detailed descriptions of CBT procedures that target the full range of criminal risk domains, see Tafrate et al. (2018).

Activity monitoring as a traditional treatment for depression involves clients keeping track of their daily actions with the overall goal of increasing pleasurable activities. For forensic clients like Mike who have a problem with use of leisure time, activity monitoring can be used to shape a more positive and prosocial use of time. For example, as a first step to obtain a snapshot of current day-to-day routines, Mike might be asked to complete a log of his typical activities from the time he wakes up until the time he goes to bed and to rate each activity along the dimensions of relative risk (how helpful is the activity in staying out of trouble) and level of enjoyment. Mike's practitioner would then work collaboratively with him to replace any high-risk activities identified with new, enjoyable, and less risky alternatives.

In many cases, advancing educational achievement and enhancing marketable job skills of forensic clients will have to be addressed directly in treatment. Assisting clients in finding employment can be challenging and will involve behaviorally supporting a range of practical issues (e.g., creating a résumé, acquiring appropriate work clothes, organizing transportation), improving positive impression and interview skills (e.g., hygiene, eye contact, rate of speech, answering questions about criminal history), and developing time management and job search strategies. A client like Mike might also benefit from ongoing behavioral coaching to help him maintain the job that he lands. Common coaching activities include practice responding to negative feedback, handling disagreements, and maintaining a high degree of integrity and honesty in work interactions.

Restructuring relationships is common in forensically oriented CBT, because altering the client's social context can significantly diminish an influential element of risk inherent in the person's lifestyle. Potential changes will typically involve relationships with close friends, family members, and romantic partners. Restructuring relationships starts with baseline monitoring and risk ratings of existing relationships. An additional ingredient, designed to foster motivation for change, is to increase awareness regarding the negative impact that high-risk relationships have on the client's life trajectory. For Mike, behavioral steps to reduce his risk may include working with him to intentionally distance himself from, or better manage the influence of, his high-risk friends. Equally important is to develop awareness, motivation, and practical steps for strengthening existing positive relationships or healthy relationships that have been dormant. For some clients, ongoing coaching aimed at improving social skills may be necessary in creating new friendships and romantic relationships. Other habitual and destructive patterns (e.g., substance misuse, anger dysregulation, and so forth) may also become the target of behavioral interventions.

4.4 Recent Innovations: The Integration of CBT into Probation

An exciting development in the use of CBT with justice-involved clients has been the migration of CBT techniques into the supervision sessions of probation and parole officers. While the education and training of community corrections officers obviously differs tremendously from that of counseling and mental health professionals, there are several reasons to see the integration of CBT into community corrections as a logical, efficient, and positive development in the field.

A groundbreaking study analyzing audio-recordings of probation supervision sessions found that they showed little adherence to fundamental RNR principles (Bonta, Rugge, Scott, Bourgon, & Yessine, 2008). For example, the content of supervision sessions rarely focused on criminal risk domains and instead was dominated by reviews of the conditions of probation. Further, sessions devoted to probation conditions were associated with higher rates of recidivism. In contrast, sessions with a higher proportion of content devoted to criminal risk domains were associated with lower rates of recidivism. A primary implication of these findings is that probation is underutilized in terms of addressing key criminal risk domains that are drivers of criminal behavior. A corollary of that implication is that if criminal risk domains are to be addressed in supervision sessions, the research base is clear that CBT strategies are the preferred modality for doing so.

A related reason to promote CBT integration into community corrections practice concerns the working alliance between community corrections officers and clients. It has been well established in the psychotherapy literature that the therapist-client relationship is an important factor in treatment success (Horvath & Symonds, 1991). In a parallel manner, research suggests that the relationship between community corrections officers and clients is an important factor in success of community supervision; clients who perceive their officer as fair, firm, and trusting have better outcomes (Kennealy, Skeem, Manchak, & Eno Louden, 2012). Therefore, providing officers with skills likely to enhance their working relationships is likely to have a positive impact on their clients' life trajectories.

The first CBT training program for community supervision officers was the Strategic Training Initiative in Community Supervision (STICS), developed in Canada (Bonta et al., 2011). Other models have subsequently been developed in the United States, including Effective Practices in Community Supervision (EPICS), Staff Training Aimed at Reducing Re-Arrest (STARR), and Forensic CBT. While the programs differ in structure, training delivery, and specific CBT techniques, they share a number of underlying similarities. Officers are trained in (1) the nature and importance of RNR principles, (2) relationship building/communication skills (such as MI), (3) how to structure supervision sessions around criminal risk domains, (4) cognitive techniques to address criminogenic thinking, and (5) behavioral techniques to alter risky patterns of behavior in criminal risk domains. CBT-oriented probation is intended to augment forensic treatment, not replace it. Supervision sessions are opportunities to reinforce the content of other programming. Unlike many forensic treatment environments, where programs are delivered in group setting, probation supervision is conducted in individual, face-to-face sessions, providing an opportunity for clients to receive focused attention on a relevant criminal risk domain by a helping professional.

As an example of how CBT-oriented probation is different from regular probation, we'll return once more to the case of Mike, for whom antisocial companions is a significant criminal risk domain. In general, regular probation interactions tend to emphasize monitoring the client's compliance with the conditions of probation. In a regular probation supervision session, Mike might be asked if he is avoiding contact with convicted felons or co-defendants. Thus, this criminal risk domain is essentially treated as a probation condition and briefly touched upon. In contrast, Mike's antisocial companions will receive significant ongoing attention in CBT-oriented probation. Cognitive interventions may explore the nature of specific risky relationships, the criminogenic thoughts that emerge when he makes decisions with these companions, and practicing less risky thoughts and better decisions in the context of his social network. Behavioral interventions might involve strategies to distance himself from the most problematic, risky friendships, reconnect with former prosocial companions, and explore opportunities to meet new prosocial peers.

Outcome data on the impact of CBT programs for community supervision officers is limited but shows promising findings in both community supervision officers and their clients. The largest and most methodologically rigorous evaluation found significant differences in analyses of audio-recorded supervision sessions between officers who participated in STICS and control group officers (Bonta et al., 2011). STICS-trained officers devoted a significantly greater proportion of supervision sessions to discussing criminal risk domains, while control group officers devoted a significantly greater proportion of supervision sessions to discussing probation conditions. STICS officers also demonstrated better relationship building skills and provided more structure to the supervision sessions. Client recidivism for officers in the STICS group declined from 47% to 25%, a significant decrease, while client recidivism for officers in the control group remained essentially the same (41% to 40% over the same time period).

The results from similar programs in the United State have also been encouraging. A small pilot study that utilized audio-recordings of supervision sessions found that EPICS-trained officers were more likely to target criminal risk domains and to challenge client's criminogenic thinking than non-EPICS-trained officers (Smith, Schweitzer, Labrecque, & Latessa, 2012). Similarly, an analysis of pre- versus post-training audio-recordings of officers in the Forensic CBT program found significant increases in supervision session content devoted to criminal risk domains on post-training recordings as well as significant increases in communication and relationship building skills (Mitchell, Tafrate, Cox, & Hogan, 2017). Further, the 6-month recidivism rate of the clients assigned to the FCBT-trained officer's caseloads dropped from 21% to 12%. Results of an evaluation of the STARR program also reported positive effects on recidivism (Lowenkamp, Holsinger, Robinson, & Alexander, 2014). The rearrest rate of medium-risk clients supervised by

STARR-trained officers was 28% at 24-month follow-up compared to 41% for non-STARR-trained officers, a difference that was not statistically significant but substantively significant in terms of its impact on reoffending.

4.5 Summary

With the underlying premise that people behave according to their thoughts and think according to their behaviors, CBT seeks to improve functioning by altering problematic thoughts and behavior patterns. Initially developed to alleviate depression and anxiety, CBT has become a popular treatment approach for a variety of mental and physical health problems and has been more recently expanded to forensic treatment. Applying CBT to forensic treatment involves focusing on the criminal risk domains most associated with recidivism, restructuring the criminogenic thinking that facilitates the client's destructive behavior, and altering risky routines, relationships, and habits. CBT has become the most empirically supported modality of treatment for offenders, with support for its effectiveness in reducing general, sexual, drug-related, and violent recidivism. The effectiveness of CBT interventions for offenders has recently led to its integration into community supervision in the form of initiatives that train community corrections officers to use CBT techniques in supervision sessions. The results of CBT-oriented probation have promise in improving officers' relationship building skills, focusing supervision on criminal risk domains, and reducing reoffending among probationers.

References

Albert Ellis Institute. (n.d.). *Welcome to the Albert Ellis Institute*. Retrieved from http://albertellis.org

Amrod, J., & Hayes, S. C. (2014). ACT for the incarcerated. In R. C. Tafrate & D. Mitchell (Eds.), *Forensic CBT: A handbook for clinical practice* (pp. 43–65). Chichester, UK: Wiley.

Andrews, D. A., Zinger, I., Hoge, R. D., Bonta, J., Gendreau, P., & Cullen, F. T. (1990). Does correctional treatment work? A clinically relevant and psychologically informed meta-analysis. *Criminology, 28*(3), 369–404. https://doi.org/10.1111/j.1745-9125.1990.tb01330.x

Aos, S., Miller, M., & Drake, E. (2006). *Evidence-based adult corrections programs: What works and what does not*. Olympia, WA: Washington State Institute for Public Policy.

Arias, E., Arce, R., & Vilariño, M. (2013). Batterer intervention programmes: A meta-analytic review of effectiveness. *Psychosocial Intervention, 22*(2), 153–160. https://doi.org/10.5093/in2013a18

Bahr, S. J., Masters, A. L., & Taylor, B. M. (2012). What works in substance abuse treatment programs for offenders? *The Prison Journal, 92*(2), 155–174. https://doi.org/10.1177/0032885512438836

Barlow, D. H., Farchione, T. J., Sauer-Zavala, S., Latin, H. M., Ellard, K. K., Bullis, J. R., … Cassiello-Robbins, C. (2017). *Unified protocol for transdiagnostic treatment of emotional disorders: Workbook* (2nd ed.). New York, NY: Oxford University Press.

Beck, A. T. (1963). Thinking and depression: I. idiosyncratic content and cognitive distortions. *Archives of General Psychiatry, 9*(4), 324–333. https://doi.org/10.1001/archpsyc.1963.01720160014002

Beck, A. T. (1967). *Depression: Causes and treatment*. Philadelphia, PA: University of Pennsylvania Press.

Beck, A. T., Davis, D. D., & Freeman, A. (Eds.). (2015). *Cognitive therapy of personality disorders* (3rd ed.). New York, NY: The Guilford Press.

Beck, A. T., Wright, F. D., Newman, C. F., & Liese, B. S. (2001). *Cognitive therapy of substance abuse*. New York, NY: The Guilford Press.

Beck Institute for Cognitive Behavior Therapy. (n.d.). *What is cognitive behavior therapy (CBT)?* Retrieved from https://beckinstitute.org/get-informed/what-is-cognitive-therapy/

Beck, J. S. (2011). *Cognitive therapy: Basics and beyond* (2nd ed.). New York, NY: The Guilford Press.

Bishop, F. M. (2001). *Managing addictions: Cognitive, emotive, and behavioral techniques*. Lanham, MD: Rowman & Littlefield Publishers Inc.

Bishop, F. M. (2014). An integrated REBT-based approach to the treatment of addicted offenders. In R. C. Tafrate & D. Mitchell (Eds.), *Forensic CBT: A handbook for clinical practice* (pp. 233–251). Chichester, UK: Wiley.

Bonta, J., & Andrews, D. A. (2017). *The psychology of criminal conduct* (6th ed.). New York, NY: Routledge.

Bonta, J., Blais, J., & Wilson, H. A. (2014). A theoretically informed meta-analysis of the risk for general and violent recidivism for mentally disordered offenders. *Aggression and Violent Behavior, 19*(3), 278–287. https://doi.org/10.1016/j.avb.2014.04.014

Bonta, J., Bourgon, G., Rugge, T., Scott, T.-L., Yessine, A. K., Gutierrez, L., & Li, J. (2011). An experimental demonstration of training probation officers in evidence-based community supervision. *Criminal Justice and Behavior, 38*(11), 1127–1148. https://doi.org/10.1177/0093854811420678

Bonta, J., Law, M., & Hanson, R. K. (1998). The prediction of criminal and violent recidivism among mentally disordered offenders: A meta-analysis. *Psychological Bulletin, 123*(2), 123–142. https://doi.org/10.1037/0033-2909.123.2.123

Bonta, J., Rugge, T., Scott, T.-L., Bourgon, G., & Yessine, A. K. (2008). Exploring the black box of community supervision. *Journal of Offender Rehabilitation, 47*(3), 248–270. https://doi.org/10.1080/10509670802134085

Butler, A. C., Chapman, J. E., Forman, E. M., & Beck, A. T. (2006). The empirical status of cognitive-behavioral therapy: A review of meta-analyses. *Clinical Psychology Review, 26*(1), 17–31. https://doi.org/10.1016/j.cpr.2005.07.003

Carpenter, J. K., Andrews, L. A., Witcraft, S. M., Powers, M. B., Smits, J. A. J., & Hofmann, S. G. (2018). Cognitive behavioral therapy for anxiety and related disorders: A meta-analysis of randomized placebo-controlled trials. *Depression and Anxiety, 35*(6), 502–514. https://doi.org/10.1002/da.22728

CBT Australia. (n.d.). *Welcome to CBT Australia*. Retrieved from https://www.cbtaustralia.com.au

Cuijpers, P., van Straten, A., Andersson, G., & van Oppen, P. (2008). Psychotherapy for depression in adults: A meta-analysis of comparative outcome studies. *Journal of Consulting and Clinical Psychology, 76*(6), 909–922. https://doi.org/10.1037/a0013075

Cullen, F. T., & Gendreau, P. (2001). From nothing works to what works: Changing professional ideology in the 21st century. *The Prison Journal, 81*(3), 313–338. https://doi.org/10.1177/0032885501081003002

Deffenbacher, J. L., & McKay, M. (2000). *Overcoming situational and general anger: A protocol for the treatment of anger based on relaxation, cognitive restructuring, and coping skills training*. Oakland, CA: New Harbinger Publications.

DiGiuseppe, R. (2008). Surfing the waves of behavior therapy. *The Behavior Therapist, 31*(8), 154–155. Retrieved from http://www.abct.org/Journals/?m=mJournal&fa=TBT

DiGiuseppe, R. A., Doyle, K. A., Dryden, W., & Backx, W. (2013). *The practitioner's guide to rational emotive behavior therapy* (3rd ed.). New York, NY: Oxford University Press.
Dobson, K. S. (1989). A meta-analysis of the efficacy of cognitive therapy for depression. *Journal of Consulting and Clinical Psychology, 57*(3), 414–419. https://doi.org/10.1037/0022-006X.57.3.414
Dowden, C., & Andrews, D. A. (2004). The importance of staff practice in delivering effective correctional treatment: A meta-analytic review of core correctional practice. *International Journal of Offender Therapy and Comparative Criminology, 48*(2), 203–214. https://doi.org/10.1177/0306624X03257765
Dutra, L., Stathopoulou, G., Basden, S. L., Leyro, T. M., Powers, M. B., & Otto, M. W. (2008). A meta-analytic review of psychosocial interventions for substance use disorders. *The American Journal of Psychiatry, 165*(2), 179–187. https://doi.org/10.1176/appi.ajp.2007.06111851
Eckhardt, C. I., Crane, C. A., & Sprunger, J. G. (2014). CBT for perpetrators of intimate partner violence: The "I^3" approach. In R. C. Tafrate & D. Mitchell (Eds.), *Forensic CBT: A handbook for clinical practice* (pp. 187–210). Chichester, UK: Wiley.
Ellis, A. (1957). Rational psychotherapy and individual psychology. *Journal of Individual Psychology, 13*(1), 38–44. Retrieved from https://utpress.utexas.edu/journals/journal-of-individual-psychology
Ellis, A. (1962). *Reason and emotion in psychotherapy*. New York, NY: Lyle Stuart.
Gardner, F. L., & Moore, Z. E. (2014). Contextual anger regulation therapy (CART): An acceptance-based treatment for domestic and non-domestic violent offenders. In R. C. Tafrate & D. Mitchell (Eds.), *Forensic CBT:A handbook for clinical practice* (pp. 161–184). Chichester, UK: Wiley.
Gardner, F. L., Moore, Z. E., Birkley, E. L., & Eckhardt, C. I. (2016). History, comparative outcomes, and future directions for intimate partner violence intervention programs. *The Behavior Therapist, 39*(5), 168–174. Retrieved from http://www.abct.org/Journals/?m=mJournal&fa=TBT
Gloaguen, V., Cottraux, J., Cucherat, M., & Blackburn, I.-M. (1998). A meta-analysis of the effects of cognitive therapy in depressed patients. *Journal of Affective Disorders, 49*(1), 59–72. https://doi.org/10.1016/S0165-0327(97)00199-7
Gould, R. A., Otto, M. W., Pollack, M. H., & Yap, L. (1997). Cognitive behavioral and pharmacological treatment of generalized anxiety disorder: A preliminary meta-analysis. *Behavior Therapy, 28*(2), 285–305. https://doi.org/10.1016/S0005-7894(97)80048-2
Hanson, R. K., Bourgon, G., Helmus, L., & Hodgson, S. (2009). The principles of effective correctional treatment also apply to sexual offenders: A meta-analysis. *Criminal Justice and Behavior, 36*(9), 865–891. https://doi.org/10.1177/0093854809338545
Hanson, R. K., Gordon, A., Harris, A. J. R., Marques, J. K., Murphy, W., Quinsey, V. L., & Seto, M. C. (2002). First report of the collaborative outcome data project on the effectiveness of psychological treatment of sex offenders. *Sexual Abuse: A Journal of Research and Treatment, 14*(2), 169–194. https://doi.org/10.1177/107906320201400207
Hayes, S. C. (2008). Avoiding the mistakes of the past. *The Behavior Therapist, 31*(8), 150–153. Retrieved from http://www.abct.org/Journals/?m=mJournal&fa=TBT
Hayes, S. C., & Smith, S. (2005). *Get out of your mind and into your life: The new acceptance and commitment therapy*. Oakland, CA: New Harbinger Publications.
Hayes, S. C., Strosahl, K. D., & Wilson, K. G. (2012). *Acceptance and commitment therapy: The process and practice of mindful change* (2nd ed.). New York, NY: The Guilford Press.
Henwood, K. S., Chou, S., & Browne, K. D. (2015). A systematic review and meta-analysis on the effectiveness of CBT informed anger management. *Aggression and Violent Behavior, 25*(Part B), 280–292. https://doi.org/10.1016/j.avb.2015.09.011
Hoffman, S. G., Asnaani, A., Vonk, I. J. J., Sawyer, A. T., & Fang, A. (2012). The efficacy of cognitive behavioral therapy: A review of meta-analyses. *Cognitive Therapy and Research, 36*(5), 427–440. https://doi.org/10.1007/s10608-012-9476-1

Hofmann, S. G., & Smits, J. A. J. (2008). Cognitive-behavioral therapy for adult anxiety disorders: A meta-analysis of randomized placebo-controlled trials. *Journal of Clinical Psychiatry, 69*(4), 621–632. https://doi.org/10.4088/JCP.v69n0415

Hollon, S. D., Shelton, R. C., & Loosen, P. T. (1991). Cognitive therapy and pharmacotherapy for depression. *Journal of Consulting and Clinical Psychology, 59*(1), 88–99. https://doi.org/10.1037/0022-006X.59.1.88

Horvath, A. O., & Symonds, B. D. (1991). Relation between working alliance and outcome in psychotherapy: A meta-analysis. *Journal of Counseling Psychology, 38*(2), 139–149. https://doi.org/10.1037/0022-0167.38.2.139

Jeglic, E. L., Hanson, R. K, & Calkins, C. (2016). Sex offender treatment: The need for cognitive behavioral therapists. *The Behavior Therapist, 39*(5), 162–167. Retrieved from http://www.abct.org/Journals/?m=mJournal&fa=TBT

Johnsen, T. J., & Friborg, O. (2015). The effects of cognitive behavioral therapy as an anti-depressive treatment is falling: A meta-analysis. *Psychological Bulletin, 141*(4), 747–768. https://doi.org/10.1037/bul0000015

Johnsen, T. J., & Thimm, J. C. (2018). A meta-analysis of group cognitive–behavioral therapy as an antidepressive treatment: Are we getting better? *Canadian Psychology/Psychologie Canadienne, 59*(1), 15–30. https://doi.org/10.1037/cap0000132

Jolliffe, D., & Farrington, D. P. (2007). *A systematic review of the national and international evidence on the effectiveness of interventions with violent offenders, Ministry of Justice research series 16/07*. London, UK: Ministry of Justice, Research Development Statistics (RDS).

Kazantzis, N., Luong, H. K., Usatoff, A. S., Impala, T., Yew, R. Y., & Hofmann, S. G. (2018). The processes of cognitive behavioral therapy: A review of meta-analyses. *Cognitive Therapy and Research, 42*(4), 349–357. https://doi.org/10.1007/s10608-018-9920-y

Kennealy, P. J., Skeem, J. L., Manchak, S. M., & Eno Louden, J. (2012). Firm, fair, and caring officer-offender relationships protect against supervision failure. *Law and Human Behavior, 36*(6), 496–505. https://doi.org/10.1037/h0093935

Keulen-de Vos, M., Bernstein, D. P., & Arntz, A. (2014). Schema therapy for aggressive offenders with personality disorders. In R. Tafrate & D. Mitchell (Eds.), *Forensic CBT: A handbook for clinical practice* (pp. 66–83). Chichester, UK: Wiley.

Knight, K., Garner, B. R., Simpson, D. D., Morey, J. T., & Flynn, P. M. (2006). An assessment for criminal thinking. *Crime & Delinquency, 52*(1), 159–177. https://doi.org/10.1177/0011128705281749

Koehler, J. A., Lösel, F., Akoensi, T. D., & Humphreys, D. K. (2013). A systematic review and meta-analysis on the effects of young offender treatment programs in Europe. *Journal of Experimental Criminology, 9*(1), 19–43. https://doi.org/10.1007/s11292-012-9159-7

Kroner, D. G., & Morgan, R. D. (2014). An overview of strategies for the assessment and treatment of criminal thinking. In R. Tafrate & D. Mitchell (Eds.), *Forensic CBT: A handbook for clinical practice* (pp. 87–103). Chichester, UK: Wiley.

Landenberger, N. A., & Lipsey, M. W. (2005). The positive effects of cognitive behavioral programs for offenders: A meta-analysis of factors associated with effective treatment. *Journal of Experimental Criminology, 1*(4), 451–476. https://doi.org/10.1007/s11292-005-3541-7

Langhinrichsen-Rohling, J., McCullars, A., & Misra, T. A. (2012). Motivations for men and women's intimate partner violence perpetration: A comprehensive review. *Partner Abuse, 3*(4), 429–468. https://doi.org/10.1891/1946-6560.3.4.429

Leahy, R. L. (2008). A closer look at ACT. *The Behavior Therapist, 31*(8), 148–150. Retrieved from http://www.abct.org/Journals/?m=mJournal&fa=TBT

Leahy, R. L., Holland, S. J. F., & McGinn, L. K. (2012). *Treatment plans and interventions for depression and anxiety disorders* (2nd ed.). New York, NY: The Guilford Press.

Lipsey, M. W., Chapman, G. L., & Landenberger, N. A. (2001). Cognitive-behavioral programs for offenders. *The Annals of the American Academy of Political and Social Science, 578*(1), 144–157. https://doi.org/10.1177/000271620157800109

Lipsey, M. W., & Cullen, F. T. (2007). The effectiveness of correctional rehabilitation: A review of systematic reviews. *Annual Review of Law and Social Science, 3*, 297–320. https://doi.org/10.1146/annurev.lawsocsci.3.081806.112833

Lipsey, M. W., Landenberger, N. A., & Wilson, S. J. (2007). Effects of cognitive-behavioral programs for criminal offenders. *Campbell Systematic Reviews, 2007*(6), 1–27. https://doi.org/10.4073/csr.2007.6

Little, G. L., & Robinson, K. D. (1986). *How to escape your prison: A moral reconation therapy workbook*. Memphis, TN: Eagle Wing Books.

Lösel, F., & Schmucker, M. (2005). The effectiveness of treatment for sexual offenders: A comprehensive meta-analysis. *Journal of Experimental Criminology, 1*(1), 117–146. https://doi.org/10.1007/s11292-004-6466-7

Lowenkamp, C. T., Holsinger, A., Robinson, C. R., & Alexander, M. (2014). Diminishing or durable treatment effects of STARR? A research note on 24-month re-arrest rates. *Journal of Crime and Justice, 37*(2), 275–283. https://doi.org/10.1080/0735648X.2012.753849

Magill, M., & Ray, L. A. (2009). Cognitive-behavioral treatment with adult alcohol and illicit drug users: A meta-analysis of randomized controlled trials. *Journal of Studies on Alcohol and Drugs, 70*(4), 516–527. https://doi.org/10.15288/jsad.2009.70.516

Mandracchia, J. T., Morgan, R. D., Garos, S., & Garland, J. T. (2007). Inmate thinking patterns: An empirical investigation. *Criminal Justice and Behavior, 34*(8), 1029–1043. https://doi.org/10.1177/0093854807301788

Marshall, W. L., & O'Brien, M. D. (2014). Balancing clients' strengths and deficits in sexual offender treatment: The Rockwood treatment approach. In R. C. Tafrate & D. Mitchell (Eds.), *Forensic CBT: A handbook for clinical practice* (pp. 281–301). Chichester, UK: Wiley.

Martinson, R. (1974). What works? – Questions and answers about prison reform. *The Public Interest, 35*, 22–54. Retrieved from https://www.nationalaffairs.com/public_interest/issues/spring-1974

McGrath, R. J., Cumming, G. F., Burchard, B. L., Zeoli, S., & Ellerby, L. (2009). *Current practices and emerging trends in sexual abuser management: The safer society 2009 North American survey*. Brandon, VT: The Safer Society Press.

McMurran, M. (2007). What works in substance misuse treatments for offenders? *Criminal Behaviour and Mental Health, 17*(4), 225–233. https://doi.org/10.1002/cbm.662

Meichenbaum, D. H., & Cameron, R. (1973). Training schizophrenics to talk to themselves: A means of developing attentional controls. *Behavior Therapy, 4*(4), 515–534. https://doi.org/10.1016/S0005-7894(73)80003-6

Miller, W. R., & Rollnick, S. (2013). *Motivational interviewing: Helping people change* (3rd ed.). New York, NY: The Guilford Press.

Mills, J. F., Kroner, D. G., & Forth, A. E. (2002). Measures of criminal attitudes and associates (MCAA): Development, factor structure, reliability, and validity. *Assessment, 9*(3), 240–253. https://doi.org/10.1177/1073191102009003003

Mitchell, D., & Tafrate, R. C. (2012). Conceptualization and measurement of criminal thinking: Initial validation of the criminogenic thinking profile. *International Journal of Offender Therapy and Comparative Criminology, 56*(7), 1080–1102. https://doi.org/10.1177/0306624X11416197

Mitchell, D., Tafrate, R. C., Cox, S. M., & Hogan, T. (2017, June). *The impact of a probation officer CBT training program on supervision sessions and client recidivism*. Poster presented at the annual meeting of the Canadian Psychological Association, Toronto, Ontario, Canada

Mitchell, D., Tafrate, R. C., & Freeman, A. (2015). Antisocial personality disorder. In A. T. Beck, D. D. Davis, & A. Freeman (Eds.), *Cognitive therapy of personality disorders* (3rd ed., pp. 346–365). New York, NY: The Guilford Press.

Morgan, R. D., Flora, D. B., Kroner, D. G., Mills, J. F., Varghese, F. P., & Steffan, J. S. (2012). Treating offenders with mental illness: A research synthesis. *Law and Human Behavior, 36*(1), 37–50. https://doi.org/10.1037/h0093964

National Institute of Corrections & Crime and Justice Institute. (2004). *Implementing evidence-based practice in community corrections: The principles of effective intervention*. Retrieved from http://nicic.gov/Library/019342

Newby, J. M., McKinnon, A., Kuyken, W., Gilbody, S., & Dalgleish, T. (2015). Systematic review and meta-analysis of transdiagnostic psychological treatments for anxiety and depressive disorders in adulthood. *Clinical Psychology Review, 40*, 91–110. https://doi.org/10.1016/j.cpr.2015.06.002

Norton, P. J., & Price, E. C. (2007). A meta-analytic review of adult cognitive-behavioral treatment outcome across the anxiety disorders. *The Journal of Nervous and Mental Disease, 195*(6), 521–531. https://doi.org/10.1097/01.nmd.0000253843.70149.9a

O'Kelly, M. E. (2010). *CBT in action: A practitioner's toolkit*. Melbourne, Australia: CBT Australia.

Parhar, K. K., Wormith, J. S., Derkzen, D. M., & Beauregard, A. M. (2008). Offender coercion in treatment: A meta-analysis of effectiveness. *Criminal Justice and Behavior, 35*(9), 1109–1135. https://doi.org/10.1177/0093854808320169

Pearson, F. S., & Lipton, D. S. (1999). A meta-analytic review of the effectiveness of corrections-based treatments for drug abuse. *The Prison Journal, 79*(4), 384–410. https://doi.org/10.1177/0032885599079004003

Phillips, H. K., Gray, N. S., MacCulloch, S. I., Taylor, J., Moore, S. C., Huckle, P., & MacCulloch, M. J. (2005). Risk assessment in offenders with mental disorders: Relative efficacy of personal, demographic, criminal history, and clinical variables. *Journal of Interpersonal Violence, 20*(7), 833–847. https://doi.org/10.1177/0886260504272898

Ronan, G. F., Maurelli, K., & Holman, K. M. (2014). A couples-based violence reduction approach to curbing intimate partner assault. In R. C. Tafrate & D. Mitchell (Eds.), *Forensic CBT: A handbook for clinical practice* (pp. 211–229). Chichester, UK: Wiley.

Ross, R. R., Fabiano, E. A., & Ross, R. D. (1986). *Reasoning and rehabilitation: A handbook for teaching cognitive skills*. Ottawa, ON, Canada: T3 Associates.

Schmucker, M., & Lösel, F. (2015). The effects of sexual offender treatment on recidivism: An international meta-analysis of sound quality evaluations. *Journal of Experimental Criminology, 11*(4), 597–630. https://doi.org/10.1007/s11292-015-9241-z

Seeler, L., Freeman, A., DiGuiseppe, R., & Mitchell, D. (2014). Traditional cognitive-behavioral therapy models for antisocial patterns. In R. C. Tafrate & D. Mitchell (Eds.), *Forensic CBT: A handbook for clinical practice* (pp. 15–42). Chichester, UK: Wiley.

Simourd, D. J. (1997). The criminal sentiments scale-modified and pride in delinquency scale: Psychometric properties and construct validity of two measures of criminal attitudes. *Criminal Justice and Behavior, 24*(1), 52–70. https://doi.org/10.1177/0093854897024001004

Singh, J. P., Kroner, D. G., Wormith, J. S., Desmarais, S. L., & Hamilton, Z. (Eds.). (2018). *Handbook of recidivism risk/needs assessment tools*. Chichester, UK: Wiley.

Skeem, J., Kennealy, P., Monahan, J., Peterson, J. K., & Appelbaum, P. (2016). Psychosis uncommonly and inconsistently precedes violence among high-risk individuals. *Clinical Psychological Science, 4*(1), 40–49. https://doi.org/10.1177/2167702615575879

Smith, P., Gendreau, P., & Swartz, K. (2009). Validating the principles of effective intervention: A systematic review of the contributions of meta-analysis in the field of corrections. *Victims & Offenders, 4*(2), 148–169. https://doi.org/10.1080/15564880802612581

Smith, P., Schweitzer, M., Labrecque, R. M., & Latessa, E. J. (2012). Improving probation officers' supervision skills: An evaluation of the EPICS model. *Journal of Crime and Justice, 35*(2), 189–199. https://doi.org/10.1080/0735648X.2012.674826

Tafrate, R. C., Hogan, T., & Mitchell, D. (in press). Integrating motivational interviewing with risk- need-responsivity based practice in community corrections: Collaboratively focusing on what matters most. In D. Polaschek, A. Day, & C. Hollin (Eds.), *The handbook of correctional psychology*. Chichester, UK: Wiley.

Tafrate, R. C., & Kassinove, H. (in press). *Anger management for everyone: Ten proven strategies to help you control anger and live a happier life* (2nd ed.). Oakland, CA: New Harbinger Publications.

Tafrate, R. C., & Luther, J. D. (2014). Integrating motivational interviewing with forensic CBT: Promoting treatment engagement and behavior change with justice-involved clients. In R. C. Tafrate & D. Mitchell (Eds.), *Forensic CBT: A handbook for clinical practice* (pp. 411–435). Chichester, UK: Wiley.

Tafrate, R. C., & Mitchell, D. (Eds.). (2014). *Forensic CBT: A handbook for clinical practice*. Chichester, UK: Wiley.

Tafrate, R. C., Mitchell, D., & Novaco, R. W. (2014). Forensic CBT: Five recommendations for clinical practice and five topics in need of more attention. In R. Tafrate & D. Mitchell (Eds.), *Forensic CBT: A handbook for clinical practice* (pp. 473–486). Chichester, UK: Wiley.

Tafrate, R. C., Mitchell, D., & Simourd, D. J. (2018). *CBT with justice-involved clients: Interventions for antisocial and self-destructive behaviors*. New York, NY: The Guilford Press.

Tangney, J. P., Steuwig, J., Furukawa, E., Kopelovich, S., Meyer, P. J., & Crosby, B. (2012). Reliability, validity, and predictive utility of the 25-item criminogenic cognitions scale (CCS). *Criminal Justice and Behavior, 39*(10), 1340–1360. https://doi.org/10.1177/0093854812451092

Taxman, F. S., Sherpardson, E. S., & Byrne, J. M. (2004). *Tools of the trade: A guide to incorporating science into practice*. Washington, DC: National Institute of Corrections, Maryland Department of Public Safety and Correctional Services.

Walters, G. D. (1995). The psychological inventory of criminal thinking styles: Part I: Reliability and preliminary validity. *Criminal Justice and Behavior, 22*(3), 307–325. https://doi.org/10.1177/0093854895022003008

Walters, G. D. (2014). Applying CBT to the criminal thought process. In R. C. Tafrate & D. Mitchell (Eds.), *Forensic CBT: A handbook for clinical practice* (pp. 104–121). Chichester, UK: Wiley.

Wampold, B. E., Minami, T., Baskin, T. W., & Callen Tierney, S. (2002). A meta-(re)analysis of the effects of cognitive therapy versus 'other therapies' for depression. *Journal of Affective Disorders, 68*(2–3), 159–165. https://doi.org/10.1016/S0165-0327(00)00287-1

Wanberg, K. W., & Milkman, H. B. (2014). Social and community responsibility therapy (SCRT): A cognitive-behavioral model for the treatment of substance-abusing judicial clients. In R. C. Tafrate & D. Mitchell (Eds.), *Forensic CBT: A handbook for clinical practice* (pp. 252–277). Chichester, UK: Wiley.

Wheeler, J., & Covell, C. (2014). Recidivism risk reduction therapy (3RT): Cognitive-behavioral approaches to treating sexual offense behavior. In R. C. Tafrate & D. Mitchell (Eds.), *Forensic CBT: A handbook for clinical practice* (pp. 302–326). Chichester, UK: Wiley.

Wilson, D. B., Bouffard, L. A., & MacKenzie, D. L. (2005). A quantitative review of structured, group-oriented, cognitive-behavioral programs for offenders. *Criminal Justice and Behavior, 32*(2), 172–204. https://doi.org/10.1177/0093854804272889

Part II
Clinical Factors Contributing to Treatment Outcome in Corrections

Chapter 5
The Role of the Therapeutic Alliance in Offender Therapy

Brandy Blasko, Geris Serran, and Jeff Abracen

5.1 Introduction

The therapeutic alliance—also referred to as the working alliance (Bordin, 1979; Horvath & Greenberg, 1989) and the helping alliance—is defined as the collaboration between client and therapist (Horvath & Symonds, 1991). General psychotherapy literature has long demonstrated that the therapeutic alliance predicts psychotherapeutic outcome (Martin, Garske, & Davis, 2000). The relationship between client and therapist is considered the foundation of therapeutic work and is viewed as one of the main tools for achieving client change (Klerman, Weissman, Rounsaville, & Chevron, 1984; Luborsky, 1994). Effect sizes of 0.22 (Martin et al., 2000) and 0.26 (Horvath & Symonds, 1991) have been associated with the influence of the therapeutic alliance on various in-treatment and posttreatment outcomes. Importantly, the therapeutic relationship features account for 30% of treatment-induced changes (Norcross, 2002), while the combined effect of specific procedures only accounted for between 7% (Flückiger et al., 2012) and 15% (Norcross, 2002) of changes.

Less research attention is paid to the therapeutic alliance in offender therapy. Developing a therapeutic relationship with offenders can be challenging, particularly with high-risk offenders. This chapter focuses specifically on the therapeutic alliance between therapists and clients in criminal justice therapy settings. The

B. Blasko (✉)
Center for Advancing Correctional Excellence, George Mason University, Fairfax, VA, USA

G. Serran
Warkworth Institution, Correctional Service Canada, Warkworth, ON, Canada
e-mail: Geris.Serran@csc-scc.gc.ca

J. Abracen
Keele Center, Correctional Service Canada, Toronto, ON, Canada
e-mail: Jeff.Abracen@csc-scc.gc.ca

E. L. Jeglic, C. Calkins (eds.), *New Frontiers in Offender Treatment*,
https://doi.org/10.1007/978-3-030-01030-0_5

general psychotherapy literature is examined and is followed by a synthesis of the offender-specific research to date. A specific section is devoted to therapeutic relationships with high-risk offenders. We conclude with suggestions for future directions in research on the therapeutic alliance within criminal justice therapy settings.

5.2 The Therapeutic Alliance in General Psychotherapy: Theory, Research, and Practice

Therapists need to be able to establish a relationship with their clients in order to increase clients' hope, enhance their expectation for change, and motivate them to maintain treatment gains. Failure to create an effective therapeutic alliance can lead to client non-compliance (Eisenthal, Emery, Lazare, & Udin, 1979), which is the typical reason given for removing clients from treatment. Eisenthal et al. (1979) demonstrated that if the quality of the therapeutic relationship is positive, the drop-out rate is markedly reduced. Thus, it is critical to examine therapist behaviors and whether they are serving to increase or decrease the therapeutic alliance.

5.2.1 Therapist Characteristics

The initial impetus for directing research to the importance of therapist qualities would be credited to the work of Carl Rogers (1965), who argued that healing occurred when a therapist displayed the three characteristics of empathy, warmth, and positive regard. While these three characteristics are no longer deemed sufficient for change, these qualities appear to be necessary for effective therapy. Beutler et al. (2004) examined a range of therapist features (e.g., gender, age, ethnicity, years of training), the majority of which had minimal effect, while positive therapist qualities were strongly predictive of outcome.

5.2.2 Features that Facilitate Change

Certain therapist qualities have been found essential to developing a positive alliance. For example, empathy, warmth, and genuineness have all been shown to influence outcome in the treatment of various psychological disorders (Keijsers, Schaap, & Hoogduin, 2000). Empathy refers to the ability of the therapist to understand and emotionally respond to the client (Bohart, Elliott, Greenberg, & Watson, 2002). In their meta-analysis, Bohart et al. (2002) found that therapist empathy alone accounted for between 7 and 10% of the variance in outcome. Display of empathy by the therapist was a positive predictor of both abstinence and controlled drinking in clients with alcohol addiction (Miller, Taylor, & West, 1980) and was related to improved coping in patients with panic disorder (Mathews et al., 1976), as well as reductions in depression (Burns & Auerbach, 1996).

Warmth is displayed as acceptance, caring, and support and serves to encourage clients to examine their problem behavior (Safran & Segal, 1990). Orlinsky and Howard (1986), in their comprehensive review, concluded that warmth displayed by the therapist was a significant predictor of positive outcome and was associated with positive client ratings. Lambert (1999) showed that warm and affirming therapists were the most effective. Genuineness, defined as the therapist being himself/herself, is associated with sincerity, consistency, nondefensiveness, comfort, honesty, and a clear display of interest (Egan, 1998). Both sincerity and respect have been linked to beneficial treatment outcome (Ford, 1978; Rabavilas, Boulougouris, & Perissaki, 1979).

Treating clients with respect has also been shown to generate positive outcomes (Rabavilas et al., 1979; Strupp, 1980). Demonstrating respect tells the client that they are valued and accepted. Being respectful is very important to sexual offender clients, who typically experience shame (Proeve & Howells, 2006) which decreases their ability to change (Tangney & Dearing, 2002). Helping offenders distinguish themselves from their behavior helps them to recover their self-respect which is importantly related to their full engagement in treatment (Marshall, Anderson, & Champagne, 1997). Adopting a reinforcing or encouraging approach increases clients' self-efficacy, enhances their expectations about the likely benefits of treatment (Miller & Rollnick, 2002), and reduces resistance and aggression (Bandura, Lipsher, & Miller, 1960). Clients should be rewarded for small steps early in treatment, whereas encouragement for more extended chains of appropriate behavior can be introduced once the client becomes more confident (Martin & Pear, 1996). Therapist's support and encouragement increases client self-efficacy, enhances positive expectations about treatment (Miller & Rollnick, 2002), and reduces aggression and resistance (Bandura et al., 1960).

Some degree of directiveness is also important in establishing a constructive working relationship with the client and results in a better outcome (Alexander, Barton, Schiaro, & Parsons, 1976; Beutler, Dunbar, & Baer, 1980; Schindler, Revenstorf, Hahlweg, & Brengelmann, 1983). Being directive does not require the therapist to tell the client how to handle a situation but rather involves offering alternatives so that a collaborative approach can be developed. Adopting a directive approach includes encouraging clients to practice skills outside of the treatment session (Schaap, Bennum, Schindler, & Hoogduin, 1993) and helps clients develop problem-solving skills (Elliott, Barker, Caskey, & Pistrang, 1982). Being directive with clients provides structure, helps establish an effective working relationship, and leads to improved therapeutic outcome (Mintz, Luborsky, & Auerbach, 1971). However, it is important to balance directiveness with reflectiveness. It has been shown, for example, that a reflective style is more successful with angry and aggressive clients, while a directive approach is effective with submissive or defensive clients (Ashby, Ford, Guerkey, Guerkey, & Snyder, 1957; Beutler, Pollack, & Jobe, 1978). Clearly, flexibility is critical, as some clients require more structure, whereas others might feel overly controlled.

Other important skills include encouraging active participation, use of humor, and some degree of self-disclosure. Encouraging active participation is associated with both successful completion of treatment and positive outcomes (Garfield & Bergin, 1986). Although Keijsers et al. (2000) argue that self-disclosure by therapists is not helpful, the evidence does not support this claim. While excessive or irrelevant self-disclosure undermines client confidence in the therapist (Curtis, 1982), appropriate self-disclosure increases trust (Braaten, Otto, & Handelsman, 1993), which in turn increases the client's ability to share their issues and feelings (McCarthy, 2001; Sermat & Smyth, 1973). Disclosure has also been associated with positive outcome (Barrett & Berman, 2001; Hill & Knox, 2001; Lilliengren & Werbart, 2005). Therapists who disclose their thoughts and feelings appropriately are modeling to client appropriate behavior and by so doing display a coping rather than a mastery model. As Mahoney and Norcross (1993) suggest, if therapists present themselves as perfectly adjusted, clients will find it difficult to identify with them and will be unlikely or unable to emulate the therapist.

Although little research has been conducted on the use of humor, Rutherford (1994) concluded that its appropriate use increases clients' interest and helps them adopt a more tolerant perspective. Humor creates a positive and open atmosphere (Greenwald, 1987) and helps relieve tension (Falk & Hill, 1992). Bates (2007) notes that the use of humor in group therapy helps group members bond with each other and encourages flexibility and openness.

A flexible approach that is adapted to each individual client is more effective than rigidly adhering to the same agenda for all clients (Ringler, 1977). Therapists who can adjust their style and tailor their approach to suit individual clients generate more positive results (Kottler, Sexton, & Whiston, 1994). Effective therapists are sensitive to clients' responses and are able to change their interactions based on this feedback (Duncan, Miller, & Sparks, 2004). Flexibility results in increased effectiveness compared to a rigid, structured approach (Ringler, 1977). Flexibility seems even more important in a group setting, where a wide range of clients with different experiences, sexual orientations, ages, and needs are present. In fact, one of the objections that has been raised about the use of highly detailed manuals is that they do not allow the flexibility essential to effective treatment (Marshall, Marshall, & Ware, 2009).

Therapist confidence and credibility are also related to beneficial changes (Seligman, 1990). Confident therapists typically display more positive therapeutic skills than do therapists who lack confidence (Alexander et al., 1976). Clients who rated their therapists as confident improved more than those who did not (McGuff, Gitlin, & Enderlin, 1996; Ryan & Gizynski, 1971). Overconfidence, however, can be problematic. Assuming an "expert role" where the therapist manifests certainty is likely to engender resistance in clients, whereas modeling a learning approach, while acknowledging limits to knowledge along with a willingness to admit to mistakes and apologize, is more likely to encourage a belief in clients that they do not have to be perfect to succeed.

In addition, the manner in which questions are asked by the therapist is important. Asking closed questions, which typically require a yes or no response, does not generate much useful information and discourages client disclosure. Open-ended questions, on the other hand, encourage the client to elaborate and, as a result, typically provide detailed responses leading to greater insight (Schaap et al., 1993). Open-ended questions are preferred by clients (Elliott, 1985) and serve to enhance the therapeutic relationship.

While confrontation (described below) seems to impede progress, supportive challenges are helpful. These supportive challenges can be used to help clients consider alternative perspectives, change unhealthy attitudes, and follow through on behavioral goals. Firm, supportive challenges produce significant reductions in depression (Teasdale & Fennell, 1982) and produce increased client awareness (Safran & Segal, 1990).

5.2.3 Features that Impede Change

Various problematic characteristics appear to reduce treatment effectiveness. The most significant of these problematic features involves aggressive confrontation by therapists. Yalom and Lieberman (1971) found that the most damaging therapist style was what they termed the "aggressive stimulator" characterized by an intrusive, aggressive approach involving harsh confrontational. Confrontation has been shown to be particularly harmful to clients at the "precontemplative" stage (DiClemente, 1991). This is particularly relevant when we consider that many sexual offenders are at this stage when they enter treatment (Marshall et al., 2008), which is discussed later in this chapter.

Patterson and Forgatch (1985) have shown that increased non-compliance with treatment is significantly related to the degree of confrontation in therapy, and Nichols and Taylor (1975) found that therapists who adopt a confrontational style had less effective outcomes compared to supportive group leaders. In the substance abuse field, Miller, Benefield, and Tonigan (1993) report that a confrontational style was predictive of client relapse at 1-year follow-up. Similarly, Miller and Sovereign (1989) found increased resistance, denial, and greater alcohol consumption in clients who are exposed to an aggressively confrontational therapist. Others found that clients who perceive the therapist as confrontational either discredit or forcefully challenge the therapist, devalue the issues, or agree on the surface but fail to make appropriate changes (Rice, Harris, & Cormier, 1992). Overall, a confrontational approach is clearly countertherapeutic and ineffective (Lieberman, Yalom, & Miles, 1973).

Other therapist variables have been associated with negative effects including rejection, lack of therapist skills, manipulating clients in order to meet therapists' needs, and lack of interest in the client (Lambert, Christensen, & DeJulio, 1983). Strupp (1980) identified therapist hostility in response to client negativism as a major indicator of poor outcome. Other researchers (Cullari, 1996; Fremont &

Anderson, 1986) found that when the therapist expressed anger toward the client, the therapeutic relationship was disrupted, and progress in treatment declined.

5.2.4 Emotion in the Therapeutic Relationship

Greenberg and Watson (2006) argue that the therapeutic relationship should facilitate emotional processing and emotional regulation, as they believe this is key to producing lasting changes. Importantly, a validating relationship with the therapist is crucial in helping clients regulate affect (Greenberg, 2007); clients with under-regulated affect have been shown to benefit from interpersonal validation as much as they do from specific techniques aimed directly at emotion regulation and distress tolerance skills (Linehan, 1993). More to the point, research indicates that successful treatment outcome is related to the degree to which clients with various disorders are given the opportunity to be emotionally expressive (Cooley & LaJoy, 1980; Orlinsky & Howard, 1986).

Empathy and acceptance by the therapists contribute to affect regulation by providing interpersonal soothing which enhances the ability to regulate emotion. The therapist's communication of emotion (through facial body and verbal expressions) creates the emotional climate, and by providing a safe and responsive emotional climate, emotional processing is facilitated. Other research has also indicated that encouraging emotional expression enhances the attainment of desired treatment change (Klein, Mathieu-Coughlan, & Kiesler, 1986; Orlinsky & Howard, 1986). Saunders (1999) demonstrated that the expression of feelings by clients determines the impact each treatment session has, and he found that these expressions were best facilitated by the emotional expressiveness of the therapist. These various studies, then, indicate that attitudes and beliefs are affected by emotional states and that interpersonal schemas, which are often strongly held by clients, are typically only accessed and ultimately changed when activated through emotional expression.

Processing information while in an emotional state leads to stable change, while intellectualizing and analyzing issues is less likely to do so (Klein et al., 1986). In fact, Lietaer (1992) notes that little progress occurs when therapists are excessively rational. Research supports this contention. For example, Saunders (1999) found that the expression of feelings by clients determined the impact of treatment sessions and that clients' emotional expression was facilitated by the emotional expressiveness of the therapist.

5.2.5 Clients' Perceptions

The clients' judgment of the therapeutic relationship is a better predictor of outcome than that of the therapist (Bedi, Davis, & Wiliams, 2005). Horvath (2001) notes that the client's perception of treatment significantly influences outcome, which is noteworthy given that Davis (1986) found that clients regard the use of procedures or techniques as of secondary importance to the influence of the therapist. McLeod (1990) observed that the most helpful therapists were those who clients said displayed interest, encouragement, and reassurance and who were able to instill hope and assist clients in improving their coping abilities. Clients' perceptions of the therapist's confidence, involvement, focus, and emotional engagement, as well as his/her display of positive feelings toward them, determined the clients' view of the value of treatment and the degree to which they were willing to engage in the therapeutic process (Saunders, 1999). When clients see therapists as directive (Schindler et al., 1983), sincere (Ford, 1978), confident, and persuasive (Ryan & Gizynski, 1971), then greater treatment benefits are generated. Furthermore, when asked what they found helpful, clients identified factors such as being able to express their feelings, as well as feeling understood, encouraged, validated, and supported (Lilliengren & Werbart, 2005). These researchers also showed that clients were more engaged in treatment when they perceived the therapist as honest and open to feedback; they also preferred therapists who offered some degree of self-disclosure and who listened to what they had to say.

Bachelor (1995) also examined the therapeutic relationship from the perspective of the client. He noted that the manner in which clinicians and clients view the alliance often differs, emphasizing how important it is for therapists to consider their clients' views of the relationship and address these issues. More specifically, Free, Green, Grace, Chernus, and Whitman (1985) showed that therapists were inaccurate in estimating client perceptions of their empathy, and yet it was the client ratings of therapist empathy that predicted treatment benefits. Similarly, Orlinsky, Grawe, and Parks (1994) reviewed various studies and found that in the majority, it was the clients' estimate of therapist features that correlated with indices of beneficial treatment outcome. Fortunately, various measures are available for clients to report their perception of specific therapist features (see Burns & Auerbach, 1996).

5.3 Research on the Therapeutic Alliance in Corrections Settings

While the therapeutic alliance has been found to significantly impact treatment outcomes in general psychotherapy (Ackerman & Hilsenroth, 2003; Horvath & Bedi, 2002; Horvath & Symonds, 1991; Lambert & Barley, 2001; Murphy, Cramer, & Lillie, 1984; Norcross & Lambert, 2006), it is only recently that researchers have begun to study the alliance among offending populations (Beech, Fisher, & Beckett, 1998; Blasko, Friedmann, Rhodes, & Taxman, 2015; Blasko & Jeglic, 2016; Fernandez, Marshall, Lightbody, & O'Sullivan, 1999; Kozar & Day, 2012; Polaschek & Ross, 2010; Ross, Polaschek, & Ward, 2008; Ross, Polaschek, & Wilson, 2011; Skeem, Louden, Polaschek, & Camp, 2007; Tatman & Love, 2010). This research is important as poor quality alliances have been shown to increase the rate of dropouts, which is particularly relevant because in offender therapy dropouts typically have higher failure rates than those who complete treatment (Abel, Becker, Cunningham-Rathner, Mittelman, & Rouleau, 1988; Seto & Barbaree, 1999).

To date, research has found that offenders can form a strong working alliance with their therapist (Blasko & Jeglic, 2016; Polaschek & Ross, 2010; Tatman & Love, 2010). In addition, several therapist factors and one client factor have been found to predict the quality of the working alliance within offender treatment (Marshall et al., 2002; Marshall, Anderson, & Fernandez, 1999; Walton, Jeglic, & Blasko, 2018). The majority of these studies have relied on the Working Alliance Inventory (WAI; Horvath & Greenberg, 1989) to assess the therapeutic alliance (see Table 5.1). The WAI subscales (goals, tasks, bond) are operationalized following Bordin's (1979, 1994) theoretical conceptualization of the working alliance.

Much of the research on the therapeutic alliance in offender therapy contexts has examined either therapist or offender characteristics. Early literature on the working alliance among offending populations placed significant focus on the therapist characteristics and behaviors associated with positive, or conversely negative, treatment outcomes (Blasko & Jeglic, 2016; Goldfried, Burckell, & Eubanks-Carter, 2003; Marshall, et al., 2003). A body of research by Marshall and colleagues has demonstrated that the therapist plays a key role in the client-therapist relationship for offending populations. In one empirical paper, Marshall et al. (2002) conducted a two-part study in an effort first to identify common therapist behaviors and then to examine the relationship between the identified therapist behaviors and client changes in sex offender treatment. Using videotapes of 2-h group treatment sessions, results showed that across 44 potential treatment targets, 4 therapist behaviors were associated with the largest number of changes—empathy, warmth, directiveness, and rewarding behaviors (Marshall et al., 2002). Specifically, when therapists created a supportive and encouraging environment, used a warm and empathic style, and encouraged improvement, the posttreatment functioning of sexual offenders was found to improve (Fernandez et al., 1999; Marshall et al., 2002). Another of their studies, using the same data, found that similar therapist characteristics were associated with positive treatment gain among sexual offenders in three areas—perspective taking, coping skills, and relationship difficulties (Marshall, Fernandez, et al., 2003)—which mirror what has been found in the general psychotherapy literature (Nissen-Lie, Monsen, & Rønnestad, 2010).

In sum, work on therapist characteristics in offender treatment has demonstrated that therapists who display empathy, warmth, and directiveness, as well as reward their client's good behavior, have been found to impact changes in the client-therapist relationship for offenders (Fernandez et al., 1999; Marshall et al., 2002). Marshall, Fernandez, et al. (2003) reported that these therapist characteristics accounted for between 30% and 60% of the variance for indices of behavior change. Conversely, when offenders perceive therapists as aggressive, critical, hostile, or sarcastic, research showed little treatment-induced change and reduced participation (Marshall, Fernandez, et al., 2003). Confrontation has been shown to be particularly harmful to offenders who enter therapy at the "precontemplative" stage (DiClemente, 1991). This is particularly relevant when we consider that many offenders are at this stage

Table 5.1 Research using the Working Alliance Inventory (WAI) in offender therapy settings

Authors	Study location	Sample	Population	CJ setting	Administration schedule	WAI total score	WAI goals scale	WAI tasks scale	WAI bond scale	Key variables
DeSorcy, Olver, and Wormith (2017)	Saskatoon, Saskatchewan, Canada	111 adult males	Sexual offenders	Multi-Level Correctional Treatment Facility, Federal Correctional Department	3 months in 6–9-month program	194.82	65.18	68.09	61.55	Psychopathy, treatment completion, recidivism (conviction)
DeSorcy et al. (2016)	Saskatoon, Saskatchewan, Canada	427 adult males	Sexual offenders	Multi-Level Correctional Treatment Facility, Federal Correctional Department	3 months in 6–9-month program	195.07	64.97	67.74	62.35	Treatment completion, recidivism (conviction), ancestry
Blasko and Jeglic (2016)	PA, USA	202 adult males	Sexual offenders	Maximum Security State Prison	3 months in 9–12 month and 18–24 months programs	206.82	69.28	69.77	68.74	Therapist gender, general and sexual risk for recidivism
Walton et al. (2018)	PA, USA	202 adult males	Sexual offenders	Maximum Security State Prison	3 months in 9–12 month and 18–24 months programs	197.88	66.05	67.41	64.41	Psychopathy, therapist and client perceptions, aftercare

Note: *WAI* Working Alliance Inventory (Horvath & Greenberg, 1989), *CJ* criminal justice when they enter treatment (Marshall, Moulden, & Marshall, 2008). Research has shown that harsh challenges at this stage of offender therapy serve to increase resistance, denial, and non-compliance as well as reduce self-esteem. Specifically, Annis and Chan (1983) found that a confrontational approach with offenders was particularly damaging to self-esteem. Further, Beech and Fordham (1997) found similar results when confrontation was used with sexual offenders. Miller and Rollnick (2002) have found that confrontational styles are common in programs targeting substance-abusing offenders.

Other than therapist behaviors, the gender of the therapist (Blasko & Jeglic, 2016) has found to impart the client's perception of their relationship with their female therapist for high-risk offenders in treatment. This is further discussed later in this chapter in discussion of high-risk offender and the alliance.

Efforts to explain client-therapist relationship factors that contribute to positive outcomes in offender therapy have largely focused on the therapists' perceptions of the alliance or the therapists' behaviors in session as perceived by independent observers (Beech et al., 1998; Fernandez et al., 1999; Marshall, 2005; Marshall et al., 2002; Marshall et al., 2003; Marshall, Fernandez, et al., 2003). Yet, aside from therapist characteristics and behaviors, the client's perception of the relationship is also impacted by client-based factors. Blasko and Jeglic (2016) used the Working Alliance Inventory (WAI; Horvath & Greenberg, 1989) to examine whether offender perceptions of the alliance varied by risk of sexual or general recidivism. Findings demonstrated that the therapeutic alliance was negatively impacted when offenders were higher risk for reoffending sexually. The next section is devoted to the role of the therapeutic alliance for high-risk offender specifically.

5.4 The Therapeutic Alliance and High-Risk Offenders in Therapy

As noted by Hervé (2007), descriptions of psychopaths as instrumentally impulsive individuals with poor behavioral controls as well as presenting with callous and unemotional traits are found across time and culture. These generalizations have understandably found their way both into the clinical literature and been incorporated into measures designed to assess for the presence of psychopathic personality (see Hare, 1991, 2003; Hervé & Yuille, 2007 for a comprehensive discussion of these issues). With the development of the Hare Psychopathy Checklist-Revised (PCL-R; Hare, 1991, 2003), an accepted definition of the construct of psychopathy was developed as well as a psychometrically sound method of assessing for the construct. The Hare PCL-R consists of 20 items each rated zero, one, or two. Those clients who score above 30 on the measure are considered to meet the clinical cutoff for psychopathy. Research, however, suggests that, for experimental purposes, a cutoff of 25 may be more acceptable, at least when samples consisting of moderate to large groups are included in research (see Abracen, Looman, & Langton, 2008 for a discussion).

Given the clinical evidence that psychopathic clients are callous and lacking in their ability to establish empathy, it is perhaps not surprising that there have been relatively few studies published on issues associated with mental health (especially conditions related to such issues as emotionally based disorders), the development of rapport with psychopathic clients, and specifically the therapeutic relationship. It is generally assumed that psychopathic clients will have a limited ability to develop rapport and that they are less likely to suffer from serious mental illness (with possible exception to substance abuse disorders and antisocial personality disorder). Nonetheless, it can be argued that such generalizations regarding psychopathic clients obscure important details about the population. Recently, Abracen and Looman (2016) published a text discussing how many high-risk sexual offenders (including those who would meet the criteria for psychopathy as defined by the PCL-R) present with numerous mental health issues and can be successfully treated given an appropriate dosage of treatment. The resulting conclusions are in line with others (e.g., Olver & Wong, 2013a; Salekin, Worley, & Grimes, 2010; Wilson & Tamatea, 2013) who have suggested that effective treatment may well be associated with reduced rates of recidivism in this population. Olver and Wong (2013b), however, are certainly reasonable in suggesting to readers that there are a variety of issues that need to be addressed among high-risk sexual offenders. While these issues were discussed earlier in this chapter as they related to offender therapy in general, this discussion turns to high-risk offenders specifically.

In particular, Olver and Wong (2013b) note that issues associated with high rates of attrition exist among such groups. For example, they cite Olver, Stockdale, and Wormith's (2011) meta-analysis of predictors of offender treatment attrition which demonstrated a non-completion rate of 27.6% for sex offender programs in general. Olver and Wong (2013b) also discuss the need for appropriately trained staff in the treatment of high-risk sexual offenders. As we will discuss below, when one looks at the available research, it is clear that sexual offenders who score high on the PCL-R present with a wide range of deficits. It, therefore, seems reasonable to assume that well-qualified staff with experience in managing issues related to both serious mental illness and the management of criminogenic needs will be required in the delivery of treatment to high-risk sexual offenders. At a minimum, an undergraduate education in a relevant mental health field should be required of professionals working with such populations.

A second issue which should be noted is that contemporary programs for offenders in general have been associated with low to moderate effect sizes when examining the impact of treatment on outcome (typically between 0.15 and 0.34; see Andrews & Bonta, 2010 as well as Wilson & Tamatea, 2013 for a discussion). Although the magnitude of such effect sizes is described as being robust across offender populations, these data simultaneously suggest that there is much room for improvement in terms of generating effective correctional outcomes. The few programs that have demonstrated significantly reduced rates of recidivism among high-risk treated sexual offenders and comparison subjects (e.g., the Regional Psychiatric

Centre, Prairies, and the Regional Treatment Centre, Ontario; see Abracen & Looman, 2016; Olver & Wong, 2013b for reviews of such programs) have included comprehensive treatment manuals, the use of cognitive-behavioral strategies, and skilled therapists with appropriate levels of professional training among other issues. Although stereotypes associated with psychopathy suggest that issues associated with the therapeutic alliance may be of tertiary relevance when working with such groups, it is our view that such issues are as important when working with high-risk groups of clients as with any other clinical population. Given the resistance that clients who score high on the PCL-R may present with, a great deal of clinical skill is required in the establishment of rapport and overcoming resistance.

Although there have only been a few studies published in relation to the therapeutic alliance with high-risk offenders (e.g., Polaschek & Ross, 2010; Walton et al., 2018), the available data suggest that there may be grounds for optimism. Contrary to the generalizations regarding psychopathy, Walton et al. (2018) found no significant associations between PCL-R scores and the Working Alliance Inventory (a measure of the therapeutic alliance) for either client or therapist ratings. Although these authors note that there are a few studies that support these findings and several that refute them, these recent data certainly present an encouraging picture in relation to the ability of treatment staff to develop rapport even with high-risk clients.

A study conducted by Looman, Abracen, Serin, and Marquis (2005) observed that psychopathic clients who received poor ratings on measures of therapeutic progress actually recidivated at significantly lower rates than those who received higher behavioral ratings on these same measures. Although such data may seem hard to explain at first glance, it is quite possible that these data are in keeping with issues discussed above regarding the therapeutic alliance. That is, staff in the program actually provided clients with sufficient information both in individual and group therapies to complete these assignments and receive high scores on these assignments. At the time it was believed that this would offer the clients attending treatment a mastery experience and provide reinforcement regarding the efforts that they were making in treatment. In choosing not to provide the information that they had discussed with these clients, these individuals would typically engage in behaviors that may be described as resistant. In retrospect, such behaviors should not be seen as surprising, especially in light of the high-risk high-need nature of the population with whom we were engaged. The more interesting issue is that, perhaps, in engaging in conversation with them about the matter (if only to disagree with our perspective regarding any number of issues), the clients may well have internalized some of the material presented in individual therapy and group. With reference to those psychopathic clients who received higher behavioral ratings, it is entirely possible that they were simply "going through the motions" and, as a result, internalized less of the material presented. The fact that all the staff delivering treatment were well-trained (most staff were registered with a professional college, be it nursing or psychology) and had adequate training in working through issues associated with resistance likely contributed to the success of the program.

The Clearwater Sex Offender Program operated at the Regional Psychiatric Centre (RPC; see Olver & Wong, 2013b, for a discussion) is another example of a high-intensity sex offender treatment program that has managed to demonstrate significant reductions in recidivism among treated offenders versus matched comparison samples. In many respects, the RPC program is similar to the RTC Sex Offender Treatment Program (RTCSOTP). Although it is beyond the scope of the present chapter to discuss the similarities and differences between these programs in detail, features that are common to both programs include the use of professional staff who are well-versed on issues associated with maintaining a therapeutic alliance with high-risk populations. Given that many clients attending high-intensity programs present with issues associated with mental illness, both programs also employ staff well-versed on the treatment of serious mental illness. Of course, both programs have also focused on criminogenic needs and other factors (e.g., deviant arousal) that the research literature suggests are directly related to increased rates of recidivism. As well, both programs are inpatient-based and employ cognitive-behavioral strategies.

Recently, Abracen and colleagues developed a treatment model that we believe provides details regarding the features associated with successful treatment programs geared to the needs of high-risk offender populations (see Abracen & Looman, 2016; Abracen, Looman, & Ferguson, 2017). In the latest version of the model, which they have called the Integrated Risk Assessment and Treatment System (IRATS) Model, they have listed three core features as well as internal and external pressures that act upon the core features as well as being influenced by these core factors. With reference to the core features of the model, the team notes that issues associated with criminal history (e.g., persistence and range of offending, antisocial peers, and attitudes) and attachment difficulties/complex trauma-related conditions (including issues associated with chronic mental illness and a history of emotional, physical, or sexual abuse) and deviant arousal (e.g., diagnosed with a paraphilic condition) are critical to the management of groups of high-risk offender populations. External pressures include such observable behaviors as intoxication, victim access, and social dislocation. Internal pressures include such factors as negative emotionality, deviant thoughts or fantasies, and intimacy deficits. It is the team's view that the IRATS Model, in keeping with the current trend to expand upon the rather narrow range of criminal behaviors associated with earlier models (e.g., the risk-need-responsivity model developed by Andrews & Bonta, 1998, 2010), lists a broader range of factors that clinicians need to attend to in integrated programs. Programs such as the RTCSOTP and the community-based programs with which Abracen, Gallo, Looman, and Goodwill (2015) have been involved (see Abracen et al., 2015, for more information) address issues related to criminal attitudes and behavior but also factors that simply can't be ignored based on the available literature. Offenders do not simply present with a range of deficits related to criminal behavior and associates. Such oversimplifications ignore the many issues that more recent literature suggests need to be addressed in high-risk populations, if better outcomes are to be achieved. Those programs that appear to have achieved the best outcomes with groups of high-risk offenders appear to be those that do not neglect such issues as attachment and serious mental illness. Rather, staff make great efforts to address the complex needs with which such clients present. Given these complex needs, issues associated with the therapeutic alliance become critical, if we are to both respect our clients and provide appropriate levels of intervention.

5.5 Conclusion and Promising Directions for Future Research

Beginning in 1990s, Marshall and colleagues called attention to the therapeutic alliance in offender treatment with their work on sexual offender treatment. This research was an opportunity to reshape the offender rehabilitation research agenda and advance offender rehabilitation studies. Despite their innovative research, empirical focus on the therapeutic alliance in the sexual offender literature soon dwindled. For correctional settings in general, policy innovations like Andrew and Bonta's risk-need-responsivity model gradually shifted the focus of criminal justice research away from process and toward classification and risk assessment. Now, nearly three decades later, history is arguably repeating itself. There is a renewed focus on the therapeutic alliance in correctional settings, and there are signs that a new wave of therapeutic alliance research is underway.

Taken together, research with offender populations has generally demonstrated that the therapeutic alliance is as important for offender therapy as it is for general psychotherapy. We propose two areas of research focus for the next generation of therapeutic alliance research in corrections settings. The first is research focused on the relationship between the therapeutic alliance criminal justice-involved clients and posttreatment outcomes. To date only one published study has examined the relationship between the therapeutic alliance and recidivism in a correctional setting (see DeSorcy, Olver, & Wormith, 2016). In addition to replicating this study, research should examine other outcomes, such as reentry success.

The second area in need of investigation is understanding how the therapeutic relationship develops over the course of offender treatment. Currently, it is not well understood how the working alliance changes over the course of treatment and what contributes to these changes. The general psychotherapy research on the therapeutic alliance has found that there are three longitudinal trajectories that the client's ratings follow. These patterns include a stable alliance, a positive linear growth, or a quadratic growth where the alliance starts high, decreases, and then increases (Gelso & Carter, 1994; Horvath & Luborsky, 1993; Kivlighan & Shaughnessy, 1995, 2000; Piper, Boroto, Joyce, McCallum, & Azim, 1995). Research on the therapeutic alliance in offender treatment has largely measured the alliance at a singular point, which may yield an unreliable assessment of the relationship (Walling, Suvak, Howard, Taft, & Murphy, 2012). As such, understanding if and how the alliance changes over the course of offender treatment is necessary to fully understand this relationship and has important implications for therapist training in corrections settings.

A recent article by Bierie and Mann (2017) on the history and future of prison psychology notes that "psychological research on imprisonment should be driven by a genuine concern for the people who live in prisons, recognizing that they deserve the best that psychology has to offer, rather than being mere research subjects for matters of academic interest" (p. 482). Bierie and Mann (2017) note that progress has been made in a variety of areas with reference to treatment in corrections settings. They also note that much research needs to be done in order to further improve upon the progress that has been made. Perhaps no greater service can be provided than to understand that our clients present with complex treatment needs and need to be treated with the same respect and dignity as would any client groups. A focus on issues associated with the therapeutic alliance is certainly in keeping with this important and necessary therapeutic goal.

References

Abel, G. G., Becker, J. V., Cunningham-Rathner, J., Mittelman, M., & Rouleau, J. L. (1988). Multiple paraphilic diagnoses among sex offenders. *Journal of the American Academy of Psychiatry and the Law Online, 16*(2), 153–168. Retrieved from jaapl.org

Abracen, J., Gallo, A., Looman, J., & Goodwill, A. (2015). Individual community-based treatment of offenders with mental illness: Relationship to recidivism. *Journal of Interpersonal Violence, 31*(10), 1842–1858. https://doi.org/10.1177/0886260515570745

Abracen, J., & Looman, J. (2016). *Treatment of high risk sexual offenders: An integrated approach.* Oxford, UK: Wiley-Blackwell.

Abracen, J., Looman, J., & Ferguson, M. (2017). Substance abuse among sexual offenders: Review of research and clinical implications. *Journal of Sexual Aggression, 23*(3), 235–250. https://doi.org/10.1080/13552600.2017.1334967

Abracen, J., Looman, J., & Langton, C. M. (2008). Treatment of sexual offenders with psychopathic traits: Recent research developments and clinical implications. *Trauma, Violence & Abuse, 9*(3), 144–166. https://doi.org/10.1177/1524838008319633

Ackerman, S. J., & Hilsenroth, M. J. (2003). A review of therapist characteristics and techniques positively impacting the therapeutic alliance. *Clinical Psychology Review, 23*(1), 1–33. https://doi.org/10.1016/S0272-7358(02)00146-0

Alexander, J. F., Barton, C., Schiaro, R. S., & Parsons, B. V. (1976). Systems-behavioral intervention with families of delinquents: Therapist characteristics, family behavior, and outcome. *Journal of Consulting and Clinical Psychology, 44*(4), 656–664. https://doi.org/10.1037/0022-006X.44.4.656

Andrews, D. A., & Bonta, J. (1998). *The psychology of criminal conduct* (2nd ed.). Cincinnati, OH: Anderson.

Andrews, D. A., & Bonta, J. (2010). *The psychology of criminal conduct* (5th ed.). New Providence, NJ: Matthew Bender & Company.

Annis, H. M., & Chan, D. (1983). The differential treatment model: Empirical evidence from a personality typology of adult offenders. *Criminal Justice and Behavior, 10*(2), 159–173. https://doi.org/10.1177/0093854883010002002

Ashby, J. D., Ford, D. H., Guerkey, B. G., Jr., Guerkey, L. F., & Snyder, W. U. (1957). Effects on clients of a reflective and a leading type of psychotherapy. *Psychological Monographs: General and Applied, 71*(24), 1–32. https://doi.org/10.1037/h0093778

Bachelor, A. (1995). Clients' perception of the therapeutic alliance: A qualitative analysis. *Journal of Counseling Psychology, 42*(3), 323–337. https://doi.org/10.1037/0022-0167.42.3.323

Bandura, A., Lipsher, D. H., & Miller, P. E. (1960). Psychotherapists approach-avoidance reactions to patients' expressions of hostility. *Journal of Consulting Psychology, 24*(1), 1–8. https://doi.org/10.1037/h0043403

Barrett, M. S., & Berman, J. S. (2001). Is psychotherapy more effective when therapists disclose information about themselves? *Journal of Consulting and Clinical Psychology, 69*(4), 597–603. https://doi.org/10.1037/0022-006X.69.4.597

Bates, S. (2007). The eight most frequent mistakes people make in front of an audience. *Business Strategy Series, 8*(4), 311–317. https://doi.org/10.1108/17515630710684367

Bedi, R. P., Davis, M. D., & Wiliams, M. (2005). Critical incidents in the formation of the therapeutic alliance from the client's perspective. *Psychotherapy: Theory, Research, Practice, Training, 42*(3), 311–323. https://doi.org/10.1037/0033-3204.42.3.311

Beech, A. R., Fisher, D., & Beckett, R. C. (1998). *An evaluation of the prison sex offender treatment programme. U.K. Home Office Occasional Report*. London, UK: Home Office.

Beech, A. R., & Fordham, A. S. (1997). Therapeutic climate of sexual offender treatment programs. *Sexual Abuse: A Journal of Research and Treatment, 9*(3), 219–237. https://doi.org/10.1007/BF02675066

Beutler, L. E., Dunbar, P. W., & Baer, P. E. (1980). Individual variation among therapists' perceptions of patients, therapy process and outcome. *Psychiatry, 43*(3), 205–210. https://doi.org/10.1080/00332747.1980.11024067

Beutler, L. E., Malik, M. L., Alimohamed, S., Harwood, T. M., Talebi, H., Noble, S., & Wong, E. (2004). Therapist variables. In M. J. Lambert (Ed.), *Bergin and Garfield's handbook of psychotherapy and behaviour change* (5th ed., pp. 227–306). New York, NY: Wiley.

Beutler, L. E., Pollack, S., & Jobe, A. (1978). Acceptance, values, and therapeutic change. *Journal of Consulting and Clinical Psychology, 46*(1), 198–199. https://doi.org/10.1037/0022-006X.46.1.198

Bierie, D. M., & Mann, R. E. (2017). The history and future of prison psychology. *Psychology, Public Policy, and Law, 23*(4), 478–489. https://doi.org/10.1037/law0000143

Blasko, B. L., Friedmann, P. D., Rhodes, A. G., & Taxman, F. S. (2015). The parolee–parole officer relationship as a mediator of criminal justice outcomes. *Criminal Justice and Behavior, 42*(7), 722–740. https://doi.org/10.1177/0093854814562642

Blasko, B. L., & Jeglic, E. L. (2016). Sexual offenders' perceptions of the client-therapist relationship: The role of risk. *Sexual Abuse: A Journal of Research and Treatment, 28*(4), 271–290. https://doi.org/10.1177/1079063214529802

Bohart, A. C., Elliott, R., Greenberg, L. S., & Watson, J. C. (2002). Empathy. In J. C. Norcross (Ed.), *Psychotherapy relationships that work: Therapist contributions and responsiveness to patients* (pp. 89–108). New York, NY: Oxford University Press.

Bordin, E. S. (1979). The generalizability of the psychoanalytic concept of the working alliance. *Psychotherapy: Theory, Research & Practice, 16*(3), 252–260. https://doi.org/10.1037/h0085885

Bordin, E. S. (1994). Theory and research on the therapeutic working alliance: New directions. In A. O. Horvath & L. S. Greenberg (Eds.), *The working alliance: Theory, research, and practice* (pp. 13–37). New York, NY: Wiley.

Braaten, E. B., Otto, S., & Handelsman, M. M. (1993). What do people want to know about psychotherapy? *Psychotherapy: Theory, Research, Practice, Training, 30*(4), 565–570. https://doi.org/10.1037/0033-3204.30.4.565

Burns, D. D., & Auerbach, A. (1996). Therapeutic empathy in cognitive-behavioral therapy: Does it really make a difference? In P. M. Salkovskis (Ed.), *Frontiers of cognitive therapy* (pp. 135–164). New York, NY: The Guilford Press.

Cooley, E. J., & Lajoy, R. (1980). Therapeutic relationship and improvement as perceived by clients and therapists. *Journal of Clinical Psychology, 36*(2), 562–570. https://doi.org/10.1002/jclp.6120360230

Cullari, S. (1996). *Treatment resistance: A guide for practitioners*. Needham Heights, MA: Allyn & Bacon.
Curtis, J. M. (1982). The effect of therapist self-disclosure on patients' perceptions of empathy, competence and trust in an analogue psychotherapeutic interaction. *Psychotherapy: Theory, Research & Practice, 19*(1), 54–62. https://doi.org/10.1037/h0088417
Davis, K. (1986). The process of problem and (re)formulation in psychotherapy. *Sociology of Health and Illness, 8*(1), 44–74. https://doi.org/10.1111/1467-9566.ep11346469
DeSorcy, D. R., Olver, M. E., & Wormith, J. S. (2016). Working alliance and its relationship with treatment outcome in a sample of aboriginal and non-aboriginal sexual offenders. *Sexual Abuse: A Journal of Research and Treatment, 28*(4), 291–313. https://doi.org/10.1177/1079063214556360
DeSorcy, D. R., Olver, M. E., & Wormith, J. S. (2017). Working alliance and psychopathy: Linkages to treatment outcome in a sample of treated sexual offenders. *Journal of Interpersonal Violence*. https://doi.org/10.1177/0886260517698822
DiClemente, C. C. (1991). Motivational interviewing and the stages of change. In W. R. Miller & S. Rollnick (Eds.), *Motivational interviewing: Preparing people to change addictive behavior* (pp. 191–202). New York, NY: The Guilford Press.
Duncan, B. L., Miller, S. D., & Sparks, J. A. (2004). *The heroic client: A revolutionary way to improve effectiveness through client-directed, outcome-informed therapy* (Rev. ed.). San Francisco, CA: Jossey-Bass.
Egan, G. (1998). *The skilled helper: A problem-management approach to helping* (6th ed.). Pacific Grove, CA: Brooks/Cole.
Eisenthal, S., Emery, R., Lazare, A., & Udin, H. (1979). Adherence and the negotiated approach to patienthood. *Archives of General Psychiatry, 36*(4), 393–398. https://doi.org/10.1001/archpsyc.1979.01780040035003
Elliott, R. (1985). Helpful and nonhelpful events in brief counseling interviews: An empirical taxonomy. *Journal of Counseling Psychology, 32*(3), 307–322. https://doi.org/10.1037/0022-0167.32.3.307
Elliott, R., Barker, C. B., Caskey, N., & Pistrang, N. (1982). Differential helpfulness of counselor verbal response modes. *Journal of Counseling Psychology, 29*(4), 354–361. https://doi.org/10.1037/0022-0167.29.4.354
Falk, D. R., & Hill, C. E. (1992). Counselor interventions preceding client laughter in brief therapy. *Journal of Counseling Psychology, 39*(1), 39–45. https://doi.org/10.1037/0022-0167.39.1.39
Fernandez, Y. M., Marshall, W. L., Lightbody, S., & O'Sullivan, C. (1999). The child molester empathy measure. *Sexual Abuse: A Journal of Research and Treatment, 11*(1), 17–31. https://doi.org/10.1177/107906329901100103
Flückiger, C., Del Re, A. C., Wampold, B. E., Symonds, D., Wampold, B. E., & Horvath, A. O. (2012). How central is the alliance in psychotherapy? A multilevel longitudinal meta-analysis. *Journal of Counseling Psychology, 59*(1), 10–17. https://doi.org/10.1037/a0025749
Ford, J. D. (1978). Therapeutic relationship in behavior therapy: An empirical analysis. *Journal of Consulting and Clinical Psychology, 46*(6), 1302–1314. https://doi.org/10.1037/0022-006X.46.6.1302
Free, N. K., Green, B. L., Grace, M. C., Chernus, L. A., & Whitman, R. M. (1985). Empathy and outcome in brief focal dynamic therapy. *The American Journal of Psychiatry, 142*(8), 917–921. https://doi.org/10.1176/ajp.142.8.917
Fremont, S., & Anderson, W. (1986). What client behaviors make counselors angry? An exploratory study. *Journal of Counseling & Development, 65*(2), 67–70. https://doi.org/10.1002/j.1556-6676.1986.tb01233.x
Garfield, S. L., & Bergin, A. E. (1986). *Handbook of psychotherapy and behavior change* (3rd ed.). New York, NY: Wiley.
Gelso, C. J., & Carter, J. A. (1994). Components of the psychotherapy relationship: Their interaction and unfolding during treatment. *Journal of Counseling Psychology, 41*(3), 296–306. https://doi.org/10.1037/0022-0167.41.3.296

Goldfried, M. R., Burckell, L. A., & Eubanks-Carter, C. (2003). Therapist self-disclosure in cognitive-behavior therapy. *Journal of Clinical Psychology, 59*(5), 555–568. https://doi.org/10.1002/jclp.10159
Greenberg, L. S. (2007). Emotion coming of age. *Clinical Psychology: Science and practice, 14*(4), 414–421. https://doi.org/10.1111/j.1468-2850.2007.00101.x
Greenberg, L. S., & Watson, J. C. (2006). *Emotion-focused therapy for depression*. Washington, DC: American Psychological Association.
Greenwald, H. (1987). The humor decision. In W. F. Fry Jr. & W. A. Salameh (Eds.), *Handbook of humor and psychotherapy: Advances in the clinical use of humor* (pp. 41–54). Sarasota, FL: Professional Resource Exchange.
Hare, R. D. (1991). *Manual for the revised psychopathy checklist*. Toronto, ON: Multi-Health Systems.
Hare, R. D. (2003). *The Hare psychopathy checklist-revised (PCL-R)* (2nd ed.). Toronto, ON: Multi-Health Systems.
Hervé, H. (2007). Psychopathy across the ages: A history of the Hare psychopath. In H. Hervé & J. C. Yuille (Eds.), *The psychopath: Theory, research, and practice* (pp. 31–56). New York, NY: Routledge.
Hervé, H., & Yuille, J. C. (Eds.). (2007). *The psychopath: Theory, research, and practice*. New York, NY: Routledge.
Hill, C. E., & Knox, S. (2001). Self-disclosure. *Psychotherapy: Theory, Research, Practice, Training, 38*(4), 413–417. https://doi.org/10.1037/0033-3204.38.4.413
Horvath, A. O. (2001). The alliance. *Psychotherapy: Theory, Research, Practice, Training, 38*(4), 365–372. https://doi.org/10.1037/0033-3204.38.4.365
Horvath, A. O., & Bedi, R. P. (2002). The alliance. In J. C. Norcross (Ed.), *Psychotherapy relationships that work: Therapist contributions and responsiveness to patients* (pp. 37–69). London, UK: Oxford University Press.
Horvath, A. O., & Greenberg, L. S. (1989). Development and validation of the Working Alliance Inventory. *Journal of Counseling Psychology, 36*(2), 223–233. https://doi.org/10.1037/0022-0167.36.2.223
Horvath, A. O., & Luborsky, L. (1993). The role of the therapeutic alliance in psychotherapy. *Journal of Consulting and Clinical Psychology, 61*(4), 561–573. https://doi.org/10.1037/0022-006X.61.4.561
Horvath, A. O., & Symonds, B. D. (1991). Relation between working alliance and outcome in psychotherapy: A meta-analysis. *Journal of Counseling Psychology, 38*(2), 139–149. https://doi.org/10.1037/0022-0167.38.2.139
Keijsers, G. P. J., Schaap, C. P. D. R., & Hoogduin, C. A. L. (2000). The impact of interpersonal patient and therapist behavior on outcome in cognitive-behavior therapy: A review of empirical studies. *Behavior Modification, 24*(2), 264–297. https://doi.org/10.1177/0145445500242006
Kivlighan, D. M., & Shaughnessy, P. (1995). Analysis of the development of the working alliance using hierarchical linear modeling. *Journal of Counseling Psychology, 42*(3), 338–349. https://doi.org/10.1037/0022-0167.42.3.338
Kivlighan, D. M., Jr., & Shaughnessy, P. (2000). Patterns of working alliance development: A typology of client's working alliance ratings. *Journal of Counseling Psychology, 47*(3), 362–371. https://doi.org/10.1037/0022-0167.47.3.362
Klein, M. H., Mathieu-Coughlan, P., & Kiesler, D. J. (1986). The experiencing scales. In L. S. Greenberg & W. M. Pinsof (Eds.), *Guilford clinical psychology and psychotherapy series. The psychotherapeutic process: A research handbook* (pp. 21–71). New York, NY: The Guilford Press.
Klerman, G. L., Weissman, M. M., Rounsaville, B., & Chevron, E. (1984). *Interpersonal psychotherapy of depression*. New York, NY: Basic Books.
Kottler, J. A., Sexton, T. L., & Whiston, S. C. (1994). *The heart of healing: Relationships in therapy*. San Francisco, CA: Jossey-Bass.

Kozar, C. J., & Day, A. (2012). The therapeutic alliance in offending behavior programs: A necessary and sufficient condition for change? *Aggression and Violent Behavior, 17*(5), 482–487. https://doi.org/10.1016/j.avb.2012.07.004

Lambert, M. J. (1999). Are differential treatment effects inflated by researcher therapy allegiance? Could clever Hans count? *Clinical Psychology: Science and Practice, 6*(1), 127–130. https://doi.org/10.1093/clipsy.6.1.127

Lambert, M. J., & Barley, D. E. (2001). Research summary on the therapeutic relationship and psychotherapy outcome. *Psychotherapy: Theory, Research, Practice, Training, 38*(4), 357–361. https://doi.org/10.1037/0033-3204.38.4.357

Lambert, M. J., Christensen, E. R., & DeJulio, S. S. (Eds.). (1983). *The assessment of psychotherapy outcome*. New York, NY: Wiley.

Lieberman, M. A., Yalom, I. D., & Miles, M. B. (1973). *Encounter groups: First facts*. New York, NY: Basic Books.

Lietaer, G. (1992). Helping and hindering processes in client-centered/experiential psychotherapy: A content analysis of client and therapist postsession perceptions. In S. G. Toukmanian & D. L. Rennie (Eds.), *Psychotherapy process research: Paradigmatic and narrative approaches* (Sage focus ed., Vol. 143, pp. 134–162). Thousand Oaks, CA: Sage Publications.

Lilliengren, P., & Werbart, A. (2005). A model of therapeutic action grounded in the patients' view of curative and hindering factors in psychoanalytic psychotherapy. *Psychotherapy: Theory, Research, Practice, Training, 42*(3), 324–339. https://doi.org/10.1037/0033-3204.42.3.324

Linehan, M. M. (1993). *Cognitive-behavioral treatment of borderline personality disorder*. New York, NY: The Guilford Press.

Looman, J., Abracen, J., Serin, R., & Marquis, P. (2005). Psychopathy, treatment change, and recidivism in high-risk high-need sexual offenders. *Journal of Interpersonal Violence, 20*(5), 549–568. https://doi.org/10.1177/0886260504271583

Luborsky, M. R. (1994). The identification and analysis of themes and patterns. In J. F. Gubrium & A. Sankar (Eds.), *Qualitative methods in aging research* (Sage focus ed., Vol. 168, pp. 189–210). Thousand Oaks, CA: Sage Publications.

Mahoney, M. J., & Norcross, J. C. (1993). Relationship styles and therapeutic choices: A commentary on the preceding four articles. *Psychotherapy: Theory, Research, Practice, Training, 30*(3), 423–426. https://doi.org/10.1037/0033-3204.30.3.423

Marshall, L. E., Marshall, W. L., Moulden, H. M., & Serran, G. A. (2008). CEU eligible article the prevalence of sexual addiction in incarcerated sexual offenders and matched community nonoffenders. *Sexual Addiction & Compulsivity, 15*, 271–283.

Marshall, W. L. (2005). Therapist style in sexual offender treatment: Influence on indices of change. *Sexual Abuse: A Journal of Research and Treatment, 17*(2), 109–116. https://doi.org/10.1177/107906320501700202

Marshall, W. L., Anderson, D., & Champagne, F. (1997). Self-esteem and its relationship to sexual offending. *Psychology, Crime & Law, 3*(3), 81–106. https://doi.org/10.1080/10683169708410811

Marshall, W. L., Anderson, D., & Fernandez, Y. (1999). *Cognitive behavioural treatment of sexual offenders*. London, UK: Wiley.

Marshall, W. L., Fernandez, Y. M., Serran, G. A., Mulloy, R., Thornton, D., Mann, R., & Anderson, D. (2003). Process variables in the treatment of sexual offenders: A review of the relevant literature. *Aggression and Violent Behavior, 8*(2), 205–234. https://doi.org/10.1016/S1359-1789(01)00065-9

Marshall, W. L., Marshall, L. E., & Ware, J. (2009). Cognitive distortions in sexual offenders: Should they all be treatment targets? *Sexual Abuse in Australia and New Zealand, 2*(1), 21–33. Retrieved from https://www.anzatsa.org/saanz-journal/

Marshall, W. L., Serran, G., Moulden, H., Mulloy, R., Fernandez, Y. M., Mann, R., & Thornton, D. (2002). Therapist features in sexual offender treatment: Their reliable identification and influence on behaviour change. *Clinical Psychology & Psychotherapy, 9*(6), 395–405. https://doi.org/10.1002/cpp.335

Marshall, W. L., Serran, G. A., Fernandez, Y. M., Mulloy, R., Mann, R. E., & Thornton, D. (2003). Therapist characteristics in the treatment of sexual offenders: Tentative data on their relationship with indices of behaviour change. *Journal of Sexual Aggression, 9*(1), 25–30. https://doi.org/10.1080/355260031000137940

Martin, D. J., Garske, J. P., & Davis, M. K. (2000). Relation of the therapeutic alliance with outcome and other variables: A meta-analytic review. *Journal of Consulting and Clinical Psychology, 68*(3), 438–450. https://doi.org/10.1037/0022-006X.68.3.438

Martin, G., & Pear, J. (1996). *Behavior modification: What it is and how to do it* (5th ed.). Upper Saddle River, NJ: Prentice Hall.

Mathews, A. M., Johnston, D. W., Lancashire, M., Munby, M., Shaw, P. M., & Gelder, M. G. (1976). Imaginal flooding exposure to real phobic situations: Treatment outcome with agoraphobic patients. *British Journal of Psychiatry, 129*, 362–371. https://doi.org/10.1192/bjp.129.4.361

McCarthy, J. (2001). Post-traumatic stress disorder in people with learning disability. *Advances in Psychiatric Treatment, 7*(3), 163–169. https://doi.org/10.1192/apt.7.3.163

McGuff, R., Gitlin, D., & Enderlin, M. (1996). Clients' and therapists' confidence and attendance at planned individual therapy sessions. *Psychological Reports, 79*(2), 537–538. https://doi.org/10.2466/pr0.1996.79.2.537

McLeod, J. (1990). The client's experience of counselling and psychotherapy: A review of the research literature. In D. Mearns & W. Dryden (Eds.), *Experiences of counselling in action* (pp. 66–79). Thousand Oaks, CA: Sage Publications.

Miller, W. R., Benefield, R. G., & Tonigan, J. S. (1993). Enhancing motivation for change in problem drinking: A controlled comparison of two therapist styles. *Journal of Consulting and Clinical Psychology, 61*(3), 455–461. https://doi.org/10.1037/0022-006X.61.3.455

Miller, W. R., & Rollnick, S. (2002). *Motivational interviewing: Preparing people for change* (2nd ed.). New York, NY: The Guilford Press.

Miller, W. R., & Sovereign, R. G. (1989). The check-up: A model for early intervention in addictive behaviors. In T. Løberg, W. R. Miller, P. E. Nathan, & G. A. Marlatt (Eds.), *Addictive behaviors: Prevention and early intervention* (pp. 219–231). Lisse, Netherlands: Swets & Zeitlinger Publishers.

Miller, W. R., Taylor, C. A., & West, J. C. (1980). Focused versus broad-spectrum behavior therapy for problem drinkers. *Journal of Consulting and Clinical Psychology, 48*(5), 590–601. https://doi.org/10.1037/0022-006X.48.5.590

Mintz, J., Luborsky, L., & Auerbach, A. H. (1971). Dimensions of psychotherapy: A factor-analytic study of ratings of psychotherapy sessions. *Journal of Consulting and Clinical Psychology, 36*(1), 106–120. https://doi.org/10.1037/h0030481

Murphy, P. M., Cramer, D., & Lillie, F. J. (1984). The relationship between curative factors perceived by patients in their psychotherapy and treatment outcome: An exploratory study. *British Journal of Medical Psychology, 57*(2), 187–192. https://doi.org/10.1111/j.2044-8341.1984.tb01599.x

Nichols, M. P., & Taylor, T. Y. (1975). Impact of therapist interventions on early sessions of group therapy. *Journal of Clinical Psychology, 31*(4), 726–729. https://doi.org/10.1002/1097-4679(197510)31:4<726::AID-JCLP2270310438>3.0.CO;2-S

Nissen-Lie, H. A., Monsen, J. T., & Rønnestad, M. H. (2010). Therapist predictors of early patient-rated working alliance: A multilevel approach. *Psychotherapy Research, 20*(6), 627–646. https://doi.org/10.1080/10503307.2010.497633

Norcross, J. C. (2002). *Psychotherapy relationships that work: Therapist contributions and responsiveness to patients*. New York, NY: Oxford University Press.

Norcross, J. C., & Lambert, M. J. (2006). The therapy relationship. In J. C. Norcross, L. E. Beutler, & R. F. Levant (Eds.), *Evidence-based practices in mental health: Debate and dialogue on the fundamental questions* (pp. 208–218). Washington, DC: American Psychological Association.

Olver, M. E., Stockdale, K. C., & Wormith, J. S. (2011). A meta-analysis of predictors of offender treatment attrition and its relationship to recidivism. *Journal of Consulting and Clinical Psychology, 79*(1), 6–21. https://doi.org/10.1037/a0022200

Olver, M. E., & Wong, S. C. P. (2013a). A description and research review of the Clearwater Sex Offender Treatment Programme. *Psychology, Crime & Law, 19*(5-6), 477–492. https://doi.org/10.1080/1068316X.2013.758983

Olver, M. E., & Wong, S. C. P. (2013b). Treatment programs for high risk sexual offenders: Program and offender characteristics, attrition, treatment change and recidivism. *Aggression and Violent Behavior, 18*(5), 579–591. https://doi.org/10.1016/j.avb.2013.06.002

Orlinsky, D. E., Grawe, K., & Parks, B. K. (1994). Process and outcome in psychotherapy: Noch einmal. In A. E. Garfield & S. L. Garfield (Eds.), *Handbook of psychotherapy and behavior change* (4th ed., pp. 270–376). Oxford, UK: Wiley.

Orlinsky, D. E., & Howard, K. I. (1986). Process and outcome in psychotherapy. In S. L. Garfield & A. E. Bergin (Eds.), *Handbook of psychotherapy and behavior change* (3rd ed., pp. 311–381). New York, NY: Riley.

Patterson, G. R., & Forgatch, M. S. (1985). Therapist behavior as a determinant for client noncompliance: A paradox for the behavior modifier. *Journal of Consulting and Clinical Psychology, 53*(6), 846–851. https://doi.org/10.1037/0022-006X.53.6.846

Piper, W. E., Boroto, D. R., Joyce, A. S., McCallum, M., & Azim, H. F. A. (1995). Pattern of alliance and outcome in short-term individual psychotherapy. *Psychotherapy: Theory, Research, Practice, Training, 32*(4), 639–647. https://doi.org/10.1037/0033-3204.32.4.639

Polaschek, D. L. L., & Ross, E. C. (2010). Do early therapeutic alliance, motivation, and stages of change predict therapy change for high-risk, psychopathic violent prisoners? *Criminal Behaviour and Mental Health, 20*(2), 100–111. https://doi.org/10.1002/cbm.759

Proeve, M. J., & Howells, K. (2006). Effects of remorse and shame and criminal justice experience on judgements about a sex offender. *Psychology, Crime & Law, 12*(2), 145–161. https://doi.org/10.1080/10683160512331316271

Rabavilas, A. D., Boulougouris, J. C., & Perissaki, C. (1979). Therapist qualities related to outcome with exposure in vivo in neurotic patients. *Journal of Behavior Therapy and Experimental Psychiatry, 10*(4), 293–294. https://doi.org/10.1016/0005-7916(79)90005-3

Rice, M. E., Harris, G. T., & Cormier, C. A. (1992). An evaluation of a maximum security therapeutic community for psychopaths and other mentally disordered offenders. *Law and Human Behavior, 16*(4), 399–412. https://doi.org/10.1007/BF02352266

Ringler, M. (1977). The effect of democratic versus authoritarian therapist behavior on success, success-expectation and self-attribution in desensitization of examination anxiety. *Zeitchrift fur Klinische Psychologie, 6*, 40–58. Retrieved from https://us.hogrefe.com/products/journals/zkp

Rogers, C. R. (1965). The therapeutic relationship: Recent theory and research. *Australian Journal of Psychology, 17*(2), 95–108. https://doi.org/10.1080/00049536508255531

Ross, E. C., Polaschek, D. L. L., & Ward, T. (2008). The therapeutic alliance: A theoretical revision for offender rehabilitation. *Aggression and Violent Behavior, 13*(6), 462–480. https://doi.org/10.1016/j.avb.2008.07.003

Ross, E. C., Polaschek, D. L. L., & Wilson, M. (2011). Shifting perspectives: A confirmatory factor analysis of the Working Alliance Inventory (short form) with high-risk violent offenders. *International Journal of Offender Therapy and Comparative Criminology, 55*(8), 1308–1323. https://doi.org/10.1177/0306624X11384948

Rutherford, K. (1994). Humor in psychotherapy. *Individual Psychology: Journal of Adlerian Theory, Research & Practice, 50*(2), 207–222.

Ryan, V. L., & Gizynski, M. N. (1971). Behavior therapy in retrospect: Patients' feelings about their behavior therapies. *Journal of Consulting and Clinical Psychology, 37*(1), 1–9. https://doi.org/10.1037/h0031293

Safran, J. D., & Segal, Z. V. (1990). *Cognitive therapy: An interpersonal process perspective.* Lanham, MD: Rowman & Littlefield Publishers.

Salekin, R. T., Worley, C., & Grimes, R. D. (2010). Treatment of psychopathy: A review and brief introduction to the mental model approach for psychopathy. *Behavioral Sciences & the Law, 28*(2), 235–266. https://doi.org/10.1002/bsl.928

Saunders, S. M. (1999). Clients' assessments of the effective environment of the psychotherapy session: Relationship to session quality and treatment effectiveness. *Journal of Clinical Psychology, 55*(5), 597–605. https://doi.org/10.1002/(SICI)1097-4679(199905)55:5<597::AID-JCLP7>3.0.CO;2-M

Schaap, C., Bennum, I., Schindler, L., & Hoogduin, K. (1993). *The therapeutic relationship in behavioral psychotherapy*. Chichester, UK: Wiley.

Schindler, L., Revenstorf, D., Hahlweg, K., & Brengelmann, J. C. (1983). Therapeutenverhalten in der Verhaltenstherapie. Entwicklung eines Instrumentes zur Beurteilung durch den Klienten [The evaluation of therapist qualities in behavior therapy]. *Partnerberatung, 20*(2-3), 149–160.

Seligman, M. E. P. (1990). Why is there so much depression today? The waxing of the individual and the waning of the commons. In R. E. Ingram (Ed.), *Contemporary psychological approaches to depression: Theory, research, and treatment* (pp. 1–9). New York, NY: Plenum Press. https://doi.org/10.1007/978-1-4613-0649-8_1

Sermat, V., & Smyth, M. (1973). Content analysis of verbal communication in the development of relationship: Conditions influencing self-disclosure. *Journal of Personality and Social Psychology, 26*(3), 332–346. https://doi.org/10.1037/h0034473

Seto, M. C., & Barbaree, H. E. (1999). Psychopathy, treatment behavior, and sex offender recidivism. *Journal of Interpersonal Violence, 14*(12), 1235–1248. https://doi.org/10.1177/088626099014012001

Skeem, J. L., Louden, J. E., Polaschek, D., & Camp, J. (2007). Assessing relationship quality in mandated community treatment: Blending care with control. *Psychological Assessment, 19*(4), 397–410. https://doi.org/10.1037/1040-3590.19.4.397

Strupp, H. H. (1980). Success and failure in time-limited psychotherapy: A systematic comparison of two cases: Comparison 2. *Archives of General Psychiatry, 37*(6), 595–603. https://doi.org/10.1001/archpsyc.1980.01780190106013

Tangney, J. P., & Dearing, R. L. (2002). *Shame and guilt*. New York, NY: The Guilford Press.

Tatman, A. W., & Love, K. M. (2010). An offender version of the Working Alliance Inventory-short revised. *Journal of Offender Rehabilitation, 49*(3), 165–179. https://doi.org/10.1080/10509671003666560

Teasdale, J. D., & Fennell, M. J. (1982). Immediate effects on depression of cognitive therapy interventions. *Cognitive Therapy and Research, 6*(3), 343–351. https://doi.org/10.1007/BF01173582

Walling, S. M., Suvak, M. K., Howard, J. M., Taft, C. T., & Murphy, C. M. (2012). Race/ethnicity as a predictor of change in working alliance during cognitive behavioral therapy for intimate partner violence perpetrators. *Psychotherapy, 49*(2), 180–189. https://doi.org/10.1037/a0025751

Walton, A., Jeglic, E. L., & Blasko, B. L. (2018). The role of psychopathic traits in the development of the therapeutic alliance among sexual offenders. *Sexual Abuse: A Journal of Research and Treatment, 30*(3), 211–229. https://doi.org/10.1177/1079063216637859

Wilson, N. J., & Tamatea, A. (2013). Challenging the "urban myth" of psychopathy untreatability: The high-risk personality programme. *Psychology, Crime & Law, 19*(5-6), 493–510. https://doi.org/10.1080/1068316X.2013.758994

Yalom, I. D., & Lieberman, M. A. (1971). A study of encounter group casualties. *Archives of General Psychiatry, 25*(1), 16–30. https://doi.org/10.1001/archpsyc.1971.01750130018002

Chapter 6
Therapist-Related Factors in Correctional Treatment

Elizabeth L. Jeglic and Kseniya Katsman

6.1 Introduction

In the general psychology literature, the importance of the therapist to treatment outcome has been extensively researched. While it was initially believed that approximately 25% of the variance in treatment outcome could be attributed to factors related to the therapist, such as therapeutic alliance (see Chap. 5) (Lambert & Bergin, 1994), more recent research puts that number closer to between 5% and 7% (Flückiger, Del Re, Wampold, Symonds, & Horvath, 2012; Saxon, Firth, & Barkham, 2017). While 5–7% may seem small, therapist-related factors account for more variance in therapy outcome than any other treatment-related variable (Webb, DeRubeis, & Barber, 2010). Additionally, it is consistently found that certain therapists achieve better results than others regardless of treatment modality and these results are more pronounced in naturalistic settings as opposed to clinical trials. In fact, one meta-analysis of therapist effects on outcome found modest therapist effects on outcome in clinical trials and large therapist effects on outcome in naturalistic settings, further suggesting that there are certain therapist qualities that make some therapists more effective than others (Baldwin & Imel, 2013). While the last several decades have shown increases in research involving therapist characteristics and how these affect treatment outcome, this area of inquiry has largely been ignored for those working in forensic contexts. Given that there are few clinical trials conducted in forensic contexts, we would anticipate that the quality of the therapists may be particularly salient to outcome in this milieu.

As the debate for what works in offender treatment still rages on (see Chap. 1), the most comprehensive research to date suggests that treatments effects remain small. In corrections, the most methodically sound research to date comes from a

E. L. Jeglic (✉) · K. Katsman
Department of Psychology, John Jay College of Criminal Justice,
City University of New York, New York, NY, USA
e-mail: ejeglic@jjay.cuny.edu; kseniya.katsman@jjay.cuny.edu

E. L. Jeglic, C. Calkins (eds.), *New Frontiers in Offender Treatment*,
https://doi.org/10.1007/978-3-030-01030-0_6

meta-analysis of sex offender-specific therapy outcomes. Schmucker and Lösel (2015) found a recidivism rate of 10.1% for individuals who completed sex offender-specific treatment ($n = 4939$) compared to 13.7% for those individuals who committed a sexual offense but did not receive treatment. While even small reductions in recidivism rates are significant, it has been argued that larger treatment effects have not been observed, as the quality of program delivery among those working with justice-involved populations has not been emphasized (Jeglic, Hanson, & Calkins, 2016). In fact, very little is known about the characteristics of therapists who provide services to those involved in the criminal justice system. In this chapter we will review what is known in the general psychotherapy literature about therapist-related factors that affect treatment outcome and present what we know about characteristics, training, burnout, vicarious traumatization, and countertransference among therapists working with criminal justice-involved clients. The chapter will conclude with recommendations for supervision and training for therapists working in the correctional milieu in order to ensure program integrity and therapist well-being.

6.2 Therapist Characteristics

As with any interpersonal relationship, there are certain therapist characteristics that can impact the bond with the client and hence the quality of the therapy. In 2006, a task force sponsored by Division 12 (Society of Clinical Psychology) of the American Psychological Association (APA) and the North American Society for Psychotherapy examined empirically derived factors that contributed to therapeutic change across a host of affective, personality, and substance abuse disorders (Castonguay & Beutler, 2006). The task found that across treatments, there were three main sources of therapeutic change that are labeled as (1) participant characteristics, including characteristics of the client and the therapist; (2) relational factors, broadly encompassing the therapeutic alliance or rapport; and (3) technical factors, referring to the techniques and skill of program delivery (Castonguay & Beutler, 2006). While many of these characteristics are discussed in Chap. 5 as they pertain to the therapeutic alliance specifically, there are several therapist characteristics that have been consistently linked to better treatment outcomes. Using multilevel modeling, Saxon et al. (2017) assessed the impact of therapist skill, therapeutic modality, therapeutic dose, and therapy ending type (drop out versus termination) on treatment outcome and found that therapist variables accounted for 5.8% of the variance in outcome. In another large analysis of data from 119 therapists and 10,786 patients referred to the United Kingdom's National Health Service Primary Care counseling and psychotherapy, Saxon and Barkham (2012) found that therapist quality accounted for 6.6% of the outcome for the average patient severity.

So, what are the characteristics that make one therapist more effective than another? Wampold (2011) compiled the best available research and practice guidelines (see Anderson, Ogles, Patterson, Lambert, & Vermeersch, 2009; APA Presidential Task Force on Evidence-Based Practice, 2006; Baldwin, Wampold, & Imel, 2007; Duncan, Miller, Wampold, & Hubble, 2010; Lambert, Harmon, Slade, Whipple, & Hawkins, 2005; Norcross, 2011 and Wampold, 2007) to provide a list of qualities and actions that exemplified those therapists that were the most effective at eliciting change among their patients. These included well-developed interpersonal skills comprising verbal fluency, interpersonal perception, affect modulation, expressiveness, and the ability to show warmth, acceptance, and empathy. Wampold (2011) emphasized that a therapist's ability to provide a solid rationale for the treatment and execute a treatment plan according to this rationale while at the same time monitoring client progress was integral to therapeutic success. Further, according to his review, effective therapists were flexible in their style, addressed difficult issues without avoidance, and communicated hope and optimism for success. Finally, responsivity issues, such as those discussed in Chap. 2 pertaining to cultural competence and using evidence-based practice, were employed by those therapists deemed to be the most effective.

Similarly, Heinonen, Lindfors, Laaksonen, and Knelt (2012) found that in short-term solution-focused or psychodynamic therapy, active, engaging, and extroverted therapists produced the greatest symptom reduction in patients seeking treatment for depression and anxiety. Another study of therapist effects on treatment outcome with non-CBT-based interventions conducted by Berglar et al. (2016) also found that some therapists were more effective than others, and this effect was maximized when the patient's presenting problems were more severe. Specifically, they found that therapists with more professional experience and better therapeutic alliance were more effective at treating patients with more severe psychopathology—yet it should be cautioned that this explained only 3.4% of the outcome variance, and thus other factors must also be considered relevant to treatment outcome (Berglar et al., 2016). Interestingly, it appears that some of the characteristics that make an effective therapist may be innate. In a prospective study, Anderson, McClintock, Himawan, Song, and Patterson (2016) surveyed 44 future graduate students prior to starting their graduate studies using the Facilitative Interpersonal Skills task (FIS) which assesses verbal fluency, emotional expression, persuasiveness, warmth/positive regard, hopefulness, empathy, alliance bond capacity, and alliance rupture-repair responsiveness. They found that among this cohort of 44 students, their scores on the FIS at the beginning of graduate school predicted client symptom change in short-term therapy later on in their studies (fewer than 8 sessions); however, this effect was not observed for longer duration therapy (greater than 16 sessions). Thus overall, research in the general therapy literature has found that there are indeed some therapists who are more effective than others at eliciting change and that factors such as verbal fluency, positive outlook, the therapists general skill at developing and following a treatment plan, and their ability to form and repair the therapeutic relationship can positively impact client outcome, particularly in short-term therapy.

6.3 Therapists in the Criminal Justice System

While we know quite a lot about what makes a good therapist in general, we know substantially less about characteristics of effective therapists who work with clients involved in the criminal justice system. Further, it is unclear whether there is a different set of characteristics required to work with those who are or were incarcerated, as there have yet to be comparative studies of therapists who work with criminal justice-involved clients and those who do not. Articles on skills necessary for forensic psychologists highlight the importance of solid training and experience, grounding in scientific theory and research, critical thinking skills, legal knowledge, clear writing and presentation skills, and the ability to maintain composure under stress (Franklin, 2014; Ward, 2013); however, none of these skills have been empirically assessed. The majority of what we do know about therapists in the criminal justice has been focused largely on therapists who work with those who have committed sex crimes, and less is known about therapists who work in other domains. For example, Marshall (2005) conducted a study in which videotapes of therapists who conducted CBT-based sexual offender treatment in HM Prison Service in the UK were rated by trained graduate-level raters with experience conducting sex offender treatment. Following training, the raters were able to accurately identify behaviors exhibited by the therapists, and Marshall (2005) found that the therapists who were rated to exhibit higher levels of empathy, warmth, rewardingness, and directiveness were positively associated with treatment outcome. Additionally, he found that using a harsh confrontational style was negatively related to treatment. In a separate study, Marshall et al. (2002) found that the combination of therapist warmth, empathy, rewardingness, directiveness, and non-confrontational style explained between 32% and 61% of treatment outcome. In addition to the aforementioned therapist characteristics, Marshall et al. (2003) also found that the appropriate amount of talking, appropriate voice tone, and the use of open-ended questioning by the therapist were associated with increases in coping skills among those who committed sexual offenses.

More recently, Sandhu and Rose (2012) reviewed the sex offender treatment literature in order to identify therapist-related factors that were associated with a therapeutic change in sex offender treatment. Based upon their review of the 15 papers, the authors identified several characteristics that were related to therapeutic change among those who have committed a sexual offense. In the context of offender treatment, Sandhu and Rose found that female gender may bear some impact on the outcome. They found that men participating in sex offender treatment may see therapeutic benefits when working with a female therapist—seeing the female perspective on their behavior has greater potential to change their perceptions, attitudes, and relationships with females. In addition, they also found that across studies, empathy, directiveness, a humane attitude toward those who have committed sexual offenses, and a supportive group leadership style were also related to therapeutic change (Sandhu & Rose, 2012). However, the authors also note that while there is evidence that the characteristics of those who engage in therapy with offending populations are related to therapeutic change, many of the studies they reviewed had small sample sizes, and thus they recommended that more methodologically sound research with larger, more diverse samples is needed. Thus, in sum, the available research on characteristics of those who provide services to individuals involved with the criminal justice system (primarily therapists who conduct therapy with those who committed sexual offenses) suggests that many of the same characteristics that make someone an effective therapist in general are also needed for a therapist to be effective when conducting treatment with those who have committed offenses.

6.4 Therapist Training

In the general psychology literature, there is a large body of research examining the effect of training on therapist skill and outcome. Those who provide mental health services are required to be licensed (or license eligible and working under supervision) by state licensing boards and to have completed state-approved training programs. These individuals can be doctoral-level clinical, counseling, or school psychologists (Ph.D., Psy.D., or Ed.D.), psychiatrists (M.D. or D.O.) and then a host of master's-level practitioners including advanced nurse practitioners with psychiatric training (A.N.Ps), licensed psychological associates (L.P.A.), licensed professional counselors (L.P.C.), licensed clinical social workers (L.C.S.W.), and licensed marriage and family therapists (L.M.F.T.). All of these licensed professionals are required to do lengthy supervised internships and demonstrate educational qualifications before attaining licensure. While Castonguay and Beutler (2006) identified therapist characteristics and the relationship with the client as two of the three elements of effective psychotherapy, it is unclear whether these elements can in fact be taught or they are affected by training and experience. In 1984 Hattie, Sharpley, and Rogers conducted an early quantitative review of the literature examining therapy outcome when treatment was conducted with professional therapists and paraprofessionals with no formal training. Based upon their review, they concluded that paraprofessionals achieved better outcomes than those with formal training. Upon further examination, Berman and Norton (1985) concluded that Hattie and colleagues' study contained methodologically flawed studies and inappropriate analyses. In an effort to rectify this error, Berman and Norton (1985) reanalyzed the data omitting the problematic studies and concluded that paraprofessionals in fact were not more effective than professional therapists, but neither were professional therapists more effective than paraprofessionals.

In a similar more recent study, Anderson, Crowley, Himawan, Holmberg, and Uhlin (2016) compared the effect of training on treatment outcome using 11 clinical psychology doctoral students with at least 2 years training and 12 graduate students in disciplines unrelated to psychology (i.e., biology, chemistry, history) who had no therapy training. Additionally, they assessed all 23 therapists' facilitative interpersonal skills (FIS), which they defined as the ability to understand and transmit interpersonal messages to others as well as the ability to communicate a rationale for the client's problems and propose effective solutions. At the conclusion of the study, no significant differences were found in client outcome between therapists with and without training. However, those therapists that were deemed to possess a high level of FIS were significantly more likely to have better treatment outcomes than those rated low on FIS, suggesting that it is innate characteristics of the individual and not training that impact the outcome.

A separate body of literature has looked at the effects of training in general. One meta-analysis found modest but consistent effect sizes for therapist training, such that therapists with more training and experience had higher client satisfaction and client improvement, and in community mental healthcare training was associated with lower client dropout rates (Stein & Lambert, 1995). In a 12-month longitudinal analysis of practicum students, predoctoral interns, and postdoctoral fellows who were working in college counseling centers, Owen, Wampold, Kopta, Rousmaniere, and Miller (2016) examined whether trainees' client outcomes improved over time. They found that across all training levels, trainees' outcomes improved over time but that this was moderated by client distress levels, such that growth was observed with less distressed clients over the 12-month period, but no change was observed with more seriously distressed clients over time. A similar longitudinal analysis using outcome data for 170 community therapists who treated 6591 clients over an average of 4.75 years found that in general there was no evidence that therapists in the community improved over time. Further, they found that patient's outcomes deteriorated for 61% of the therapists over time, while 39% of the therapists improved over time (Goldberg et al., 2016). Together these findings suggest that there appears to be minimal effect on psychotherapy outcome based upon therapist training and experience.

6.5 Correctional Therapist Training and Experience

There is little to no research focusing specifically on factors related to training and experience for those who work in corrections. Further, the majority of those who work as therapists within the criminal justice system do not have any specific forensic training. It was only in 2001 that forensic psychology was recognized as a specialty by the APA. In recent years, 3–7% of doctoral-level psychology internships were situated in correctional settings (Association of Psychology Postdoctoral and Internship Centers, 2012, 2015, 2016). There are now several master's- and doctoral-level clinical and mental health counseling programs that are geared toward training clinicians to work with criminal justice-involved individuals, but there is currently no approved curriculum or special licensure for those who work with forensic clientele. There are certification programs for forensic subspecialties (like the provision of services to those who have committed sexual offenses), but these are not regulated by the APA. To regulate this ever-expanding field, the APA has issued *Specialty Guidelines for Forensic Psychology* which were first developed and published in

1991 and then revised and republished in 2013 (American Psychological Association, 2013). APA determined that the field of forensic psychology differed in several important ways from more traditional areas of psychological practice and thus required separate guidelines. The APA specifies that the guidelines should apply to all issues in which psychologists provide expertise. The field of forensic psychology and consequently training in the specialty remains in its naissance, and at present there are few front-line correctional therapists in the USA and Canada who have obtained doctoral degrees. Many providers only have high school or Bachelor's degrees, with minimal training in the theory and application of behavior change (Jeglic et al., 2016).

Magaletta, Patry, Dietz, and Ax (2007) identified several core knowledge areas necessary to deliver effective interventions within correctional settings. The authors indicated that thorough knowledge of psychopathology was the most important, followed by closely related knowledge areas such as suicide prevention, working with individuals suffering from mental illness in special housing units (SHU), and psychopharmacology. Other knowledge areas highlighted by Magaletta et al. (2007) included confrontation avoidance, safety, knowledge of interdepartmental relations in prison, and ethics. The authors emphasized that while professionals practicing in correctional settings can be expected to initially possess the academic knowledge of these core areas, such as psychopathology-related fields and professional ethics, aspects that involve day-to-day correctional work (e.g., managing individuals with mental illness in segregation, safety on the job, avoiding confrontation) were not routinely covered in graduate academic education (Magaletta et al., 2007). In addition, Magaletta and colleagues recommended that an understanding of general correctional policy and specific policies for various positions within the criminal justice system is an important aspect of professional training for those who want to work with incarcerated individuals (Magaletta et al., 2016). While one study found that therapists who worked with those convicted of sexual offenses were familiar with evidence-based practices, it was also revealed that the delivery of the interventions was flawed (Moon & Shivy, 2008). Another study looked at the relationship between three domains of correctional staff quality (staff characteristics, staff training, and staff supervision) and program treatment effectiveness in community correctional facilities (Makarios, Lovins, Latessa, & Smith, 2016). The authors concluded that staff characteristics and staff training were significantly related to decrease in recidivism, while staff supervision had weaker effects. In total, the study found that those three domains explained 28% in the variance of treatment effect size, suggesting that the relationship between staff quality and program effectiveness is not a simple one (Makarios et al., 2016). The only other studies that have explored the effect of training and experience of correctional therapists examined how they impact attitudes toward those who have committed a sexual offense. Several studies have found that training (Hogue, 1995), exposure (Lea, Auburn, & Kibblewhite, 1999), and experience (Nelson, Herlihy, & Oescher, 2002) working with those who committed a sexual offense resulted in increased positive attitudes toward them, and it was speculated that this translated to better treatment outcomes (Harkins & Beech, 2007). Thus, while it appears that education and training can result in more positive attitudes toward forensically involved clients, it remains unclear whether specialized training and education are required and how experience factors into treatment outcome with criminal justice-involved clients.

6.6 Burnout

Burnout has consistently been found to be an issue among those who provide care to others (Dyrbye et al., 2017). It is estimated that between 21% and 67% of those in the mental health field may be experiencing high levels of burnout (Morse, Salyers, Rollins, Monroe-DeVita, & Pfahler, 2012). Burnout among therapists is often believed to be comprised of three dimensions: (1) emotional exhaustion (feeling worn-out, overextended, and tired); (2) depersonalization or cynicism (having negative attitudes toward clients and work); and (3) reduced personal accomplishment (a negative appraisal of ability and effectiveness) (Maslach, 2017). Most studies of burnout used a measure developed by Maslach and her colleagues based upon this three-dimensional model entitled the Maslach Burnout Inventory (MBI; Maslach, Jackson, & Leiter, 1996). Burnout among therapists has been found to be related to less control over the working environment, longer hours, high levels of paperwork/administrative duties, and dealing with clients who experienced more negative behaviors (Rupert & Morgan, 2005). Among mental health professionals, burnout has been associated with depression, anxiety, insomnia, memory impairment, and substance abuse (Peterson et al., 2008). It has also been associated with physical pain, flu-like symptoms, and symptoms of gastroenteritis (Acker, 2010; Peterson et al., 2008). Further, burnout is associated with more negative attitudes toward clients and consequently poorer treatment outcomes (Garman, Corrigan, & Morris, 2002; Gowdy, Carlson, & Rapp, 2003; Holmqvist & Jeanneau, 2006). Finally, burnout was related to job turnover (Schwab, Jackson, & Schuler, 1986; Smoot & Gonzales, 1995), which in turn is associated with poorer adherence to evidence-based practices (Rollins, Salyers, Tsai, & Lydick, 2010) and higher costs to recruit and train new staff (Gilbody et al., 2006).

6.7 Burnout Among Therapists in the Criminal Justice System

While burnout may be common among clinicians who provide therapy in general, burnout may be particularly prevalent among those involved in the treatment of criminal justice-involved clients as therapists often have to work with mandated clients who are not engaged in treatment; in addition, the content of the treatment is often difficult and disturbing. These difficulties can be further exacerbated by environments that are not supportive of rehabilitation and high workloads. However, at present, research on burnout among therapists in the criminal justice system remains sparse, and there are no known estimates of the prevalence of burnout specifically for those who work with offending populations. What we do know comes primarily from studies of those who work with individuals who have committed sexual offenses. One study of burnout using the MBI in a sample of 86 sex offender treatment providers found that high caseloads were related to depersonalization but not emotional exhaustion or reduced personal accomplishments (Adams, 2017). Further, no relationship was found between gender, coping styles, and years of experience and burnout. Another study compared MBI levels of 86 sex offender therapists to norms for mental health professional and found that those who provided services to offenders who committed sexual crimes reported higher scores on all three dimensions of the MBI than mental healthcare professional in general (Shelby, Stoddart, & Taylor, 2001). It was also suggested that the prison environment may affect burnout rates: correctional counselors who worked in maximum security environments experienced higher levels of burnout compared to those who provided treatment to forensically involved clients in less restricted settings (Carrola, Olivarez, & Karcher, 2016). Other factors that are related to burnout among correctional treatment providers include vague role and responsibility descriptions, disconnect from correctional administrators, insufficient training prior to starting the position, and inadequate work and group space (Garland, 2002). Given the implications of burnout to the therapist themselves and the effectiveness of the treatment they deliver, more research regarding burnout among correctional treatment providers is needed. Two concepts that are closely related to burnout—vicarious traumatization and countertransference—are discussed below.

6.7.1 Vicarious Traumatization

In the last several decades, it has become generally accepted that treatment providers who work with victims of trauma may themselves begin to experience symptoms of trauma, as they are repeatedly exposed to explicit details of the crime (Alexander & Atcheson, 1998). This is known as vicarious traumatization, since those afflicted have themselves not personally been victimized. The symptoms of vicarious traumatization may include changes in relationships, identity, capacity for dealing with affective tensions, cognitive frame of reference, and psychological well-being (Moulden & Firestone, 2007). Vicarious traumatization was previously found to co-occur and sometimes lead to eventual burnout and decline in professional efficacy, particularly when it was not identified and treated (Cieslak et al., 2014; Munger, Savage, & Panosky, 2015). Vicarious traumatization can be considered as an occupational hazard; thus, aspiring and early-career professionals can benefit from engaging in discussion about this topic and how to develop preventative strategies (Salston & Figley, 2003). Optimism, spirituality, institutional support, proper supervision, peer consultation, and utilization of personal coping strategies in the workplace were named as some of the potentially effective approaches for dealing with vicarious traumatization (Branson, 2018; Cohen & Collens, 2013).

While early research on vicarious traumatization focused on those who provided services to victims, more recently the focus has shifted to examining vicarious traumatization among those who provide services to perpetrators of trauma, namely, offenders who have committed sexually based crimes. As a part of the therapeutic process, sex offender therapists are exposed to plethora of graphic details of often heinous crimes. Many sex offender treatments require that offenders describe their crimes in an effort for them to accept responsibility and demonstrate remorse for what they have done (Moster, Wnuk, & Jeglic, 2008). In addition, therapists often need to analyze detailed police records and victim statements to better evaluate what their clients did, so that they may challenge their cognitive distortions and erroneous beliefs in treatment. Continuous exposure to such explicit material can be deeply traumatic. Several studies have found that approximately half of sex offender therapists reported clinically significant trauma symptoms (Steed & Bicknell, 2001; Way, VanDeusen, Martin, Applegate, & Jandle, 2004). In one of the first studies examining vicarious trauma among sex offender therapists, Farrenkopf (1992) found that about one third of his sample described feelings of hypervigilance and fear for their own safety, while others reported emotional hardening, anger, and irritability. Another study found that sex offender therapists reported feelings of depression, anxiety, vulnerability, decreased trust, and isolation (Rich, 1997). Some research has suggested that early- and late-career therapists have higher levels of vicarious traumatization compared to the therapists in the middle of their career (Steed & Bicknell, 2001). Further, working in a correctional setting (as opposed to the community) and having negative coping skills also increased the risk of developing trauma (Ennis & Horne, 2003; Way et al., 2004). The responsibility of protecting public safety and inability to discuss the explicit details of the daily routine contribute to increased stress among those working with individuals who offended sexually (Catanese, 2010). While the majority of these studies were uncontrolled, the findings suggest that working with individuals who committed sex crimes may have a significant negative impact on the well-being of therapists and therefore may impact their ability to provide effective services to their clients (Moulden & Firestone, 2007).

6.7.2 Countertransference

Countertransference is defined as the therapist's emotional entanglement with the client at both the conscious and unconscious level (Mitchell & Melikian, 1995). Each therapist brings with them a host of personal characteristics and past experiences that can affect their perceptions and reactions to the client. While countertransference was originally associated with psychoanalysis, it is now a concept that is addressed in psychotherapy across all therapeutic modalities including cognitive behavioral therapy—countertransference can emerge in treatment regardless of clinician's theoretical orientation or belief about the process (Betan, Heim, Zittel Conklin, & Westen, 2005). Countertransference is a frequent occurrence in therapy and can negatively affect treatment, although proper management may promote therapeutic effectiveness (Hayes, Gelso, & Hummel, 2011). Once viewed as an unfortunate and bothersome mistake on the part of the therapist, it is now acknowledged as a ubiquitous part of a therapeutic process that can help the clinician to better understand the client and facilitate meaningful change (Berzoff & Kita, 2010). However, simply intellectualizing countertransference does not improve it—in order to cope with these feelings, therapists should engage in self-care practices while combining their reaction to the client with their theoretical framework in order to understand and effectively manage the evoked emotions (Hayes et al., 2011). Although countertransference is frequently discussed in the literature, there remains a dearth of empirical studies examining how countertransference impacts outcome generally and how it can impact both the therapist and the treatment when conducting therapy with criminal justice-involved clients.

Treating individuals who committed a crime may elicit strong reactions during treatment from both the therapist and client. Clients in the criminal justice system are often mandated to treatment, either as a requirement of their sentence or as a means to improve their chances of release. Thus, their motivation to change may be low (see Chap. 11 for a discussion of motivational interviewing with court-ordered clients), they may not be forthcoming with important information about their past and their crimes that would be needed for change which can be frustrating for the therapist, and they may be verbally or even physically aggressive to the therapist or other clients. Further, many of the topics discussed in treatment with those who have committed offenses can be difficult and disturbing. Clients may share details of crimes where they have hurt, degraded, and abused others, including children which can elicit strong emotions in the therapist. According to Mitchell and Melikian (1995), negative reactions from the therapist directed toward the client may include sadistic thoughts and feelings, as well as anger and aggression. The authors postulated that sadistic thoughts may arise toward clients who have committed heinous crimes and show little to no empathy or remorse for their actions. Consequently, therapists may feel the desire to avenge the victims. Similarly, a lack of empathy for victims may lead to feelings of anger and aggression, as the therapist may find themselves wanting to hurt or punish the offender for what they have done. These types of feelings may be particularly distressing for clinicians whose job it is to be empathetic and to help the offender change for the better. These feelings may be further exacerbated if the therapist has children and the client has committed offenses against minors. Thus, the authors recommend that such feelings and emotions are discussed in supervision and normalize them in the context of providing treatment to those involved with the criminal justice system (Mitchell & Melikian, 1995).

Gerber (1995) cautions that another countertransference reaction that can be extremely distressing to therapists of individuals who have committed sex crimes is having feelings of sexual arousal or attraction to the client. The author states that since sex offender-specific therapy often includes discussion of material and topics that are highly sexual in nature, this may provoke intense emotions. Gerber suggests that in some cases, these emotions can impact the therapeutic process, as the therapist may be repulsed by them, or—more dangerously—act on them, resulting in ethical violations. As these feelings of sexual arousal or attraction go against what is societally and ethically acceptable, the therapist may feel shame and be reluctant to discuss them in supervision. Gerber recommends that disclosures of these emotions in supervision should be encouraged and normalized, so as not to damage the therapeutic relationship and hinder treatment progress.

Countertransference can also arise in treatment with those in the criminal justice system based upon experiences and traumas that the therapist themselves may have experienced in the past. For example, a significant proportion of sex offender service providers have been victims of abuse (Moulden & Firestone, 2007). One study of therapists who provided services to victims and perpetrators of sexual violence found that 75% of all service providers reported a history of childhood sexual abuse (Way et al., 2004). Additionally, Edmunds (1997) found that 54% of her sample of sex offender therapists reported that they had experienced abuse (psychological, physical, and sexual) at some point in their lives. However, another study of members of the Association for the Treatment of Sexual Abusers (ATSA) found that only about one quarter of the therapists reported past traumatic experiences (Ennis & Horne, 2003). Regardless of the exact number, these studies suggest that a significant portion of sex offender therapists have a history of abuse. It is still unclear how such a history can affect the therapist's relationship with clients who have perpetrated sex crimes and whether this can impact their effectiveness. Kassam-Adams (1995) has suggested that clinicians who are interested in treating victims and perpetrators of sexual abuse may be doing so in an effort to heal themselves of their own abuse histories. If Kassam-Adams is correct, then countertransference may arise more frequently in this context, as therapists may be working through their own issues as they work with their clients. While little empirical evidence exists on the topic, Moulden and Firestone (2007) caution that such countertransference may have negative implications for the formation of rapport with the client, and thus therapists who are experiencing countertransference reactions should partake in ongoing supervision and self-care.

6.8 Conclusions and Recommendations

While there has been a dearth of research investigating therapist-related factors among those who work in corrections, some conclusions and recommendations may be drawn from the research on therapists in general. Specifically, the research suggests several avenues for training and supervision that can increase therapist effectiveness. The following are recommendations based upon what is known from the general and offender-specific literature on treatment providers.

1. Those working with offending populations should maintain reasonable caseloads with minimal administrative and documentation requirements. Both these factors were related to burnout and job retention. Thus, by assuring better working conditions for treatment providers, there will be less turnaround, which will keep training and recruiting costs down and increase treatment outcome.
2. Those providing services to offending populations should receive regular weekly individual or small group supervision in which issues pertaining to self-care, stress management, and coping are discussed to prevent burnout. Further, supervision meetings should include discussing and addressing individual cases and issues pertaining to vicarious traumatization and countertransference.
3. Training programs that focus on preparing trainees for work with offending populations should work to standardize curriculum focused on evidence-based practices and importance of program delivery, and thus they will be able to better study how training can impact service provision and treatment outcome among therapists in forensic settings.
4. Training programs should take into consideration the nature of correctional settings and provide specific education regarding aspects that professionals will encounter, including knowing general correctional policy and specific role policies, interdepartmental communications, safety in correctional settings, and providing effective assistance in corrections-specific environment (e.g., managing individuals with mental illness in SHUs).
5. There appear to be a set of core characteristics of effective therapists that can be identified by the FIS that supersedes even content-specific training as it relates to treatment outcome. Given the importance to public safety of providing effective treatment, programs that train providers for the criminal justice system should consider screening candidates based upon FIS criteria prior to admission.

The ultimate goal of offender treatment is to stop the offending behavior by teaching skills and helping the individual lead a prosocial life therein assuring community safety. The role of the therapist in offender treatment has been found to be the largest catalyst for change; however, working with criminal justice-involved clients can be challenging. The current research suggests that certain therapist characteristics such as empathy, warmth, rewardingness, and directiveness positively impact treatment outcome, while adversarial challenging of the client could hinder progress. What complicates the picture is that while training and education may impact attitudes, it appears that many of the skills needed for successful treatment outcome may not be able to be taught. Additionally, those who work with criminal justice-involved clients are at increased risk for burnout and can experience vicarious traumatization and countertransference, which when not addressed can negatively impact both the therapist and their ability to provide effective treatment. Finally, treatment is as good as its providers—meaning that in order to accurately assess the effectiveness of offender treatment, we need to ensure proper program delivery. The research-based recommendations presented in this chapter may assist clinicians, administrators, and researchers in promoting the high quality of service provided to criminal justice-involved clients.

References

Acker, G. M. (2010). The challenges in providing services to clients with mental illness: Managed care, burnout and somatic symptoms among social workers. *Community Mental Health Journal, 46*(6), 591–600. https://doi.org/10.1007/s10597-009-9269-5

Adams, S. A. (2017). *Coping and work-related correlates of burnout for counselors of sex offenders* (Doctoral dissertation). Retrieved from https://scholarworks.waldenu.edu/dissertations (Order 4121)

Alexander, D. A., & Atcheson, S. F. (1998). Psychiatric aspects of trauma care: Survey of nurses and doctors. *Psychiatric Bulletin, 22*(3), 132–136. https://doi.org/10.1192/pb.22.3.132

American Psychological Association. (2013). Specialty guidelines for forensic psychology. *American Psychologist, 68*(1), 7–19. https://doi.org/10.1037/a0029889

Anderson, T., Crowley, M. E. J., Himawan, L., Holmberg, J. K., & Uhlin, B. D. (2016). Therapist facilitative interpersonal skills and training status: A randomized clinical trial on alliance and outcome. *Psychotherapy Research, 26*(5), 511–529. https://doi.org/10.1080/10503307.2015.1049671

Anderson, T., McClintock, A. S., Himawan, L., Song, X., & Patterson, C. L. (2016). A prospective study of therapist facilitative interpersonal skills as a predictor of treatment outcome. *Journal of Consulting and Clinical Psychology, 84*(1), 57–66. https://doi.org/10.1037/ccp0000060

Anderson, T., Ogles, B. M., Patterson, C. L., Lambert, M. J., & Vermeersch, D. A. (2009). Therapist effects: Facilitative interpersonal skills as a predictor of therapist success. *Journal of Clinical Psychology, 65*(7), 755–768. https://doi.org/10.1002/jclp.20583

APA Presidential Task Force on Evidence-Based Practice. (2006). Evidence-based practice in psychology. *American Psychologist, 61*(4), 271–285. https://doi.org/10.1037/0003-066X.61.4.271

Association of Psychology Postdoctoral and Internship Centers. (2012). *2012 APPIC match: Survey of internship applicants, part 2: Summary of applicant placement by applicant and program characteristics*. Retrieved from https://www.appic.org/Internships/Match/Match-Statistics

Association of Psychology Postdoctoral and Internship Centers. (2015). *2015 APPIC match: Survey of internship applicants, part 2: Summary of applicant placement by applicant and program characteristics*. Retrieved from https://www.appic.org/Internships/Match/Match-Statistics

Association of Psychology Postdoctoral and Internship Centers. (2016). *2016 APPIC match: Survey of internship applicants, part 2: Summary of applicant placement by applicant and program characteristics*. Retrieved from https://www.appic.org/Internships/Match/Match-Statistics

Baldwin, S. A., & Imel, Z. E. (2013). Therapist effects: Findings and methods. In M. J. Lambert (Ed.), *Bergin and Garfield's handbook of psychotherapy and behavior change* (6th ed., pp. 258–297). New York, NY: Wiley.

Baldwin, S. A., Wampold, B. E., & Imel, Z. E. (2007). Untangling the alliance-outcome correlation: Exploring the relative importance of therapist and patient variability in the alliance. *Journal of Consulting and Clinical Psychology, 75*(6), 842–852. https://doi.org/10.1037/0022-006X.75.6.842

Berglar, J., Crameri, A., von Wyl, A., Koemeda-Lutz, M., Köhler, M., Staczan, P., … & Tschuschke, V. (2016). Therapist effects on treatment outcome in psychotherapy: A multilevel modelling analysis. *International Journal of Psychotherapy, 20*(2), 61–80. Retrieved from http://www.ijp.org.uk/

Berman, J. S., & Norton, N. C. (1985). Does professional training make a therapist more effective? *Psychological Bulletin, 98*(2), 401–407. https://doi.org/10.1037/0033-2909.98.2.401

Berzoff, J., & Kita, E. (2010). Compassion fatigue and countertransference: Two different concepts. *Clinical Social Work Journal, 38*(3), 341–349. https://doi.org/10.1007/s10615-010-0271-8

Betan, E., Heim, A. K., Zittel Conklin, C., & Westen, D. (2005). Countertransference phenomena and personality pathology in clinical practice: An empirical investigation. *The American Journal of Psychiatry, 162*(5), 890–898. https://doi.org/10.1176/appi.ajp.162.5.890

Branson, D. C. (2018). Vicarious trauma, themes in research, and terminology: A review of literature. *Traumatology*. https://doi.org/10.1037/trm0000161

Carrola, P. A., Olivarez, A., & Karcher, M. J. (2016). Correctional counselor burnout: Examining burnout rates using the Counselor Burnout Inventory. *Journal of Offender Rehabilitation, 55*(3), 195–212. https://doi.org/10.1080/10509674.2016.1149134

Castonguay, L. G., & Beutler, L. E. (2006). Principles of therapeutic change: A task force on participants, relationships and technique factors. *Journal of Clinical Psychology, 62*(6), 631–638. https://doi.org/10.1002/jclp.20256

Catanese, S. A. (2010). Traumatized by association: The risk of working sex crimes. *Federal Probation Journal, 74*(2), 36–38. Retrieved from http://www.uscourts.gov/statistics-reports/publications/federal-probation-journal

Cieslak, R., Shoji, K., Douglas, A., Melville, E., Luszczynska, A., & Benight, C. C. (2014). A meta-analysis of the relationship between job burnout and secondary traumatic stress among workers with indirect exposure to trauma. *Psychological Services, 11*(1), 75–86. https://doi.org/10.1037/a0033798

Cohen, K., & Collens, P. (2013). The impact of trauma work on trauma workers: A metasynthesis on vicarious trauma and vicarious posttraumatic growth. *Psychological Trauma Theory Research Practice and Policy, 5*(6), 570–580. https://doi.org/10.1037/a0030388

Duncan, B. L., Miller, S. D., Wampold, B. E., & Hubble, M. A. (Eds.). (2010). *The heart and soul of change: Delivering what works in therapy* (2nd ed.). Washington, DC: American Psychological Association.

Dyrbye, L. N., Shanafelt, T. D., Sinsky, C. A., Cipriano, C. F., Bhatt, J., Ommaya, A., … & Meyers, D. (2017). Burnout among health care professionals: A call to explore and address this underrecognized threat to safe, high-quality care. *NAM Perspectives*. Discussion Paper, National Academy of Medicine, Washington, DC. https://doi.org/10.31478/201707b

Edmunds, S. B. (1997). The personal impact of working with sex offenders. In S. B. Edmunds (Ed.), *Impact: Working with sexual abusers* (pp. 11–26). Brandon, VT: Safer Society Press.

Ennis, L., & Horne, S. (2003). Predicting psychological distress in sex offender therapists. *Sexual Abuse, 15*(2), 149–157. https://doi.org/10.1177/107906320301500205

Farrenkopf, T. (1992). What happens to therapists who work with sex offenders. *Journal of Offender Rehabilitation, 18*(3-4), 217–224. https://doi.org/10.1300/J076v18n03_16

Flückiger, C., Del Re, A. C., Wampold, B. E., Symonds, D., & Horvath, A. O. (2012). How central is the alliance in psychotherapy? A multilevel longitudinal meta-analysis. *Journal of Counseling Psychology, 59*(1), 10–17. https://doi.org/10.1037/a0025749

Franklin, K. (2014, September 15). Forensic psychology: Is it the career for me? *Psychology Today*. Retrieved from https://www.psychologytoday.com/us/blog/witness/201409/forensic-psychology-is-it-the-career-me

Garland, B. (2002). Prison treatment staff burnout: Consequences, causes and prevention. *Corrections Today, 64*(7), 116–121. Retrieved from http://www.aca.org/

Garman, A. N., Corrigan, P. W., & Morris, S. B. (2002). Staff burnout and patient satisfaction: Evidence of relationships at the care unit level. *Journal of Occupational Health Psychology, 7*(3), 235–241. https://doi.org/10.1037/1076-8998.7.3.235

Gerber, P. N. (1995). Commentary on counter-transference in working with sex offenders: The issue of sexual attraction. *Journal of Child Sexual Abuse, 4*(1), 117–121. https://doi.org/10.1300/J070v04n01_12

Gilbody, S., Cahill, J., Barkham, M., Richards, D., Bee, P., & Glanville, J. (2006). Can we improve the morale of staff working in psychiatric units? A systematic review. *Journal of Mental Health, 15*(1), 7–17. https://doi.org/10.1080/09638230500512482

Goldberg, S. B., Rousmaniere, T., Miller, S. D., Whipple, J., Nielsen, S. L., Hoyt, W. T., & Wampold, B. E. (2016). Do psychotherapists improve with time and experience? A longitudinal analysis of outcomes in a clinical setting. *Journal of Counseling Psychology, 63*(1), 1–11. https://doi.org/10.1037/cou0000131

Gowdy, E. A., Carlson, L. S., & Rapp, C. A. (2003). Practices differentiating high-performing from low-performing supported employment programs. *Psychiatric Rehabilitation Journal, 26*(3), 232–239. https://doi.org/10.2975/26.2003.232.239

Harkins, L., & Beech, A. R. (2007). A review of the factors that can influence the effectiveness of sexual offender treatment: Risk, need, responsivity, and process issues. *Aggression and Violent Behavior, 12*(6), 615–627. https://doi.org/10.1016/j.avb.2006.10.006

Hattie, J. A., Sharpley, C. F., & Rogers, H. J. (1984). Comparative effectiveness of professional and paraprofessional helpers. *Psychological Bulletin, 95*(3), 534–541. https://doi.org/10.1037/0033-2909.95.3.534

Hayes, J. A., Gelso, C. J., & Hummel, A. M. (2011). Managing countertransference. *Psychotherapy, 48*(1), 88–97. https://doi.org/10.1037/a0022182

Heinonen, E., Lindfors, O., Laaksonen, M. A., & Knelt, P. (2012). Therapists' professional and personal characteristics as predictors of outcome in short- and long-term psychotherapy. *Journal of Affective Disorders, 138*(3), 301–312. https://doi.org/10.1016/j.jad.2012.01.023

Hogue, T. E. (1995). Training multidisciplinary teams to work with sex offenders: Effects on staff attitudes. *Psychology Crime and Law, 1*(3), 227–235. https://doi.org/10.1080/10683169508411958

Holmqvist, R., & Jeanneau, M. (2006). Burnout and psychiatric staff's feelings toward patients. *Psychiatry Research, 145*(2-3), 207–213. https://doi.org/10.1016/j.psychres.2004.08.012

Jeglic, E. L., Hanson, R. K., & Calkins, C. (2016). Sex offender treatment: The need for cognitive behavioral therapists. *Behavior Therapist, 39*(5), 162–168. Retrieved from http://www.abct.org/Journals/?m=mJournal&fa=TBT

Kassam-Adams, N. (1995). The risks of treating sexual trauma: Stress and secondary trauma in psychotherapists. In B. H. Stamm (Ed.), *Secondary traumatic stress: Self-care issues for clinicians, researchers, and educators* (pp. 37–48). Baltimore, MD: The Sidran Press.

Lambert, M., & Bergin, A. E. (1994). The effectiveness of psychotherapy. In A. E. Bergin & S. L. Garfield (Eds.), *Handbook of psychotherapy and behavior change* (pp. 143–189). New York, NY: Wiley.

Lambert, M. J., Harmon, C., Slade, K., Whipple, J. L., & Hawkins, E. J. (2005). Providing feedback to psychotherapists on their patients' progress: Clinical results and practice suggestions. *Journal of Clinical Psychology, 61*(2), 165–174. https://doi.org/10.1002/jclp.20113

Lea, S., Auburn, T., & Kibblewhite, K. (1999). Working with sex offenders: The perceptions and experiences of professionals and paraprofessionals. *International Journal of Offender Therapy and Comparative Criminology, 43*(1), 103–119. https://doi.org/10.1177/0306624X99431010

Magaletta, P. R., Cermak, J. N., Anderson, E. J., Norcross, C. M., Olive, B., Shaw, S. A., & Butterfield, P. (2016). An exploratory study of experiences and training needs of early-career correctional psychologists. *Professional Psychology: Research and Practice, 47*(4), 278–286. https://doi.org/10.1037/pro0000075

Magaletta, P. R., Patry, M. W., Dietz, E. F., & Ax, R. K. (2007). What is correctional about clinical practice in corrections? *Criminal Justice and Behavior, 34*(1), 7–21. https://doi.org/10.1177/0093854806290024

Makarios, M., Lovins, L., Latessa, E., & Smith, P. (2016). Staff quality and treatment effectiveness: An examination of the relationship between staff factors and the effectiveness of correctional programs. *Justice Quarterly, 33*(2), 348–367. https://doi.org/10.1080/07418825.2014.924546

Marshall, W. L. (2005). Therapist style in sexual offender treatment: Influence on indices of change. *Sexual Abuse: A Journal of Research and Treatment, 17*(2), 109–116. https://doi.org/10.1007/s11194-005-4598-6

Marshall, W. L., Serran, G. A., Fernandez, Y. M., Mulloy, R., Mann, R. E., & Thornton, D. (2003). Therapist characteristics in the treatment of sexual offenders: Tentative data on their relationship with indices of behaviour change. *Journal of Sexual Aggression, 9*(1), 25–30. https://doi.org/10.1080/355260031000137940

Marshall, W. L., Serran, G. A., Moulden, H., Mulloy, R., Fernandez, Y. M., Mann, R. E., & Thornton, D. (2002). Therapist features in sexual offender treatment: Their reliable identification and influence on behaviour change. *Clinical Psychology & Psychotherapy, 9*(6), 395–405. https://doi.org/10.1002/cpp.335

Maslach, C. (2017). Burnout: A multidimensional perspective. In W. B. Schaufeli, C. Maslach, & T. Marek (Eds.), *Professional burnout: Recent developments in theory and research* (pp. 19–32). New York, NY: Routledge.

Maslach, C., Jackson, S. E., & Leiter, M. P. (1996). *MBI: Maslach burnout inventory*. Sunnyvale, CA: CPP.

Mitchell, C., & Melikian, K. (1995). The treatment of male sexual offenders: Countertransference reactions. *Journal of Child Sexual Abuse, 4*(1), 87–94. https://doi.org/10.1300/J070v04n01_06

Moon, A. E., & Shivy, V. A. (2008). Treatment fidelity in sex offender programming: Assessing delivery across community providers. *Victims and Offenders, 3*(1), 45–74. https://doi.org/10.1080/15564880701864135

Morse, G., Salyers, M. P., Rollins, A. L., Monroe-DeVita, M., & Pfahler, C. (2012). Burnout in mental health services: A review of the problem and its remediation. *Administration and Policy in Mental Health and Mental Health Services Research, 39*(5), 341–352. https://doi.org/10.1007/s10488-011-0352-1

Moster, A., Wnuk, D. W., & Jeglic, E. L. (2008). Cognitive behavioral therapy interventions with sex offenders. *Journal of Correctional Health Care, 14*(2), 109–121. https://doi.org/10.1177/1078345807313874

Moulden, H. M., & Firestone, P. (2007). Vicarious traumatization: The impact on therapists who work with sexual offenders. *Trauma, Violence & Abuse, 8*(1), 67–83. https://doi.org/10.1177/1524838006297729

Munger, T., Savage, T., & Panosky, D. M. (2015). When caring for perpetrators becomes a sentence: Recognizing vicarious trauma. *Journal of Correctional Health Care, 21*(4), 365–374. https://doi.org/10.1177/1078345815599976

Nelson, M., Herlihy, B., & Oescher, J. (2002). A survey of counselor attitudes towards sex offenders. *Journal of Mental Health Counseling, 24*(1), 51–67. Retrieved from http://amhcajournal.org/

Norcross, J. C. (Ed.). (2011). *Psychotherapy relationships that work: Evidence-based responsiveness* (2nd ed.). New York, NY: Oxford University Press.

Owen, J., Wampold, B. E., Kopta, M., Rousmaniere, T., & Miller, S. D. (2016). As good as it gets? Therapy outcomes of trainees over time. *Journal of Counseling Psychology, 63*(1), 12–19. https://doi.org/10.1037/cou0000112

Peterson, U., Demerouti, E., Bergström, G., Samuelsson, M., Åsberg, M., & Nygren, Å. (2008). Burnout and physical and mental health among Swedish healthcare workers. *Journal of Advanced Nursing, 62*(1), 84–95. https://doi.org/10.1111/j.1365-2648.2007.04580.x

Rich, K. (1997). Vicarious traumatization: A preliminary study. In S. B. Edmunds (Ed.), *Impact: Working with sexual abusers* (pp. 75–88). Brandon, VT: Safer Society Press.

Rollins, A. L., Salyers, M. P., Tsai, J., & Lydick, J. M. (2010). Staff turnover in statewide implementation of ACT: Relationship with ACT fidelity and other team characteristics. *Administration and Policy in Mental Health and Mental Health Services Research, 37*(5), 417–426. https://doi.org/10.1007/s10488-009-0257-4

Rupert, P. A., & Morgan, D. J. (2005). Work setting and burnout among professional psychologists. *Professional Psychology: Research and Practice, 36*(5), 544–550. https://doi.org/10.1037/0735-7028.36.5.544

Salston, M.-D., & Figley, C. R. (2003). Secondary traumatic stress effects of working with survivors of criminal victimization. *Journal of Traumatic Stress, 16*(2), 167–174. https://doi.org/10.1023/A:1022899207206

Sandhu, D. K., & Rose, J. (2012). How do therapists contribute to therapeutic change in sex offender treatment: An integration of the literature. *Journal of Sexual Aggression, 18*(3), 269–283. https://doi.org/10.1080/13552600.2011.566633

Saxon, D., & Barkham, M. (2012). Patterns of therapist variability: Therapist effects and the contribution of patient severity and risk. *Journal of Consulting and Clinical Psychology, 80*(4), 535–546. https://doi.org/10.1037/a0028898

Saxon, D., Firth, N., & Barkham, M. (2017). The relationship between therapist effects and therapy delivery factors: Therapy modality, dosage, and non-completion. *Administration and Policy in Mental Health and Mental Health Services Research, 44*(5), 705–715. https://doi.org/10.1007/s10488-016-0750-5

Schmucker, M., & Lösel, F. (2015). The effects of sexual offender treatment on recidivism: An international meta-analysis of sound quality evaluations. *Journal of Experimental Criminology, 11*(4), 597–630. https://doi.org/10.1007/s11292-015-9241-z

Schwab, R. L., Jackson, S. E., & Schuler, R. S. (1986). Educator burnout: Sources and consequences. *Educational Research Quarterly, 10*(3), 14–30. Retrieved from http://erquarterly.org/

Shelby, R. A., Stoddart, R. M., & Taylor, K. L. (2001). Factors contributing to levels of burnout among ex offender treatment providers. *Journal of Interpersonal Violence, 16*(11), 1205–1217. https://doi.org/10.1177/088626001016011006

Smoot, S. L., & Gonzales, J. L. (1995). Cost-effective communication skills training for state hospital employees. *Psychiatric Services, 46*(8), 819–822. https://doi.org/10.1176/ps.46.8.819

Steed, L., & Bicknell, J. (2001). Trauma and the therapist: The experience of therapists working with the predators of sexual abuse. *The Australasian Journal of Disaster and Trauma Studies, 1*, 527–540. Retrieved from http://trauma.massey.ac.nz

Stein, D. M., & Lambert, M. J. (1995). Graduate training in psychotherapy: Are therapy outcomes enhanced? *Journal of Consulting and Clinical Psychology, 63*(2), 182–196. https://doi.org/10.1037/0022-006X.63.2.182

Wampold, B. E. (2007). Psychotherapy: The humanistic (and effective) treatment. *American Psychologist, 62*(8), 857–873. https://doi.org/10.1037/0003-066X.62.8.857

Wampold, B. E. (2011). *Qualities and actions of effective therapists*. Washington, DC: American Psychological Association. Retrieved from https://www.apa.org/education/ce/effective-therapists.pdf

Ward, J. T. (2013). What is forensic psychology? *Psychology student network, September 2013*. Retrieved from http://www.apa.org/ed/precollege/psn/2013/09/forensic-psychology.aspx

Way, I., VanDeusen, K. M., Martin, G., Applegate, B., & Jandle, D. (2004). Vicarious trauma: A comparison of clinicians who treat survivors of sexual abuse and sexual offenders. *Journal of Interpersonal Violence, 19*(1), 49–71. https://doi.org/10.1177/0886260503259050

Webb, C. A., DeRubeis, R. J., & Barber, J. P. (2010). Therapists' adherence/competence and treatment outcome: A meta-analytic review. *Journal of Consulting and Clinical Psychology, 78*(2), 200–211. https://doi.org/10.1037/a0018912

Chapter 7
Diversity Considerations in the Application of Evidence-Based Interventions with Forensic Clients

Alejandro Leguizamo, Paige A. Beliveau, Julia M. Uber, Sarah Burnham, Matthew Conrad, and Nicholas Zike

7.1 Introduction

Mental health professionals in forensic or correctional settings are likely to encounter individuals from various backgrounds and cultures in their practice (American Psychiatric Association, 2016; Diamond, Wang, Holzer, Thomas, & Cruser, 2001). Gramlich (2018) reported that while the gap between White and African American prisoners in the USA is shrinking, minorities remain overrepresented in the justice system. He indicated that in 2016, Whites accounted for 64% of adults but only 30% of prisoners. On the other hand, the author stated that African Americans accounted for 12% of the adults but 33% of prisoners. Likewise, Latinos accounted for 16% of adults and 23% of prisoners (Gramlich, 2018). Meyer et al. (2017) found that the incarceration rate for men and women who identified as lesbian, gay, or bisexual was three times that of the general population. They found that 9.3% of men in prison, 6.2% of men in jail, 42% of women in prison, and 35.7% of women in jail were sexual minorities. Other populations that professionals will encounter include military veterans, individuals from diverse socioeconomic strata, and religious minorities (American Psychiatric Association, 2016; Hamm, 2009).

The American Psychological Association (APA) has stressed the need to take into consideration the various cultural identities as well as ecological context of clients, with a particular focus on intersectionality (APA, 2017) and that evidence-based practice is "… the integration of the best research with clinical expertise in the context of patient characteristics, culture, and preferences" (American Psychological

A. Leguizamo (✉)
Psychology Department, Roger Williams University, Bristol, RI, USA
e-mail: aleguizamo@rwu.edu

P. A. Beliveau · J. M. Uber · S. Burnham · M. Conrad · N. Zike
Roger Williams University, Bristol, RI, USA
e-mail: Pbeliveau799@g.rwu.edu; Juber629@g.rwu.edu; Sburnham259@g.rwu.edu; Mconrad580@g.rwu.edu; Nzike839@g.rwu.edu

E. L. Jeglic, C. Calkins (eds.), *New Frontiers in Offender Treatment*,
https://doi.org/10.1007/978-3-030-01030-0_7

Association, Presidential Taskforce on Evidence-Based Practice, 2006, p. 273). Therefore, unless otherwise noted, we intend for "diverse" clients to encompass as many cultural identities as possible including but not limited to ethnicity, gender identity, sexual orientation, and religious affiliation.

In this chapter, we present a framework for mental health professionals to increase their consideration of cultural issues in treatment with forensic/correctional populations. We will review the multicultural competencies developed by Sue and Sue (2015) and the Layered Ecological Model of the Multicultural Guidelines based on Bronfenbrenner (1977) developed by the American Psychological Association (2017). We will then present the evidence of the importance of the therapeutic relationship and group cohesiveness in the treatment of diverse individuals. We will also review the extant literature with respect to the application of evidence-based treatments (EBTs) in a multicultural context. Finally, we will provide recommendations based on the literature regarding the process through which to consider the application of EBTs with diverse clients in forensic and correctional settings, for whom these treatments have not been empirically validated.

7.2 Multicultural Competence

Sue and Sue (2015) described three multicultural competencies in need of development in order to provide diverse clients with sensitive and effective treatment. These competencies are awareness, knowledge, and skills. Utilizing an expanded Layered Ecological Model of the Multicultural Guidelines (APA, 2017) is recommended to assist in providing clinicians with a more thorough understanding of themselves and their clients. We suggest this as a framework through which to consider Sue and Sue's Multicultural Competencies. The Layered Ecological Model of the Multicultural Guidelines implements Bronfenbrenner's (1977) Ecological Model of Development and urges clinicians to take into consideration a variety of forces that influence their clients, such as individual, familial, community, institutional, and societal, such as immigration status, potential employment discrimination (Solinas-Saunders, Stacer, & Guy, 2015), housing discrimination (Kras, Pleggenkuhle, & Huebner, 2016), or voting disenfranchisement (Ruth, Matusitz, & Simi, 2017), and how these relate to outcomes. We would add that, in seeking to increase their cultural sensitivity or multicultural competence, clinicians should use this ecological approach as well.

The first multicultural competency, as identified by Sue and Sue (2015), is awareness. This competency assists in developing a greater awareness of clinicians' cultural identities, values, beliefs, biases, and detrimental attitudes (e.g., classism, homophobia, heterosexism, sexist, racism). Importantly, these characteristics are examined with respect to how they influence clinicians' perceptions, interactions, and treatment of their clients. In addition, clinicians must be sensitive to circumstances that may raise the need to refer the client to a different mental health professional (Sue & Sue, 2015). As clinicians work on developing a greater self-awareness, it could be helpful for them to explore the various forces that forged their beliefs, attitudes, and biases from an ecological perspective, as described by the APA (2017). Therefore, clinicians should consider their own individual context when assessing their competency, such as personality, therapeutic style, communication style, and comfort with individuals different from them broadly speaking (i.e., ethnically, geographical origin, religion, sexual orientation, among others). In addition, clinicians should be cognizant of the impact their families had on the development on these attitudes and beliefs. Questions to consider are: To what extent was their family comfortable with diversity? What messages, overt or covert, were received from family members about people different from them? Moreover, clinicians need to consider the influences and messages about diversity they received from their communities (neighborhood, schools, including higher education), including the towns/cities in which they have lived. Societal messages in general (from the media, political entities, etc.) are also very important in this context. This much needed introspection could lead clinicians to become more aware of themselves, their biases, and how they may impact their interactions with diverse clients.

The second multicultural competence is knowledge (Sue & Sue, 2015). This competency entails becoming familiar with the cultural groups with whom the clinician works, including their histories, customs, communication styles, experience of oppression, and utilization and experience with the mental health system. Moreover, this knowledge base must include an understanding of the sociopolitical systems that affect one's clients. In particular, Sue and Sue (2015) argued that the therapeutic interaction is inherently a sociopolitical interaction in which societal forces (such as oppression and power differentials) can greatly impact the process. Other authors have contended that psychotherapy as we know it may be inherently ethnocentric and could be harmful to diverse clients (Wendt, Gonc, & Nagata, 2015). Therefore, clinicians must be careful not to assume they understand their clients' experiences based on knowledge gathered about their cultural identities. In other words, they must be open to understanding their clients' individual history, context, and viewpoint while taking into consideration potential historical and sociopolitical influences.

The third multicultural competence is skills (Sue & Sue, 2015). This competency entails the provision of culturally effective assessment of treatment of clients; effective communication with diverse clients, both verbally and nonverbally; proper utilization of assessment methods appropriately normed; and structured treatment plans that are sensitive to cultural factors. These elements are key to providing culturally effective assessment and treatment. Moreover, Sue and Sue note that clinicians must also be willing to advocate for their clients in their interactions with larger systems and to implement environmental or institutional interventions when warranted. Their recommendation is consistent with the APA's (2017) multicultural guidelines and requires that clinicians not only conceptualize cases from a multisystemic viewpoint but also stresses that helping to improve clients' functioning requires that clinician venture out of individual/group treatment.

Understandably, there is evidence that perceived clinician multicultural competence is related to the development of a stronger therapeutic alliance, client satisfaction, perceived general competence, session depth, and treatment outcome to a lesser extent (Tao, Owen, Pace, & Imel, 2015). It is particularly important for mental health professionals to work on cultural sensitivity and multicultural competence as almost 84% of psychologists, 54.5% of social workers, and 59% of mental health counselors are White (DataUSA, n.d.; APA, 2015). In sum, a multiculturally competent clinician is one who engages in considerable, and consistent, self-reflection, is knowledgeable of the populations they serve, is open to learning from their clients and their experiences, and designs and implements interventions that are culturally sensitive, appropriate, and therefore the most useful to their clients.

7.3 The Therapeutic Relationship, Group Cohesion, and Diverse Clients

As part of a movement toward EBTs, Sue and Sue (2015) called for the consideration of empirically based relationships, a concept created by the authors. This concept stresses the importance of the therapeutic relationship in working with diverse clients. The therapeutic relationship, or alliance, reflects the nature and quality of engagement between the therapist and the client. Through this relationship, rapport is built, and therapeutic tasks are undertaken (Orlinsky, Ronnestad, & Willutzki, 2004). Moreover, there is strong evidence that the therapeutic relationship is an important factor in successful therapy outcomes (Vasquez, 2007). Furthermore, treatment methods do not work in isolation from but rather in conjunction with it (Norcross & Lambert, 2011). Group cohesion is considered its counterpart in group therapy (Burlingame, Fuhriman, & Johnson, 2002). Group cohesion is more complicated since it is composed of the relationships and connections between and among group members and the leader (Burlingame, McClendon, & Alonso, 2011). This paradigm exists even when more than one group leader is involved. Burlingame et al. (2011) also observed that group cohesion is positively related to treatment outcome, especially among younger clients, in interpersonal-focused groups, where cohesion is emphasized, and in groups that are interactive, as opposed to problem-specific.

While Rogers (1957) proposed that empathy, unconditional positive regard, and congruence, or genuineness, were necessary and sufficient for therapeutic change, these conditions are seen as necessary to develop a strong therapeutic relationship but are not in themselves sufficient (Norcross & Lambert, 2011). Empathy, which involves the understanding of the client's experience and conveying such understanding to the client, has been found to be positively related to treatment outcome regardless of treatment format, client severity, or therapist theoretical orientation (Elliot, Bohart, Watson, & Greenberg, 2011). Positive regard has been found to be related to treatment success and is communicated through respect, care, positive attitude, and affirmation of clients' inherent worth (Farber & Doolin, 2011). Congruence, or genuineness, refers to the authenticity of the therapist in treatment and their ability to communicate with the client in a forthcoming manner that includes appropriate self-disclosure, particularly with respect to the process in treatment (Kolden, Klein, Wang, & Austin, 2011). Congruence increases attachment in treatment, models genuineness for the client, and may be ever more important in group treatment (Kolden et al., 2011).

There are also a number of therapist attributes that have been found to contribute to a strong therapeutic relationship (Ackerman & Hilsenroth, 2003) including with respect to group cohesiveness (e.g., with individuals who sexually offended, Serran & Marshall, 2010). Empathy, warmth, flexibility, respectfulness, confidence, trustworthiness, and openness have been found to be valuable in correctional settings. Moreover, the ability to be appropriately directive with offenders convicted of sex crimes, challenging, supporting and encouraging, and emphasizing emotional expression, also contributes to strong therapeutic relationships with that population.

Developing a strong therapeutic relationship with diverse client entails an individualized adaptation to the clients' cultural style. This involves consistent assessment of one's own biases (Vasquez, 2007). As Vasquez noted, some clients may respond better to a directive approach (as has been also recommended by Sue & Sue, 2015), whereas others may react negatively. Clinicians using a cognitive behavioral approach need to consider the roles of oppression and racism on their clients' cognitions and attributions; otherwise, they may erroneously assess them to be the result of cognitive distortions instead of valid experiences (Vasquez, 2007). In addition, the author emphasized that the more a clinician understands their client's worldview and perspective, the more likely they are to foster a good therapeutic relationship. She also stated that this effort involves learning about their clients' expectations, values, and norms without relying on stereotypes.

With respect to the treatment of diverse clients, we must understand that clinicians are not free from biases, societal influences, and may be unaware of their privilege if they are White/European, potentially leading to problems forming a therapeutic relationship (Sue & Sue, 2015; Vasquez, 2007). Furthermore, clinicians who are not aware of their biases and hold negative stereotypes about their clients' competence could have difficulty empathizing with them or helping them cope with discrimination or experiences with which the clinician is not familiar (Vasquez, 2007). There is evidence that individuals experience less empathy, both cognitive and emotional, for others who experience distress from events related to cultural issues. Such decrease in empathy is often mediated by problems in assuming the perspective of the individual who is the target (Nelson & Baumgarte, 2004). In the case of clinicians working with clients from different ethnicities, gender, sexual orientation, socioeconomic status, ideologies, or political leanings, they are more likely to fail to empathize with their clients and react accordingly (Comas-Díaz, 2006).

Another threat to forming and maintaining a therapeutic relationship with clients involves the commission of microaggressions (Sue & Sue, 2015; Vasquez, 2007). Microaggressions are defined as "... the everyday slights, put-downs, invalidations, and insults directed to socially devalued group members by well-intention people who are unaware that they have engaged in such biased and harmful behaviors. A lifetime of *microaggressions* can have a major harmful impact on the psychological well-being of victims [emphasis in the original]" (Sue & Sue, 2015, p. 16). Ethnic and sexual minorities, as well as women, frequently experience these microaggressions based on their ethnicity, gender, and sexual orientation (Velez, Moradi, & DeBlaere, 2015). Microaggressions can be very subtle, such as expressing surprise, even nonverbally, when learning that a member of an ethnic minority has a high academic degree or that a woman works in a field seen as a "male" field. In addition, it is also found when it is assumed that a person with a Latin American surname speaks Spanish or when a client's perception of having perhaps been discriminated against is dismissed without first validating their feelings and exploring the events.

Various authors have also found that racial microaggressions are fairly common in counseling (e.g., Constantine, 2007; Hook et al., 2016; Owen, Tao, Imel, Wampold, & Rodolfa, 2014). However, there is a dearth of studies in which other types of microaggressions in counseling are explored (e.g., based on religion, geographical origin). In a qualitative study, Shelton and Delgado-Romero (2013) found that lesbian, gay, bisexual, and queer clients report the experience of microaggressions based on their sexual orientation. All in all, microaggressions are reported to have a negative impact on treatment. This presents itself in the perception of general, as well as multicultural, competence on the part of the clinician, the working alliance, and satisfaction with treatment.

Microaggressions could be conceptualized as being part of the what Pérez Foster (1998) called "cultural countertransference." She defined the term as "[c]omprising both cognitive and affective elements within the therapist... [it] is a complex and interacting set of: culturally derived personal life values; academically based theoretical/practice beliefs; emotionally driven biases about ethnic groups; and feelings about their own ethnic self identity" (p. 256). Further, Pérez Foster argued that cultural countertransference exists in clinicians at varying degrees of consciousness. This, however, is often disavowed by clinicians, greatly impacts treatment, and is nevertheless perceived by the client. Although there are other more systemic issues that contribute to the underutilization of mental health services by ethnic minorities, such as language barriers, immigration status, and stigma around mental illness and seeking psychological help (e.g., Anglin, Link, & Phelan, 2006; Sue & Sue, 2015) and having higher dropout rates than Whites (e.g., Maura & Weisman de Mamani, 2017), the failure to connect with the client in a meaningful and therapeutic manner creates a barrier for continued treatment.

Similar patterns are present in correctional/forensic settings. Although formal research into microaggressions in forensic and correctional settings remains nonexistent, anecdotal clinical evidence points to several different types of microaggressions being committed by mental health professionals working therein. These include, but are not limited to, ignoring or dismissing how systemic issues may have contributed to the development of the presenting problem; pathologizing behaviors that could be interpreted as adaptive to the person's specific environment or an accepted cultural experience, overt or covert unwillingness to address issues of sexual orientation, or same-sex relationships that affect clients; and subtly or openly imposing white middle-class values onto clients. Unsurprisingly, ethnic minorities are less likely to request mental health services compared to Whites (Diamond, Magaletta, Harzke, & Baxter, 2008). Working with individuals from ethnic groups that have historically been persecuted by the criminal justice system poses significant challenges. For example, they may be less receptive to treatment if they view the practitioner as an extension of an unjust system (Hicks, 2004). Many defendants and inmates will have little to no choice with respect to who is assigned to work with them; as such, it is the responsibility of the practitioner to be aware of potential challenges they may experience when working with those of different ethnicities and cultural backgrounds.

Furthermore, ethnic differences in satisfaction with care have been found among forensic and civil inpatients (Shiva, Haden, & Brooks, 2009). When patients experienced problems with staff, African Americans and Latinos were less likely than Whites to be satisfied with the overall quality of care. The researchers suggested that such ratings may be related to differences in ethnicity between staff and patients. Additional research in this area suggests that African Americans may be less trusting of treatment providers than inmates of other ethnicities (Durrah, 2013).

Disruptions to therapeutic relationships happen frequently during the course of treatment (Safran, Muran, & Eubanks-Carter, 2011). This occurs even if clinicians are multiculturally competent, establish a therapeutic relationship with a client, or reach a stage of cohesion in a group treatment setting. As Safran and colleagues note, minor tensions to major breakdowns can take place within one particular session or during the course of treatment. They also reported that repairing these ruptures in the relationship is associated with positive treatment outcomes. Therefore, it is imperative that clinicians are mindful of such ruptures and take much care in repairing them. Safran et al. (2011) recommended that clinicians respond in a nondefensive manner to clients' negative feelings about treatment and that they accept responsibility for their actions and errors and validate their clients' experience.

7.3.1 Special Considerations for LGBTQ Individuals in Correctional Settings

Compared to heterosexual and cisgender (gender-conforming) inmates, LGBTQ individuals experience ten times more sexual victimization by other inmates and three times more sexual victimization by staff (American Psychiatric Association, 2016). Of those who were sexually victimized by inmates or staff, nearly 75% sustained physical injuries, many of which went either unreported or untreated (Whitman, 2017). There is a wide range of differences in issues and experiences within LGBTQ groups. For example, lesbians may encounter sexism, gay men have especially high rates of sexually transmitted infections and illicit drug use, and bisexuals sometimes find incomplete acceptance within either LGBTQ or heterosexual communities (American Psychiatric Association, 2016). Another source of distress is choosing to stay "closeted" because of safety concerns (American Psychiatric Association, 2016). LGBTQ inmates face different issues and require different treatment than their heterosexual and cisgender counterparts.

Transgender and Gender-Nonconforming (TGNC) Individuals in Correctional Settings In correctional settings, TGNC individuals are housed according to genitalia rather than their gender identity (Whitman, 2017). Lack of clear protocols and accountability in housing placement policies for these individuals contributes to discrimination and victimization of TGNC inmates, which can range from derogatory slurs to gang rape, with impacts ranging from mild depression or anxiety to suicide attempts (American Psychiatric Association, 2016; Whitman, 2017). While incarcerated, TGNC individuals have been found to report repeated incidents of harassment, discrimination, and revictimization (Whitman, 2017). As a result of the few structured protocols or protections in place for transgender inmates, TGNC individuals will typically be placed in isolation as a protective measure for an unspecified amount of time (Whitman, 2017). As a result, clinicians working in forensic or correctional settings need to increase their awareness of issues faced by ethnic and minority clients at a societal level with an emphasis on the institutional environment. Moreover, they must remain aware of intersectionality and of all forms of oppression with respect to clients with multiple minority identities. Focusing on a particular identity simply due to its salience can have a detrimental effect on other that may be less salient (Croteau & Constantine, 2005).

7.4 Evidence-Based Treatments (EBTs) with Diverse Clients

Research in which the effectiveness of EBTs with diverse clients is assessed is somewhat sparse and fraught with methodological issues. First, studies that assess the effectiveness of treatment methods seldom include diverse clients or report such information about their participants (Sue & Sue, 2015). Second, there is a significant need to recruit more diverse clients into this type of research (Bernal & Sáez-Santiago, 2006). Third, randomized clinical trials used to examine the efficacy of treatment methods tend not to investigate their ecological validity (Bernal & Adames, 2017). Fourth, conventional treatment approaches, based on Western values, tend to ignore cultural issues and other types of healing methods and pathologize the behavior of ethnic and sexual minorities (Hegarty, 2018; Sue, Zane, Nagayama-Hall, & Berger, 2009). Fifth, very little consideration is awarded to studies that focus on the treatment of a specific disorder and contextual, cultural, and environmental variables (Sue, 2015). Finally, while this area of research does not take into consideration the importance of the therapeutic relationship (Sue & Sue, 2015), there is an emerging body of literature in which cultural adaptations of accepted EBTs are assessed. Some examples are presented next.

7.4.1 Cultural Adaptation of EBTs with African Americans

Calls to infuse EBTs with Afrocentric elements have been made by a number of authors (e.g., Cunningham, Foster, & Warner, 2010; Gilbert, Harvey, & Belgrave, 2009). These cultural elements include interdependence, collectivism, transformation, and spirituality. To start, Longshore and Grills (2000) tested the effectiveness of a cultural adaptation of motivational interviewing in a rare random sample field study comprised of 364 African American individuals who abused substances recruited from various settings. Participants were randomly divided between a control group (traditional motivational techniques were used) and an intervention group (counseling congruent with the cultural values of communalism and group process). The single intake and counseling session for both groups lasted, on average, more than 2 h. In the intervention condition, drug use was framed as a personal and community problem rooted in cultural and power inequalities between the African American and the dominant communities. In addition, the individual's life experiences, including as an African American, were discussed. Change was encouraged not only as beneficial for the person alone but also for the community. The peer shared personal experiences which was intended to show that recovery was possible. In addition, a video was used in order to help the participant to acknowledge the consequences of use for themselves and others on an emotional level (Longshore & Grills, 2000). The authors reported a significant difference in drug use at 1-year follow-up between those in the culturally adapted intervention (54.3%) and those in the control group (70.5%). This finding is remarkable in light of the fact that others have found African Americans who participated in an unadapted motivational enhancement program for substance use to report an *increase* in drug use after treatment (Montgomery, Burlew, Kosinski, & Forcehimes, 2011).

7.4.2 Cultural Adaptations of EBTs with Latinos

Adaptations targeting Latinxs center on the inclusion of discussions relevant to this particular group and the particular values are emphasized. Lee et al. (2011) utilized a culturally adapted version of motivational interviewing in a pilot study that included 25 community participants who were Latinx and met criteria for heavy drinking. Their adaptations included discussions of the participants' specific social context, the impact of their drinking on their families, engaging support networks to help change their drinking habits, and providing information about the health impact of drinking. While Lee et al. (2011) did not assess actual change in drinking patterns, they noted that participants reported an appreciation of cultural discussions as part of the program and that the intervention was helpful.

Burrow-Sanchez and Wrona (2012) assessed the effectiveness of a manualized adapted cognitive behavioral program for adolescents with substance use issues. Both the control and intervention groups, each with 19 participants, took part in a 12-week group-based treatment program. The manual used with the intervention group contained an additional module in which ethnic identity and adjustment were addressed. The remaining modules were modified in order to be more culturally congruent. In addition, therapists increased their contact with the participants' parents. The authors reported that participants in the adapted condition reported lower rates of substance use compared to the control group, especially participants who had higher levels of ethnic identity and focus on their family. Burrow-Sanchez and Wrona (2012) also noted high rates of retention in their samples, which they attributed to their therapists' ability to address participants in their preferred language (English) as well as the parents' (Spanish).

7.4.3 Cultural Adaptations of EBTs with Asian Americans

Pan, Huey, and Hernandez (2011) tested a culturally adapted, one-session treatment method for phobias with a sample of East Asian participants. Their study compared this method with a standard one-session treatment and a group who used self-help techniques. The cultural adaptations they implemented included addressing issues of acculturation, how the problem was conceptualized, normalization of the program, emphasis on confidentiality, emphasizing and facilitating emotional control, taking advantage of participants' view of the therapist as an authority figure, and using extensive psychoeducation (Pan et al., 2011). Although their samples were small (culturally adapted treatment, standard treatment, and self-help), these authors reported that the culturally adapted treatment was more effective than the other two methods both at posttreatment and at a 6-month follow-up, particularly for less acculturated participants, for general fear, and for catastrophic thinking. Moreover, they found that the cultural elements, along with the therapeutic alliance, were predictive of positive treatment outcomes.

7.4.4 Cultural Adaptations of EBTs with Native Americans

Venner et al. (2016) adapted two EBTs to use for substance abuse treatment for American Indians from a Southwest tribe. They adapted motivational interviewing and a community reinforcement approach to include culturally appropriate greetings and introductions that incorporated spirituality in social interactions. Additionally, conversations about how the counselor and the client could be connected by clan and use of spirituality if appropriate and of kinship relationships to increase motivation for change were included. Moreover, the treatment team included two American Indian counselors that were fluent in their native language, which they could use with participants who spoke it. In this pilot study involving 8 individuals who participated in 16–20 individual sessions, Venner and her colleagues found significant increases in percent days of abstinence at an 8-month follow-up and suggested that cultural adaptations could be helpful in the treatment of substance use issues among American Indians.

7.4.5 EBTs with Lesbian, Gay, Bisexual, Transgender, and Queer Individuals

Cognitive behavioral treatments are becoming available for adult LGBTQ individuals (e.g., Panchankis, Hatzenbuehler, Rendina, Safren, & Parsons, 2015) and adolescents (Craig & Austin, 2016). These approaches aim to affirm sexual and gender minorities' identities and increase their ability to cope with identity-related stress (e.g., external and internalized homophobia and rejection). Both in individual

(Panchankis et al., 2015) and in group formats (Craig & Austin, 2016), these methods have been effective in improving psychological functioning and coping and decreasing depressive symptoms (for both adult and adolescents), alcohol use, and sexually risky behaviors.

7.4.6 EBTs and Socioeconomic Status (SES)

Low socioeconomic status is related to poor psychiatric health (e.g., Martin-Carrasco et al., 2016); however, those researching evidence-based clinical treatments rarely take socioeconomic status into account. For example, Callahan, Heath, Aubuchon-Endsley, Collins, and Herbert (2013) found that only 1.2% of 338 empirical articles assess treatment efficacy and SES. Nonetheless, low-SES participants show improvement from evidence-based treatment (Santiago, Kaltman, & Miranda, 2013). Low-SES women have been found to benefit from treatment for depression (e.g., Miranda et al., 2006) and panic disorder (e.g., Roy-Byrne et al., 2006). However, this has not been found for types of interventions such as smoking cessation, given environmental challenges like higher stress levels, dependence, and exposure to other smokers (Sheffer et al., 2012). Moreover, low-SES participants have been found to drop out of treatment prematurely (DeRubeis et al., 2005; Miranda et al., 2006).

7.5 Adapting EBTs for Use with Diverse Clients in Forensic or Correctional Settings

Morales and Norcross (2010) expanded on the APA's (2006) definition of EBTs, presented earlier in this chapter, by explaining,

> ... By definition, the wholesale imposition of research without attending to the clinician or patient is *not* EBT, conversely, the indiscriminate disregard of available research is *not* EBT. Second, the definition requires integrating these three evidentiary sources [research, clinical expertise, and patient characteristics, culture, and preferences]. The integration flows seamlessly and uncontested when the three evidentiary sources agree; the integration becomes flawed and contested when the three sources disagree. Third, not all three pillars are equal: Research assumes priority in EBT. Clinicians begin with research and then integrate it with their expertise and patient's values. Fourth, patient assumes a more active, prominent position in that 'patient values' were elevated to 'patient characteristics, culture, and preferences.' The APA definition deliberately invoked cultural sensitivity. Put bluntly, clinical practice without attending to culture cannot be characterized as EBT. (emphasis in the original, p. 824)

Morales and Norcross (2010) also stressed the need to balance fidelity with EBT methods and fit with the client(s) at hand. The clinician must first rely on the EBT and then on research that addresses cultural adaptation of an EBT with a particular population. Next, clinicians need to assess whether or not their client(s) would fit the characteristics of participants in such research. Finally, clinicians need to determine if there is a need to abandon the EBT if their client(s) do not improve, seems to be deteriorating, threatens to drop out of treatment, refuses to continue, or insists on a different approach (Norcross, Beutler, & Levant, 2006).

While cultural adaptions of EBTs have been found to be a moderately strong benefit (Griner & Smith, 2006), no such research is available with respect to forensic or correctional populations. Without such literature, recommendations with respect to how to apply EBTs with diverse populations in forensic or correctional settings are somewhat tentative. Nonetheless, based on the available literature, as presented above, we can offer that treatment of diverse individuals, whether in individual or group formats, could and should be made more relevant and effective with those populations.

Increasing Multicultural Competence/Sensitivity As mental health professionals, we first need to acknowledge our need to improve how sensitive we are with respect to cultural issues, to strive to identify our biases, and to work on keeping them in check. This is a consistent task, since we are all subject to unconscious biases and therefore are likely to commit microaggressions on others (Sue & Sue, 2015). Consequently, as Sue and Sue recommended, we need to become more aware of ourselves, more knowledgeable of those we treat, and more skilled in developing and implementing culturally appropriate interventions. Such endeavor requires us to engage in long-term efforts to gain more competence/sensitivity through increased connections with individuals different from ourselves. We also need to familiarize ourselves with cultures different from ours through various media (literature, nonfiction, films, etc.) and participation in continuing education programs that address cultural and diversity issues. Finally, we need to pay particular attention to learning and interacting with groups with whom we are the most uncomfortable doing so.

Focusing on the Therapeutic Relationships Whether in individual or group counseling, we need to focus on developing and maintaining strong relationships with our clients. That means we must be able to connect with our clients based on their cultural context. Given long histories of oppression and mistrust, establishing rapport and developing a therapeutic relationship may take longer with clients different from ourselves, especially when we are members of the cultural majority and they are not (Sue & Sue, 2015). These authors also recommend that cultural differences between clinicians and clients must be addressed before treatment begins in order to acknowledge those differences. Clinicians then should assess the level of comfort of the client and create a safe space in which the client and the clinician will be willing to consider and address cultural issues in treatment. In group counseling, cohesion is built by encouraging group members to share information with others and to highlight similarities in order to facilitate connections within the group (Yalom & Leszcz, 2008). We also need to be painfully aware when we affect the therapeutic relationship with microaggressions or other slights and when group cohesion is lost (e.g., through breaches of confidentiality, conflict, etc.). We need to acknowledge these events and take steps to rebuild the alliance or group cohesion (Safran et al., 2011; Yalom & Leszcz, 2008).

Incorporating Cultural Elements into Treatment as Needed The studies on cultural adaptations of EBTs presented in this chapter have a number of features in common. First, all were respectful, accepting, and affirming of the participants' identities, whether based on ethnicity (Venner et al., 2016) or sexual orientation (Panchankis et al., 2015). It is of utmost importance to treat clients with respect and as people with an inherent value, particularly in forensic and correctional settings where the person's sense of worth can be diminished. Second, we need to follow our clients' lead with respect to how much cultural adaptation should be implemented in the EBT being used. We cannot assume our clients' needs in this respect, and we should seek their input, otherwise we could risk having our efforts become microaggressions (e.g., assuming that Latinx or African American clients will want to incorporate religion into treatment or that Latinx will speak Spanish and will need treatment in that language). Third, we should consult with our clients, other professionals, or community organizations with respect to what cultural elements could, or should be, included in treatment. Fourth, we need to be open to our clients' need to incorporate elements of their culture into treatment (e.g., Latino men shaking hands with the therapist when greeting them, which is a sign of respect, or using religious or spiritual elements in treatment).

On the other hand, we also need to be aware of instances in which our clients' cultural values need to be explored and challenged, as in the case of immigrant offenders who committed sex crimes who may rationalize offenses against young teenagers as being normative in their country of origin. We would recommend exploring those norms and providing clients with psychoeducation in order to encourage change while not holding the individual person responsible for their cultural values.

7.6 Conclusions

The time has come for mental health professionals to utilize EBTs and to take cultural issues into careful consideration (APA, 2017, 2006). Given the overrepresentation of ethnic and sexual minorities in forensic and correctional setting (Meyer et al., 2017; Miller, 2010) and their considerable mental health needs (e.g., Fuehrlein, Jha, Brenner, & North, 2014), it is imperative that mental health professionals in those settings work to increase their multicultural competence and sensitivity. Sue and Sue (2015), as well as the American Psychological Association (2017), have developed frameworks professionals can use to achieve that goal. Working with diverse clients in forensic or correctional settings requires that professionals strive to develop strong therapeutic relationships with diverse clients under difficult circumstances, to implement EBTs in those settings, and to incorporate cultural elements or adaptations in those EBTs in order to maximize the success of treatment.

References

Ackerman, S. J., & Hilsenroth, M. J. (2003). A review of therapist characteristics and techniques positively impacting the therapeutic alliance. *Clinical Psychology Review, 23*(1), 1–33. https://doi.org/10.1016/S0272-7358(02)00146-0

American Psychiatric Association. (2016). *Psychiatric services in correctional facilities* (3rd ed.). Arlington, VA: American Psychiatric Association.

American Psychological Association. (2015). *Demographics of the U.S. psychology workforce: Findings from the American Community Survey*. Washington, DC: Author.

American Psychological Association. (2017). *Multicultural guidelines: An ecological approach to context, identity, and intersectionality*. Retrieved from http://www.apa.org/about/policy/multicultural-guidelines.aspx

American Psychological Association, Presidential Task Force on Evidence-Based Practice. (2006). Evidence-based practice in psychology. *American Psychologist, 61*(4), 271–285. https://doi.org/10.1037/0003-066X.61.4.271

Anglin, D. M., Link, B. G., & Phelan, J. C. (2006). Racial differences in stigmatizing attitudes toward people with mental illness. *Psychiatric Services, 57*(6), 857–862. https://doi.org/10.1176/ps.2006.57.6.857

Bernal, G., & Adames, C. (2017). Cultural adaptations: Conceptual, ethical, contextual, and methodological issues for working with ethnocultural and majority-world populations. *Prevention Science, 18*(6), 681–688. https://doi.org/10.1007/s11121-017-0806-0

Bernal, G., & Sáez-Santiago, E. (2006). Culturally centered psychosocial interventions. *Journal of Community Psychology, 34*(2), 121–132. https://doi.org/10.1002/jcop.20096

Bronfenbrenner, U. (1977). Toward an experimental ecology of human development. *American Psychologist, 32*(7), 513–531. https://doi.org/10.1037/0003-066X.32.7.513

Burlingame, G. M., Fuhriman, A., & Johnson, J. (2002). Cohesion in group psychotherapy. In J. C. Norcross (Ed.), *Psychotherapy relationships that work* (pp. 71–87). New York, NY: Oxford University Press.

Burlingame, G. M., McClendon, D. T., & Alonso, J. (2011). Cohesion in group psychotherapy. In J. C. Norcross (Ed.), *Psychotherapy relationships that work: Evidence-based responsiveness* (2nd ed., pp. 110–131). New York, NY: Oxford University Press.

Burrow-Sanchez, J. J., & Wrona, M. (2012). Comparing culturally accommodated versus standard group CBT for Latino adolescents with substance use disorders: A pilot study. *Cultural Diversity and Ethnic Minority Psychology, 18*(4), 373–383. https://doi.org/10.1037/a0029439

Callahan, J. L., Heath, C. J., Aubuchon-Endsley, N. L., Collins, F. J., & Herbert, G. L. (2013). Enhancing information pertaining to client characteristics to facilitate evidence-based practice. *Journal of Clinical Psychology, 69*(12), 1239–1249. https://doi.org/10.1002/jclp.21995

Comas-Díaz, L. (2006). Cultural variation in the therapeutic relationship. In C. D. Goodheart, A. E. Kazdin, & R. J. Sternberg (Eds.), *Evidence-based psychotherapy: Where practice and research meet* (pp. 81–105). Washington, DC: American Psychological Association.

Constantine, M. G. (2007). Racial microaggressions against African American clients in cross-racial counseling relationships. *Journal of Counseling Psychology, 54*(1), 1–16. https://doi.org/10.1037/0022-0167.54.1.1

Craig, S. L., & Austin, A. (2016). The AFFIRM open pilot feasibility study: A brief affirmative cognitive behavioral coping skills group intervention for sexual and gender minority youth. *Children and Youth Services Review, 64*, 136–144. https://doi.org/10.1016/j.childyouth.2016.02.022

Croteau, J. M., & Constantine, M. G. (2005). Race and sexual orientation in multicultural counseling. In J. M. Croteau, J. S. Lark, M. A. Lidderdale, & Y. B. Chung (Eds.), *Deconstructing heterosexism in the counseling professions* (pp. 159–185). Thousand Oaks, CA: Sage.

Cunningham, P. B., Foster, S. L., & Warner, S. E. (2010). Culturally relevant family-based treatment for adolescent delinquency and substance abuse: Understanding within-session processes. *Journal of Clinical Psychology, 66*(8), 830–846. https://doi.org/10.1002/jclp.20709

DataUSA. (n.d.). Retrieved from https://datausa.io/profile/cip/511508/?compare=440701

DeRubeis, R. J., Hollon, S. D., Amsterdam, J. D., Shelton, R. C., Young, P. R., Salomon, R. M., ... Gallop, R. (2005). Cognitive therapy vs medications in the treatment of moderate to severe depression. *Archives of General Psychiatry, 62*(4), 409–416. https://doi.org/10.1001/archpsyc.62.4.409

Diamond, P. M., Magaletta, P. R., Harzke, A. J., & Baxter, J. (2008). Who requests psychological services upon admission to prison? *Psychological Services, 5*(2), 97–107. https://doi.org/10.1037/1541-1559.5.2.97

Diamond, P. M., Wang, E. W., Holzer, C. E., Thomas, C., & Cruser, D. A. (2001). The prevalence of mental illness in prison. *Administration and Policy in Mental Health and Mental Health Services Research, 29*(1), 21–40. https://doi.org/10.1023/A:1013164814732

Durrah, D. A. (2013). *Understanding African American male inmates' decisions to seek mental health treatment while incarcerate* (Unpublished doctoral dissertation). Marquette University, Milwaukee, Wisconsin. Retrieved from https://epublications.marquette.edu/dissertations_mu/300/

Elliot, R., Bohart, A. C., Watson, J. C., & Greenberg, L. S. (2011). Empathy. In J. C. Norcross (Ed.), *Psychotherapy relationships that work: Evidence-based responsiveness* (2nd ed., pp. 132–152). New York, NY: Oxford University Press.

Farber, B. A., & Doolin, E. M. (2011). Positive regard and affirmation. In J. C. Norcross (Ed.), *Psychotherapy relationships that work: Evidence-based responsiveness* (2nd ed., pp. 168–186). New York, NY: Oxford University Press.

Fuehrlein, B. S., Jha, M. K., Brenner, A. M., & North, C. S. (2014). Availability and attitudes toward correctional psychiatry training: Results of a national survey of training directors. *Journal of Behavioral Health Services and Research, 41*(2), 244–250. https://doi.org/10.1007/s11414-013-9336-0

Gilbert, D. J., Harvey, A. R., & Belgrave, F. Z. (2009). Advancing the Africentric paradigm shift discourse: Building toward evidence-based Africentric interventions in social work practice with African Americans. *Social Work, 54*(3), 243–252. https://doi.org/10.1093/sw/54.3.243

Gramlich, J. (2018, January 12). The gap between the number of blacks and whites in prison is shrinking. *Pew Research Center*. Retrieved from http://www.pewresearch.org/fact-tank/2018/01/12/shrinking-gap-between-number-of-blacks-and-whites-in-prison/

Griner, D., & Smith, T. B. (2006). Culturally adapted mental health interventions: A meta-analytic review. *Psychotherapy: Theory, Research, Practice, Training, 43*(4), 531–548. https://doi.org/10.1037/0033-3204.43.4.531

Hamm, M. S. (2009). Prison Islam in the age of sacred terror. *British Journal of Criminology, 49*(5), 667–685. https://doi.org/10.1093/bjc/azp035

Hegarty, P. (2018). *A recent history of lesbian and gay psychology: From homophobia to LGBT*. New York, NY: Routledge.

Hicks, J. W. (2004). Ethnicity, race, and forensic psychiatry: Are we color-blind? *Journal of the American Academy of Psychiatry and the Law Online, 32*(1), 21–33. Retrieved from http://jaapl.org/content/32/1/21.long

Hook, J. N., Farrell, J. E., Davis, D. E., DeBlaere, C., Van Tongeren, D. R., & Utsey, S. O. (2016). Cultural humility and racial microaggressions in counseling. *Journal of Counseling Psychology, 63*(3), 269–277. https://doi.org/10.1037/cou0000114

Kolden, G. G., Klein, M. H., Wang, C.-C., & Austin, S. B. (2011). Congruence/genuineness. In J. C. Norcross (Ed.), *Psychotherapy relationships that work: Evidence-based responsiveness* (2nd ed., pp. 187–202). New York, NY: Oxford University Press.

Kras, K. R., Pleggenkuhle, B., & Huebner, M. B. (2016). A new way of doing time on the outside: Sex offenders' pathways in and out of a transitional housing facility. *International Journal of Offender Therapy and Comparative Criminology, 60*(5), 512–534. https://doi.org/10.1177/0306624X14554194

Lee, C. S., López, S. R., Hernández, L., Colby, S. M., Caetano, R., Borrelli, B., & Rohsenow, D. (2011). A cultural adaptation of motivational interviewing to address heavy drinking among

Hispanics. *Cultural Diversity and Ethnic Minority Psychology, 17*(3), 317–324. https://doi.org/10.1037/a0024035

Longshore, D., & Grills, C. (2000). Motivating illegal drug use recovery: Evidence for a culturally congruent intervention. *Journal of Black Psychology, 26*(3), 288–301. https://doi.org/10.1177/0095798400026003002

Martin-Carrasco, M., Evans-Lacko, S., Dom, G., Christodoulou, N. G., Samochowiec, J., González-Fraile, E., … Wasserman, D. (2016). EPA guidance on mental health and economic crises in Europe. *European Archives of Psychiatry and Clinical Neuroscience, 266*(2), 89–124. https://doi.org/10.1007/s00406-016-0681-x

Maura, J., & Weisman de Mamani, A. (2017). Mental health disparities, treatment engagement, and attrition among racial/ethnic minorities with severe mental illness: A review. *Journal of Clinical Psychology in Medical Settings, 24*(3-4), 187–210. https://doi.org/10.1007/s10880-017-9510-2

Meyer, I. H., Flores, A. R., Stemple, L., Romero, A. P., Wilson, B. D. M., & Herman, J. L. (2017). Incarceration rates and traits of sexual minorities in the United States: National inmate survey, 2011–2012. *American Journal of Public Health, 107*(2), 267–273. https://doi.org/10.2105/AJPH.2016.303576

Miller, L. L. (2010). The invisible black victim: How American federalism perpetuates racial inequality in the criminal justice system. *Law and Society Review, 44*(3-4), 805–842. https://doi.org/10.1111/j.1540-5893.2010.00423.x

Miranda, J., Green, B. L., Krupnick, J. L., Chung, J., Siddique, J., Belin, T., & Revicki, D. (2006). One-year outcomes of a randomized clinical trial treating depression in low-income minority women. *Journal of Consulting and Clinical Psychology, 74*(1), 99–111. https://doi.org/10.1037/0022-006X.74.1.99

Montgomery, L., Burlew, A. K., Kosinski, A. S., & Forcehimes, A. A. (2011). Motivational enhancement therapy for African American substance users: A randomized clinical trial. *Cultural Diversity and Ethnic Minority Psychology, 17*(4), 357–365. https://doi.org/10.1037/a0025437

Morales, E., & Norcross, J. C. (2010). Evidence-based practices with ethnic minorities: Strange bedfellow no more. *Journal of Clinical Psychology, 66*(8), 821–829. https://doi.org/10.1002/jclp.20712

Nelson, D. W., & Baumgarte, R. (2004). Cross-cultural misunderstandings reduce empathic responding. *Journal of Applied Social Psychology, 34*(2), 391–401. https://doi.org/10.1111/j.1559-1816.2004.tb02553.x

Norcross, J. C., Beutler, L. E., & Levant, R. F. (Eds.). (2006). *Evidence-based practices in mental health: Debate and dialogue on the fundamental questions*. Washington, DC: American Psychological Association.

Norcross, J. C., & Lambert, M. J. (2011). Evidence-based therapeutic relationships. In J. C. Norcross (Ed.), *Psychotherapy relationships that work: Evidence-based responsiveness* (2nd ed., pp. 3–21). New York, NY: Oxford University Press.

Orlinsky, D. E., Ronnestad, M. H., & Willutzki, U. (2004). Fifty years of psychotherapy process-outcome research: Continuity and change. In M. J. Lambert (Ed.), *Bergin and Garfield's handbook of psychotherapy and behavioral change* (5th ed., pp. 307–390). New York, NY: Wiley.

Owen, J., Tao, K. W., Imel, Z. E., Wampold, B. E., & Rodolfa, E. (2014). Addressing racial and ethnic microaggressions in therapy. *Professional Psychology: Research and Practice, 45*(4), 283–290. https://doi.org/10.1037/a0037420

Pan, D., Huey, S. J., & Hernandez, D. (2011). Culturally-adapted versus standard exposure treatment for phobic Asian Americans: Treatment efficacy, moderators, and predictors. *Cultural Diversity and Ethnic Minority Psychology, 17*(1), 11–22. https://doi.org/10.1037/a0022534

Panchankis, J. E., Hatzenbuehler, M. L., Rendina, H. J., Safren, S. A., & Parsons, J. T. (2015). LGB-affirmative cognitive-behavioral therapy for young adult gay and bisexual men: A randomized controlled trial of a transdiagnostic minority stress approach. *Journal of Consulting and Clinical Psychology, 83*(5), 875–889. https://doi.org/10.1037/ccp0000037

Pérez Foster, R. (1998). The clinician's cultural countertransference: The psychodynamics of culturally competent practice. *Clinical Social Work Journal, 26*(3), 253–270. https://doi.org/10.1023/A:1022867910329
Rogers, C. R. (1957). The necessary and sufficient conditions of therapeutic personality change. *Journal of Consulting Psychology, 21*(2), 95–103. https://doi.org/10.1037/h0045357
Roy-Byrne, P., Sherbourne, C., Miranda, J., Stein, M., Craske, M., Golinelli, D., & Sullivan, G. (2006). Poverty and response to treatment among panic disorder patients in primary care. *The American Journal of Psychiatry, 163*(8), 1419–1425. https://doi.org/10.1176/ajp.2006.163.8.1419
Ruth, T., Matusitz, J., & Simi, D. (2017). Ethics of disenfranchisement and voting rights in the U.S.: Convicted felons, the homeless, and immigrants. *American Journal of Criminal Justice, 42*(1), 56–68. https://doi.org/10.1007/s12103-016-9346-6
Safran, J. D., Muran, J. C., & Eubanks-Carter, C. (2011). Repairing alliance ruptures. In J. C. Norcross (Ed.), *Psychotherapy relationships that work: Evidence-based responsiveness* (2nd ed., pp. 224–238). New York, NY: Oxford University Press.
Santiago, C. D., Kaltman, S., & Miranda, J. (2013). Poverty and mental health: How do low-income adults and children fare in psychotherapy? *Journal of Clinical Psychology, 69*(2), 115–126. https://doi.org/10.1002/jclp.21951
Serran, G. A., & Marshall, W. L. (2010). Therapeutic process in the treatment of sexual offenders: A review article. *The British Journal of Forensic Practice, 12*(3), 4–16. https://doi.org/10.5042/bjfp.2010.0421
Sheffer, C. E., Stitzer, M., Landes, R., Brackman, S. L., Munn, T., & Moore, P. (2012). Socioeconomic disparities in community-based treatment of tobacco dependence. *American Journal of Public Health, 102*(3), e8–e16. https://doi.org/10.2105/AJPH.2011.300519
Shelton, K., & Delgado-Romero, E. A. (2013). Sexual orientation microaggressions: The experience of lesbian, gay, bisexual, and queer clients in psychotherapy. *Psychology of Sexual Orientation and Gender Diversity, 1*(S), 59–70. https://doi.org/10.1037/2329-0382.1.S.59
Shiva, A., Haden, S. C., & Brooks, J. (2009). Psychiatric civil and forensic inpatient satisfaction with care: The impact of provider and recipient characteristics. *Social Psychiatry and Psychiatric Epidemiology, 44*, 979–987. https://doi.org/10.1007/s00127-009-0019-3
Solinas-Saunders, M., Stacer, M. J., & Guy, R. (2015). Ex-offender barriers to employment: Racial disparities in labor markets with asymmetric information. *Journal of Crime and Justice, 38*(2), 249–269. https://doi.org/10.1080/0735648X.2013.870492
Sue, D. W. (2015). Therapeutic harm and cultural oppression. *The Counseling Psychologist, 43*(3), 359–369. https://doi.org/10.1177/0011000014565713
Sue, D. W., & Sue, D. (2015). *Counseling the culturally diverse: Theory and practice* (7th ed.). Hoboken, NJ: Wiley.
Sue, S., Zane, N., Nagayama-Hall, G. C., & Berger, L. K. (2009). The case of cultural competency in psychotherapeutic intervention. *Annual Review of Psychology, 60*, 525–548. https://doi.org/10.1146/annurev.psych.60.110707.163651
Tao, K. W., Owen, J., Pace, B. T., & Imel, Z. E. (2015). A meta-analysis of multicultural competencies and psychotherapy process and outcome. *Journal of Counseling Psychology, 62*(3), 337–350. https://doi.org/10.1037/cou0000086
Vasquez, M. J. T. (2007). Cultural difference and the therapeutic alliance: An evidence-based analysis. *American Psychologist, 62*(8), 878–885. https://doi.org/10.1037/0003-066X.62.8.878
Velez, B. L., Moradi, B., & DeBlaere, C. (2015). Multiple oppressions and the mental health of sexual minority Latina/o individuals. *The Counseling Psychologist, 43*(1), 7–38. https://doi.org/10.1177/0011000014542836
Venner, K. L., Greenfield, B. L., Hagler, K. J., Simmons, J., Luppe, D., Homer, E., ... Smith, J. E. (2016). Pilot outcome results of culturally adapted evidence-based substance use disorder treatment with a Southwest Tribe. *Addictive Behaviors Reports, 3*, 21–27. https://doi.org/10.1016/j.abrep.2015.11.002

Wendt, D. C., Gone, J. P., & Nagata, D. K. (2015). Potentially harmful therapy and multicultural counseling: Bridging two disciplinary discourses. *The Counseling Psychologist, 43*(3), 334–358. https://doi.org/10.1177/0011000014548280

Whitman, C. N. (2017). Transgender criminal justice: Ethical and constitutional perspectives. *Ethics & Behavior, 27*(6), 445–457. https://doi.org/10.1080/10508422.2016.1183490

Yalom, I. D., & Leszcz, M. (2008). *The theory and practice of group psychotherapy* (5th ed.). New York, NY: Basic Books.

Part III
Adaptation of Evidence Based Treatment to Corrections

Chapter 8
Adapting Dialectical Behavior Therapy for Use in Correctional Settings

Michele Galietta

8.1 Introduction

Over two million people are currently incarcerated in the United States (Wagner & Sawyer, 2018). Many of these individuals have been diagnosed with mental illnesses or will develop mental illnesses while incarcerated. Studies have consistently demonstrated high rates of mental illness in the correctional samples (e.g., Fazel, Hayes, Bartellas, Clerici, & Trestman, 2016; Fazel & Seewald, 2012). Of all the mental disorders affecting incarcerated individuals, borderline personality disorder has been noted to be one of the most prevalent and the most problematic for systems (Trestman, 2000).

For years, advocates and correctional administrators alike have argued that correctional environments are not appropriate for many individuals with mental illness. Jamie Fellner (2004), former Senior Advisor for US Human Rights Watch, explained:

> It is rare to find police, sheriffs, prosecutors, defense attorneys, judges, prison officials and human rights activists all on the same page. But across the criminal justice spectrum there is a striking consensus that something has gone painfully awry: the nation's jails and prisons have become mental health facilities—a role for which they are singularly ill equipped. (para. 1)

However, despite diversion programs, specialty courts and the like, the number of incarcerated individuals with serious mental illness continues to remain high. In fact, the largest mental health facilities in the United States today are jails (see Ford, 2015). High numbers of mentally ill individuals, combined with the fact that jails and prisons are often under-resourced and underprepared to provide comprehensive treatment, have resulted in systems that tend to be more responsive to crises than proactive with regard to treatment. Perhaps the group most negatively affected by

M. Galietta (✉)
John Jay College of Criminal Justice, New York, NY, USA
e-mail: mgalietta@jjay.cuny.edu

E. L. Jeglic, C. Calkins (eds.), *New Frontiers in Offender Treatment*,
https://doi.org/10.1007/978-3-030-01030-0_8

this predicament are individuals who exhibit symptoms of BPD. In many cases, policies designed to manage crises, in the absence of effective concomitant treatment, actually make such individuals sicker. Problems like suicidality and intentional self-harm create ethical and pragmatic dilemmas that overwhelm many correctional environments. Thus, effective treatments, particularly those that target suicide and self-harm are critical.

Dialectical behavior therapy (DBT) is a cognitive behavioral therapy originally developed to treat individuals with chronic suicidal behavior in an outpatient setting (Linehan, 1993). With over 40 randomized controlled trials, the treatment has considerable empirical support (Linehan, 2013). DBT is a third-wave behavioral therapy that combines eastern principles of mindfulness and standard cognitive and behavioral techniques within a dialectical framework. The term dialectics describes "a method of examining and discussing opposing ideas in order to find the truth" (Merriam-Webster's Dictionary, 2018). One of the functions of dialectics in DBT is to balance and synthesize behaviorism (which is rigid, structured, and change-oriented) with Zen principles (which stress acceptance, validation, and flexibility). DBT is a comprehensive treatment that includes four primary components that each fulfill an important function in the treatment: (1) individual therapy motivates clients; (2) group skills training enhances the capabilities of clients; (3) coaching works to generalize skills in service of solving problems in the client's life; and (4) a weekly consultation meeting for therapists designed to enhance the skills of therapists and maintain their motivation to work with challenging clients. DBT in residential settings adds components that serve to structure the environment so that treatment is possible (Swenson, Sanderson, Dulit, & Linehan, 2001).

DBT was originally designed to treat very high-risk individuals who, at the time, had extremely poor prognoses. Patients in the original DBT trial had numerous diagnoses, but all met criteria for borderline personality disorder (BPD) and had recent suicidal behaviors (Linehan, Armstrong, Suarez, Allmon, & Heard, 1991). Because of its unprecedented success with that complex and multi-diagnostic group, DBT was quickly adapted for other challenging patient populations. An inpatient hospital adaptation was developed (Swenson et al., 2001), as well as one for forensic hospitals (McCann, Ball, & Ivanoff, 2000). More recently, there has been a surge of interest in the application of DBT to correctional settings (Douglas, Nicholls, & Brink, 2017). This chapter will begin with a rationale for applying DBT to patients in correctional environments. Next, a review of the literature on DBT in correctional settings will be presented. A thorough description of standard DBT will be followed by recommended adaptations for use in correctional environments.

8.2 Why Correctional DBT?

Among many reasons why DBT is an appealing approach for correctional environments is its emphasis on resolving tensions between conflicting positions. The priorities and obligations of those in correctional leadership are often at odds with mental health professionals working in the same facilities. Multiple conflicts arise as correctional professionals strive to maintain safety and mental health professionals attempt to provide therapeutic treatment. DBT provides an effective framework to resolve conflicts around security and treatment and to foster collaborative relationships among those who work within correctional environments.

8.2.1 Compatibility with Existing Models of Correctional Treatment

The most widely researched and accepted model for the treatment of offenders is the risk-needs-responsivity (RNR) model developed by Andrews et al. (1990). The authors identified principles of effective treatment empirically from their landmark meta-analysis of offender treatment (see Chap. 2). The first principle, *risk*, stipulates that individuals with the greatest risk receive the highest intensity of services. Several programs have adjusted the intensity of DBT to the level of risk (Blanchette, Flight, Verbrugge, Gobeil, & Taylor, 2011; Ferreira, 2012). Moreover, because DBT uses an individualized case formulation that prioritizes treatment targets based on risk, multiple ancillary treatment components can be added for high-risk clients. This also meets the *needs* principle particularly well, as intervention strategies are tailored to address specific factors maintaining violence and criminality for each client. DBT skills can theoretically be provided in modular form, with targeted elements differentially applied to categories of offenders (e.g., those with poor controls vs. those with cold, callous traits). Finally, DBT is strong in terms of its *responsivity* to individual differences in clients. DBT employs a host of motivational strategies and a variety of CBT tools that may be tailored to meet the particular interests, learning styles, and strengths of any client. Skills may be delivered individually or in groups and have been successfully adapted for individuals with significant cognitive impairment (Brown, Brown, & Dibiasio, 2013; Sakdalan, Shaw, & Collier, 2010). Thus, DBT aligns well with all of the RNR principles.

A second model gaining traction in offender treatment is the Good Lives Model (GLM; Ward, Yates, & Willis, 2012) (see Chap. 3). Ward developed the GLM in response to criticisms of the RNR approach (Ward, Melser, & Yates, 2007). They described the RNR approach as "theoretically impoverished" (Ward et al., 2007, p. 210) and argued that its narrow focus on risk neglects motivational, personal, and relationship factors relevant to therapeutic alliance and treatment success. Ward has described the GLM as, "a strengths-based rehabilitation theory that aims to equip clients with internal and external resources to live a good or better life—a life that is socially acceptable and personally meaningful" (Ward et al., 2012, p. 95). This model conceptualizes criminogenic needs (i.e., dynamic risk factors) as barriers toward living a good life (Ward et al., 2012). They argue that attending to RNR principles is "*necessary* but insufficient for successful rehabilitation" (Ward et al., 2007, p. 210.).

DBT was one of the first treatments to conceptualize motivational deficits as a target of treatment. DBT utilizes validation and commitment strategies to engage clients in the beginning and throughout the course of treatment. In DBT, each client identifies their "life worth living." Primary treatment targets are conceptualized as obstacles to obtaining the client's life worth living or as new, adaptive behaviors necessary for achieving a life worth living. There are many principles in DBT that enable a therapist to connect to the whole client rather than simply address their psychopathology or offense history. This is extremely important in correctional settings, where people are classified and often housed according to their offense(s) or their psychopathology. As in GLM, the emphasis in correctional DBT is on creating a meaningful life that is incompatible with violence and criminality.

A third model that is well-established in community settings, but just beginning to shape correctional treatment, is trauma-informed care (TIC) (see Chap. 9). Miller and Najavits (2012) outlined important elements for trauma-informed correctional care (TICC). They discussed the need for effective interventions to address PTSD symptoms and recommended "present-focused, cognitive-behavioral, and coping skills treatments with strong educational components" (Miller & Najavits, 2012, p. 5).

Many problems in correctional environments (e.g., refusal to participate in pat downs) are related to trauma that has not been addressed. The biosocial theory in DBT provides a way for individuals to connect past trauma to their present situation and to present ineffective behaviors. The experience of trauma is validated in DBT by therapists explicitly in pretreatment and continually throughout treatment. In stage one DBT, trauma is addressed with psychoeducation and problem-solving around trauma-related problems (e.g., sleep, nightmares). Skills are taught that assist clients to distract from situations that cause distress (e.g. using *Wise Mind Accepts* to distract from unpleasant ruminations) as well as to accept painful realities (i.e., radical acceptance). Formal processing of trauma (using exposure) occurs only when skills have been established and crisis behaviors are under control. Thus, DBT, a present-focused type of CBT rich with skills education, aligns nicely with the aims of TICC (Miller & Najavits, 2012).

8.2.2 Ability to Address Most Serious Behavioral Issues

Of all mental disorders, personality disorders are among the most prevalent and problematic disorders in correctional samples (Trestman, 2000). Estimates of BPD in female prisoners range from 20% to 45% (Sansone & Sansone, 2009; Singleton, Meltzer, & Gatward, 1998), compared with 2% in the general public, and between 6% and 42% in clinical samples (Gunderson, Weinberg, & Choi-Kain, 2013). While women are diagnosed with BPD at far higher rates than men in clinical samples, males with BPD are overrepresented in correctional settings (Sansone & Sansone, 2009). Conn et al. (2010) reported rates of BPD in males between 23% and 31% across correctional samples, comparable to estimates in female correctional samples.

People with BPD utilize health services and emergency services at disproportionately higher rates compared to others (Gunderson et al., 2013). Prisoners with BPD have higher rates of suicide and self-harm and significant comorbidity with antisocial personality disorder (ASPD) (Black et al., 2007; Black, Gunter, Loveless, Allen, & Sieleni, 2010). There is a growing literature on emotional deficits in individuals with ASPD and those high in psychopathic traits (see Galietta, Fineran, Fava, & Rosenfeld, 2010; Raine & Yang, 2006; Skeem, Polaschek, Patrick, & Lilienfeld, 2011), suggesting similarities between BPD and ASPD.

Inmates with severe personality disorders have been noted to be among those most difficult to manage in correctional settings (Trestman, 2000). Such individuals often require enhanced watch status and extensive physical health interventions to correct self-harm and are often implicated in staff injuries and burnout. DBT was the first empirically supported treatment for BPD (Linehan et al., 1991) and remains the treatment with the largest body of scientific support for treating BPD (Gunderson et al., 2013).

DBT offers advocates a proactive, rather than a crisis-driven approach toward suicide and violence. Complex cases are formulated, and clients are offered consistent support to treat the underlying causes of problem behaviors. Rather than simply blocking or managing suicidal behaviors, the specific factors maintaining high-risk behaviors for each client are targeted in treatment. Ironically, while correctional systems have gotten better at assessing and managing suicidal behaviors, the techniques used to manage risk (e.g., one-to-one watch status) often unintentionally drive up suicidal threats and behaviors. High-risk clients in some settings dictate specific officers who will watch them, and administrators comply in order to avert crises. It is absolutely essential to screen for suicide and to keep individuals safe until risk subsides, but if underlying problems driving suicidality are not clinically addressed, such individuals often overburden systems. With regard to violence, many of the same patterns can be observed. The typical institutional response to violence is punitive segregation. Individuals with mental illnesses present unique ethical and practical challenges in this regard. Punitive segregation may in fact make comorbid individuals worse and increase the frequency and severity of violence. DBT has been shown to reduce anger and aggression (Douglas et al., 2017). When emotionally dysregulated, suicidal, and aggressive clients are effectively treated, costs in correctional systems go down (e.g., reduced overtime, reduced medical care costs, fewer staff injuries). When staff are provided with tools to effectively regulate such clients, staff injuries decrease (Galietta, Rosenfeld, & Ivanoff, 2003), and burnout decreases (McCann et al., 2000).

8.2.3 Decreasing Recidivism

Another reason to consider DBT is the possibility that treating emotion dysregulation will decrease recidivism. Rehabilitation is a stated goal of correctional institutions, though given the number of individuals with severe mental health needs in prison, proactive interventions to prevent future violence often give way to immediate, acuter behavioral problems. There is preliminary evidence that DBT reduces recidivism (Drake & Barnoski, 2006; Rosenfeld et al., 2007). Tomlinson (2018) compared DBT programs for offenders that used recidivism or reduction in risk for future offending as outcome measures. She concluded that programs that adapted content to target criminogenic needs, followed an RNR approach, and maintained higher fidelity to the treatment model produced the greatest reductions in recidivism and risk for future criminal behavior.

8.2.4 Human Rights Concerns

Finally, DBT has appeal because it is compassionate and addresses human rights concerns involved with detaining and isolating individuals in correctional environments. It has the capacity to address the most complex individuals in care, as well as to provide evidence-based intervention to those at risk for developing problems while incarcerated. The debate about where individuals who are mentally ill and violent belong has existed since the 1800s (Goodman, Page, & Phelps, 2017), and it will likely continue. However, as long as there are individuals with severe mental health needs in correctional institutions, an ethical obligation to treat them exists. It has been argued that the standard of care for treatment should be the same for incarcerated individuals as for those in the community (Fazel et al., 2016). Providing DBT treatment in corrections accomplishes this goal. For all these reasons, DBT seems a reasonable choice for correctional treatment.

8.3 Evidence Base for DBT in Corrections

While there is widespread agreement that the evidence base for DBT in general is very strong (Douglas et al., 2017; Gunderson et al., 2013; Linehan, 2013), research on the efficacy of DBT for corrections is growing but still limited. Conducting high-quality psychotherapy outcome studies in such settings is possible (Rosenfeld, Byars, & Galietta, 2011) but extremely challenging for a host of reasons. Not surprisingly, a number of studies that investigated forensic and correctional applications of DBT have suffered from significant methodological shortcomings including small sample size, the absence of random assignment, and designs that lack appropriate control or comparison groups. Despite these limitations, it is important to understand this body of research.

In 2004, Berzins and Trestman reviewed forensic and correctional applications of DBT and declared it a promising practice. In 2009, their group (Shelton, Sampl, Kesten, Zhang, & Trestman, 2009) published results of their trial of DBT-CM (an adapted version of DBT). They found significant reductions of aggression before and after treatment (Shelton et al., 2009). More recently, Frazier and Vela (2014) examined published 21 articles on the use of DBT for reducing anger or aggression. While many were pre-post designs, nine randomized control trials were reviewed. The authors concluded that DBT is an effective intervention for reducing aggression, even in some cases where it was significantly modified (Frazier & Vela, 2014).

However, not all modifications have been effective. Tomlinson (2018) identified 34 programs in Australia, Canada, Iran, New Zealand, the Netherlands, the United Kingdom, and the United States that employed DBT within forensic and correctional settings, comparing program elements and outcomes for each. Only 22 programs formally evaluated outcomes. Three studies used random assignment and control groups, 6 programs included nonrandomly assigned control or comparison groups, and the remaining 14 programs used pre-post or cross-sectional designs (Tomlinson, 2018). Seven of the studies with outcome evaluations were implemented in forensic hospital settings, while the rest addressed correctional settings. Rosenfeld et al. (2007) examined DBT with a pre- and post-adjudication sample of individuals charged with stalking and living in the community.

A total of ten studies included adult participants in correctional environments. Nine studies containing male, female, and mixed samples examined DBT in adult correctional settings (Asmand, Mami, & Valizadeh, 2015; Black, Blum, McCormick, & Allen, 2013; Blanchette et al., 2011; Ferreira, 2012; Gee & Reed, 2013; Lemmon, 2008), while Shelton et al. (2009), Shelton, Kesten, Zhang, and Trestman (2011) used a combined sample that included adults and juveniles. The most problematic is the fact that operationalization and standardization of "DBT" varied tremendously across these studies, making interpretation difficult. Level of risk and degree of psychopathology also varied across samples.

Of the adult correctional studies completed to date, only four studies employed comprehensive DBT. Aside from one study conducted in Iran, which was poorly described (Asmand et al., 2015), the remaining samples came from Correctional Services of Canada (see Blanchette et al., 2011). The Canadian adaptation of DBT included adapting skills for reading level, as well as criminogenic needs. They utilized a non-experimental pre-post design and found improvements in institutional function (e.g., fewer disciplinary tickets), decreases in psychiatric symptoms, and increases in clinical measures (e.g., mood, coping skills, self-control; Blanchette et al., 2011).

Two correctional studies used a hybrid form of DBT that included skills but lacked one or more elements of comprehensive DBT (Gee & Reed, 2013; Shelton et al., 2009, 2011). Gee and Reed (2013) included individual DBT, skills training, and consultation team, but no coaching. They found significant decreases in risk and trending but nonsignificant effects on self-harm and violence. Shelton and colleagues utilized DBT-CM, including skills training, a therapist consultation team, and coaching by DBT-trained officers. Following the skills intervention, participants were randomized to an individual skills coaching condition or a comparison (case management); however, both conditions were delivered by the same DBT-trained clinicians. They found significant reductions in aggression, behavioral tickets, impulsivity, and hostility while also observing improvements in psychiatric symptoms and coping in those who received DBT. However, they found no differences between coaching and case management conditions.

The majority of correctional studies to date have used a skills-only version of DBT with mixed results (Black et al., 2013; Ferreira, 2012; Lemmon, 2008; Moore et al., 2018; Wahl, 2011). Ferreira (2012) found increases in coping, Lemmon (2008) and Moore and colleagues (Moore et al., 2018) had trending but nonsignificant difference results pre-post, and Wahl (2011) found significant decreases in anger, rule infractions, and psychiatric symptoms and increases in mindfulness (quasi-experimental pre-post-design). Thus, the results were mixed. In trying to understand all of these studies, it is clear that longer studies that were more thoughtfully adapted (e.g., with greater fidelity) had the best outcomes.

8.4 Overview of General DBT

Standard DBT is comprised of a package of treatment components. First, all providers must be participating on a consultation team. Consultation teams meet for 1–2.5 h depending on the number of clients treated. The focus of consultation is therapist behaviors. The team uses dialectical communication, validation, and behavioral strategies to hold each other to fidelity to the model, to enhance their skills as providers, and to maintain their motivation to treat challenging clients. Clients in DBT receive individual psychotherapy for approximately 1 h weekly. Clients participate in 2.5 h of skills training each week. Standard DBT involves 6 months of weekly skills training that is often repeated for a total of 1 year of skills classes. The skills taught include mindfulness, distress tolerance, emotion regulation, and interpersonal effectiveness. Some programs include a newer model originally developed for adolescents called "middle path skills" which teach dialectically balanced skills of behavior change principles (e.g., reinforcement) and validation. The second edition of the skills manual (Linehan, 2015a, 2015b) also includes numerous supplemental skills that may be used as needed, including skills designed specifically for substance abuse. All clients in standard DBT receive skills coaching from their individual therapist via telephone in the outpatient model. Clients may contact their therapist for help applying skills any time they need to. This is perhaps one of the most feared aspects of DBT for therapists aspiring to apply the model. However, when practicing with fidelity to the model, providers find that clients call less than desired, not more. For those who call too frequently, this is often a temporary problem; therapists shape clients toward applying skills, and the frequency of calls dissipates.

8.4.1 Stages of Treatment

DBT was designed to treat individuals of all levels of severity (Dimeff & Linehan, 2001). DBT has four stages of treatment, each with different goals and treatment targets. The main goal of the Stage one DBT is to move from behavioral dyscontrol to behavioral control. Behaviors such as suicide attempts, cutting, substance abuse, and disordered eating are common in Stage one. The goal of the second stage of DBT is to reduce misery associated with negative emotions. While patients have learned a great deal about their emotions and how to manage them in Stage one, they frequently continue to suffer emotionally with sequelae of past trauma. Stage two clients have been described as living lives of quiet desperation (Linehan, 1993). Stage two DBT utilizes formal exposure to treat PTSD symptoms and emotional avoidance with the goal of increasing non-traumatic emotional experiencing. The goal of Stage three DBT is to resolve issues related to normal happiness and unhappiness. Therapists utilize problem-solving, validation, and a dialectical framework to assist clients in building a life and resolving normal issues as they arise (e.g., creating satisfying relationships, vocational issues). Stage four involves self-actualization. Stage four may involve therapy or may include spiritual direction or practices, such as yoga or mindfulness, designed to cultivate and enhance the experiences of joy. It should be noted that the majority of published DBT literature describes Stage one DBT.

Clients are considered to pretreatment before beginning any stage of DBT (Manning, 2007). In order to move from pretreatment to Stage one DBT, several things must occur: (1) the client must be oriented to the biosocial theory and its relationship to their personal history; (2) the therapist helps the client to identify treatment goals consistent with the client's notion of a life worth living; (3) the therapist and client must clarify agreements (e.g., length of treatment, to work on the treatment relationship when needed), and most importantly, the client must agree to work on eliminating suicide and self-harm; (4) the client must be oriented to all of the elements of the treatment and their respective purposes; and (5) the therapist uses validation and DBT commitment strategies to obtain or strengthen the client's commitment to engage in DBT treatment. Clients engage in a similar pretreatment phase and make a commitment before beginning each new stage of DBT.

8.4.2 Elements of Treatment

Individual Therapy DBT is both a highly structured and principle-driven treatment. Individual therapy is structured through an individualized case formulation. Careful assessment of a client's history and current problem behaviors is essential for creating a sound DBT case formulation. Both nomothetic and idiographic data are used to assess risk and to derive the appropriate treatment targets. Careful attention is paid to demographic and past behavioral risk factors for suicide using structured suicide risk tools. Developmental information is viewed from the lens of biosocial theory which looks for the ways in which biological sensitivity of the client and elements of the environment transacted over time to produce increased sensitivity on the part of the client and repeated invalidation from the environment. Chain analyses of maladaptive behaviors elucidate maintaining factors for such behaviors.

Primary Treatment Targets Treatment targets in individual therapy are organized hierarchically in three categories. Level 1 treatment targets include all life-threatening behaviors (e.g., suicide behaviors, suicide planning activity, suicide urges), as well as intentional self-injury that is not undertaken with intent to die. Level 2 treatment targets include any behaviors by the client or therapist that interfere with the success of the treatment. Common treatment-interfering behaviors of clients include non-completion of between-session practice, failing to complete diary cards, calling between sessions and refusing to accept coaching, and dissociation. Common treatment-interfering behaviors of therapists include being late for sessions, taking calls during session, or being judgmental in their interactions with clients. Level 3 targets are those which affect the client's quality of life (e.g., drinking and driving, anxiety symptoms, lack of friends, disordered eating). Behaviors are prioritized from the most to the least serious within each category. All the while, the therapist is working on increasing skillful behaviors in order to help to shape more effective behaviors.

Therapists make hypotheses about maintaining factors for each behavior on the hierarchy of targeted behaviors from the case formulation and patterns observed in ongoing chain analyses. Specific interventions are determined for each targeted behavior using standard CBT tools (e.g., skills training, exposure, contingency management, contingency clarification, cognitive restructuring).

Secondary Treatment Targets Clients in DBT have often been described pejoratively as "loving drama." Secondary targets involve unbalanced styles of experiencing emotions and associated patterns of rigid problem-solving and maladaptive behaviors that function to avoid or escape emotional pain. While not directly causal of problem behaviors, secondary targets often contribute to dysfunctional behaviors and make treatment difficult. Linehan (1993) identified the following patterns in the lives of individuals diagnosed with BPD: emotional vulnerability vs. self-invalidation, active passivity vs. apparent competence, and unrelenting crises vs. inhibited grieving.

The primary dialectical tension in the lives of individuals in Stage one DBT has to do with the inability to experience emotions. Individuals with BPD have learned that strong emotions prompt them to act in ways they later regret. Similarly, many have been told that they make too much of emotions, that they are dramatic, and that they should just calm down. Emotional vulnerability describes the phenomenon of experiencing one's own emotions as being out of control, overwhelming, and dangerous. This experience often maintains dysfunctional behaviors that help people avoid or escape painful emotions (e.g., experiencing sadness as intolerable frequently leads to cutting). The opposite of this heightened attention and sensitivity to emotions is called self-invalidation which involves ignoring emotions or downplaying their significance (e.g., "everyone has problems, I just need to deal with them."). Often people may bounce between these two extremes, unable to experience or tolerate emotions.

The second common pattern derives from the panic that ensues in the face of life problems. Clients experience themselves as trapped and in need of help. Even clients who are capable in some contexts may use a passive problem-solving style, having no faith in their own ability to manage problems. They will often engage in extreme behaviors that function to motivate others to solve problems on their behalf (e.g., "You need to call my case manager, or I will lose housing"). Clients often experience therapists' push to have clients solve their own problems as cruel, believing that if a therapist cared enough, they would save the client by helping them. The opposite pole of this dilemma is a person who is completely shut off from communicating distress or seeking help either, because they believe they should solve their own problems or because they avoid thinking about them (e.g., "I'm fine, there is nothing wrong, my family always fails to show...I'm used to it").

The third common dialectical pattern is unrelenting crisis vs. inhibited grieving. Inhibited grieving involves escaping emotional pain through impulsive behaviors (e.g., substance abuse, impulsive unsatisfying sex). Unrelenting crises may be understood as making poor decisions in the present context because of an inability to tolerate the present moment and its problems (e.g., a mother who has lost her children because of substance abuse desperately wants them back but uses on a court date because of the pain of being without them and shame of having lost them due to her behavior). When they appear in therapy sessions in stage one DBT, secondary targets are managed with dialectical strategies like metaphors and treated through informal exposure to emotion in session (e.g., a client is asked to do a chain and says "That's in the past, I'm fine now, why do we need to discuss this?"). When the therapist continues with the chain, the client looks down and becomes overwhelmed with shame. The therapist would validate that this is hard, remind the client why it is essential to complete the chain, and ask the client to make eye contact repeating the phrase which preceded the client becoming overwhelmed.

The individual therapy component of DBT is complex and requires careful attention, solid knowledge of the treatment, and adept application of the principles and strategies in DBT in order to keep the client balanced, collaborating, and working toward change. Individual sessions use an agenda, where the therapist checks in on other modes of treatment (e.g., skills); therapist and client use the client's diary card which tracks the client's emotions, skill use, urges, and target behaviors in order to determine agenda items consistent with the DBT Stage one treatment hierarchy (life-threatening, therapy interfering, quality of life, and ongoing skill use).

Skills Training The skills component of DBT is protocol-driven and fairly easy to train providers to deliver. The skills schedule is chosen based on the client population. A standard, once-weekly skills course takes 6 months to complete. The main objective of skills group is to teach the client skills in an engaging manner. The group is led by a skills trainer whose primary job is to provide didactic information in a dynamic and engaging manner. Behavioral shaping, storytelling, and humor draw out even reluctant participants. Role playing and practice are essential to good skills training. Groups also have a co-lead who watches the process in the room and coaches clients having difficulty. The co-lead provides examples or uses dialectical strategies when polarization occurs. The only time skills groups are stopped are when treatment destroying behavior occurs (e.g., a fire, self-harm by a client, violence ensues). Other than that, the focus remains on teaching. Even when behaviors that are distracting or annoying take place, new teaching takes precedence. Behaviors that simply make teaching and learning more difficult (identified as treatment-interfering behaviors) are typically ignored, as more effective behaviors are drawn out and reinforced.

Client Coaching Client coaching in DBT occurs via telephone in outpatient settings and live (in vivo) from staff in the environment in residential and inpatient settings. The primary function of this mode of treatment is to assist clients in generalizing skills learned in group to problems they encounter in their daily lives. Coaching calls are brief interactions lasting 10–15 min at most. The same is true for coaching in vivo (these are not therapy sessions). They are focused on skill employment, rather than support. A therapist typically receives a call and inquiries about the problem, validates the person's experience, and invites them to engage in a particular problem-solving strategy that involves using a skill. In inpatient environments, staff may observe a client being withdrawn, making threats, or on the verge of engaging in violence. A similar coaching process would occur whereby the staff assesses the situation, validates the individual (conveys understanding of the problem and its reasonableness), and offers suggestions for how to employ skills. After the client employs a skill, the staff reinforces skill use and often checks in again later. This can be contrasted with common practices of "redirecting" which often involves separation without creating new learning on the part of the client.

Consult Team The consultation team is an essential part of DBT treatment. All providers (individual therapists, skills trainers, and coaches) require the support and ongoing learning afforded by this weekly meeting. The meeting is designed to keep individuals close to the model, to keep them in a nonjudgmental stance, and to keep them motivated to treat clients. The team begins with mindfulness practice, an agenda is created, and all members keep to DBT agreements.

8.4.3 *Inpatient Adaptation*

When DBT was adapted for inpatient settings, the function of structuring the environment took on increased importance. Things like having and adhering to a program schedule and having ways to deal with crises as they arose became essential if providers were to be able to deliver DBT effectively in a closed setting. Structuring the environment requires that policies, procedures, and practices allow and support the consistent, careful delivery of DBT components. For instance, the common practice of transferring one patient to another unit if they get into a fight is inconsistent with providing good treatment to both patients. DBT favors structuring the unit for safety to afford both clients the opportunity to practice skills and manage their environment, rather than escaping or avoiding as a consequence of crisis behavior. In many inpatient settings, dangerous behaviors by patients often trigger "emergency meetings." Existing programming is frequently delayed or canceled in service of responding to the crisis. Aside from the obvious consequences for other patients in the milieu related to missing treatment, emergency meetings often maintain escalation of staff emotions and result in impulsive or ill-conceived responses to the crisis and the client who caused it.

Egregious Behaviors Protocol DBT employs a protocol called the egregious behavior protocol (EBP) to structure the environment. The purpose of the EBP protocol is to provide a systematic approach that aids in the management and treatment of *serious* individual behaviors such as self-harm, physical aggression, and destruction of the milieu. The protocol reduces the need for "emergency meetings" and allows regular treatment to continue in the milieu, even when programs are faced with behaviors that are upsetting and potentially profoundly disruptive. Having a consistent institutional response also allows staff to regulate their own emotions about such behaviors.

The steps in EBP steps are as follows: (1) manage safety first (e.g., stop violence or self-harm, keep others safe, treat any medical needs); (2) when calm and willing, the patient is handed a form that guides them through completion of a behavioral chain analysis (BCA) of the incident (clients with cognitive limitations may be assisted by staff to complete the BCA); (3) staff meet with the client and collaborate to create an overcorrection plan that is presented to the unit; and (4) they initiate the plan and return to normal programming (including incentives if present in the environment). The EBP is a form of behavioral treatment that takes precedence over other modalities of treatment following an egregious behavior. Clients do not participate in regular programming; rather they work on steps of the protocol.

The behavioral technique applied in the EBP is called "overcorrection." It is a mildly aversive behavioral technique involving two components: (1) restitutional overcorrection where the person *repairs* or corrects the damage done to themselves, others, and the unit milieu, if possible making the environment better than before, and (2) *positive practice* where the person practices the correct or desired behavior (or some approximation of it). In other words, the individual must practice a new behavior that, if in their behavioral repertoire, would prevent such a behavior from occurring in the future. Overcorrection is a well-established behavioral technique that has shown success even in individuals with severe cognitive impairment.

The timing of the chain analysis and team meeting ensures that interventions with the client are based on client data and scientifically sound behavioral principles and that interventions are delivered in a therapeutic manner. This counteracts impulsive, emotion-driven responses to severe behavior (e.g., changing medication protocols before adequately testing previous ones, shaming or punishing patients in treatment team meetings). This protocol functions as a teaching tool for clients and staff, as important information is discovered about the factors that maintain these behaviors in particular clients, as well as and the new skills necessary to change these problem behaviors. It requires that clients practice new behaviors, rather than just talking about the behavior or simply apologizing for them. This form of behavioral treatment takes precedence over other modalities of treatment following an egregious behavior. Information from EBP often results in changes to the individual's overall treatment plan and in the ways in which staff respond to the client. Ethically, EBPs are used in environments where skills teaching and coaching are present and observable.

8.5 Adaptations to DBT in the Correctional Model

8.5.1 Biosocial Theory

While individuals with BPD experience emotions intensely, many individuals in correctional populations experience almost nothing. Some experience shallow or superficial emotions. Others experience all of the highs and lows of traditional BPD but also have significant antisocial traits. The biosocial theory is used in DBT to conceptualize the treatment and to communicate to patients the origins of their emotional and behavioral problems and conveys to them that their behaviors are not an inevitable part of their life. This is essential for the engagement and motivation of the client. Thus, in order to be effective with patients in the correctional environment, the biosocial theory must be adapted to fit all of the variations of emotional and cognitive dysfunction seen in the population. McCann et al. (2000) described the type of invalidating environment that contributes to the development of antisocial behavior as one that fails to effectively model acts of care and which may even invalidate or punish acts of care or attachment. In such environments, antisocial behavior is both modeled and reinforced. A clinical example of this was a young woman who met criteria for both BPD and ASPD. When she was young, she recalled crying about a disagreement with a sibling. Her father, who was drunk at the time, told her to "stop crying" or he would "give her something to cry about." He then stomped her kitten to death. Care and attachment have literally been punished out of her experience.

In our work on psychopathy (Galietta & Rosenfeld, 2012), we have included information about the development of psychopathic traits in our explanation of the biosocial theory to clients. There appear to be multiple biological underpinnings for psychopathy (see Skeem et al., 2011). We conceptualize biological vulnerabilities as having two components: (1) *disinhibition/impulsivity* refers to emotional sensitivity and reactivity (similar to standard DBT), and (2) *deficits in emotional experiencing* refers to cold, callous or unemotional traits, low sensitivity, and reactivity. Disinhibition is associated with secondary psychopathy and recidivism and also associated with substance abuse and suicide, while deficits in emotional experiencing are associated with primary psychopathy (Skeem et al., 2011). Individuals can have one or both as separate vulnerabilities transacting with the invalidating environment described by McCann et al. (2000).

From an RNR perspective, factor 2 traits are the most relevant to correctional treatment because of their relationship to violence, suicide, and recidivism. However, factor 1 traits have significant interpersonal consequences which make the treatment relationship challenging. Our lab investigated the effect of psychopathic traits on DBT. Clients higher in factor 1 were less likely to complete treatment; client behaviors were not associated with dropout. Interestingly, *therapy-interfering behaviors by therapists* and clinician perceptions that clients were "unmotivated" were associated with higher factor 1 scores and dropout; therapist behaviors appeared to mediate the relationship between factor 1 and completion of treatment (Stern, Galietta, Rosenfeld, & Curtis, 2014). Thus, it appears that modifications to the treatment for psychopathic traits are warranted for correctional populations.

8.5.2 Treatment Targets

Treatment targets need to be modified in corrections to include violent behaviors, urges, and thoughts as level 1 targets. Common level 2 treatment targets (treatment interfering) include lying, contraband, and engaging in rule infractions. Quality of life targets include reducing behaviors that create suffering in the present, as well as increasing behaviors necessary to forge a noncriminal life worth living (e.g., vocational training or leisure activities to decrease boredom might be a much higher treatment targets in correctional patients than in the general DBT).

8.5.3 Skills Training

Almost all correctional programs with good outcomes made significant modifications to the skills treatment component in order to address the needs of a correctional population. The average reading level in prison and jail is considerably lower than in the general public. Thus, the first adaptation to necessary for skills is to simplify the language. In addition, prison slang varies regionally, and these variations should be incorporated into examples as well as written materials.

Delivering Training Effectively In addition to editing original skills for reading level, most programs edited for content as well. It is notable that with the exception of adding modules on criminal thinking, the actual skills themselves have needed little modification for correctional populations. However, the examples used to teach skills require extensive modification in order to be effective in correctional environments. Many of the examples used in the standard skills manual include activities that are not possible in a highly controlled environment (e.g., take a bubble bath, fix your car). Examples relevant to the lives of correctional inmates must be used in order to make the material salient and understandable.

Mindfulness is a universal experience, but rather than listening to nature, a correctional example might be to listen to the sound of doors locking or keys jingling without judgment or attachment. Distress tolerance examples often focus on the pain of isolation, difficult telephone interactions with family, or missed visits. Radical acceptance, the choice to accept a painful situation and one's feelings about it through body posture and breath, assists inmates with long sentences, those who receive bad news from court and those who will remain in prison for life.

Interactive role-plays involving application of these skills and resolution of inmate dilemmas are essential. Leaders must have an engaging and interactive approach. Props and materials must be screened for safety and permissibility but are included to increase effectiveness of teaching.

Many of the correctional studies have shortened the time spent on skills compared to standard DBT. Studies on correctional adaptations and RNR findings suggest that longer durations of treatment produce better outcomes. Shortening time for covering content is not recommended. For settings with shorter length of stays, it might make sense to cover fewer skills in adequate depth (e.g., jails may wish to focus on select skills only).

Content Adaptations Our lab has created new distress tolerance skills for avoiding acting on obsessions or remaining stuck in ruminations (Rosenfeld et al., 2007). We have modified emotion regulation skills to address affective blunting/shutting down, as well as traditional emotional lability. We have made modification for individuals high in psychopathic traits (Galietta & Rosenfeld, 2012); we developed skills for boredom and skills for shaping normative emotional experiences. With regard to interpersonal effectiveness skills, we have added activities for identifying and creating values and skills for apologizing authentically and countering urges to take advantage of others. Difficulties dealing with authority feature prominently in examples we use for interpersonal effectiveness. Because of deficits in that regard, we added middle path skills dealing specifically with avoiding power struggles in correctional environments and learning to validate others. Inmates often experience tension between moving toward one's own goals by walking away from trouble and being compelled to fight in order to avoid losing face or "being punked." Additional skills designed to target antisocial beliefs (e.g., "suckers deserve to get taken advantage of") feature in our model and in most correctional DBT models.

Lastly, skills designed to create prosocial behaviors are important. McCann et al. (2000) added random acts of kindness. We have emphasized using body posture skills to reduce willfulness, oppositionality, and judgments, as well as to increase compassion for others. Finally, skills developed for individuals who abuse substances are quite helpful in corrections, given the high rate of substance abuse in the population. Skills like "urge surfing," using mindfulness as a way to manage urges to use drugs and tolerating cravings, are quite helpful (Linehan, 2015a, 2015b). Of note, we have recommended not including the "alternate rebellion" skill in order to avoid reinforcing the satisfaction individuals high in psychopathic traits often derive from deceiving others.

8.5.4 Consultation Team

Working with violent, suicidal inmates is extremely challenging. Consultation team focuses on reviewing assumptions about clients (e.g., "clients are doing the best that they can"), resolving dialectical tensions in the treatment milieu, and most importantly on maintaining a nonjudgmental stance. The way therapists talk about and think about clients impacts their behaviors in session, and the team protects treatment and fights burnout. It is a priority that this group meets weekly for 1–2 h depending on the number of clients in a program.

8.5.5 Staff Education and Support Meeting

Because of tour schedules, many officers are unable to consistently attend consult team. Therefore, it is recommended that an additional mode called SES (for staff education and support) occurs once or twice weekly. This meeting meets the function of consultation team for officers, but they may drop in as they are able. The meeting begins with brief mindfulness practice and asks attendees to briefly describe their most difficult interaction of the week. Validation is provided, as is review and practice of DBT principles that might have been effective. It is important that no supervisors attend this meeting and that the leader is well-versed in DBT and well-respected by officers.

8.5.6 Skills Coaching

Coaching clients becomes a difficult task in correctional environments. Typically, officers are trained to coach skills (and sometimes to deliver or co-lead skills groups as well), but in one setting, Women's Huron Valley, inmate mentors received extensive training and were paid to provide skills coaching to residents in a DBT Program. Equipping officers (or anyone) to provide effective coaching requires considerable training, ongoing educational support and feedback, and institutional buy-in. Framing the job of the officer as maintaining safety *and* supporting new learning is important and often requires culture change. The phrase "approach and coach" embodies the way coaching should work. In other words, even when there is no observable problem, officers should be close, engaged, and validating. This creates the context for officers to be able to offer skills coaching at times when the inmate is facing a problem and dysregulated.

8.5.7 Milieu Structures

EBP The egregious behavior, discussed previously, requires little modification. Finally, structuring the program to support treatment is challenging. Peers may not be skillful enough to provide effective feedback, and information shared may be used against individuals at a future time. Thus, it is often best to have the individual present their EBP to the treatment team only, as it is important that individuals are not shamed or punished once they have engaged in self-reflection.

Level Systems Overcoming the negative effects of authoritarian control requires some consideration. Community DBT is voluntary. In corrections, it is important to enhance the perception of voluntariness. Swenson et al. (2001) described the "program within a program" concept. In correctional environments, individuals may choose to participate or not, but those who choose to commit to treatment should receive more privileges than those who do not. Some correctional DBT programs include a level system that offers increased privileges for moving from pretreatment to commitment, more privileges for those who attempt skills and accept coaching, more privileges for those who demonstrate independent skill use, and the highest privileges for those who consistently model skillful behavior and coach others in the environment.

Daily Incentive Programs In the community, skillful behaviors generally bring positive reinforcement. This is not always the case in corrections. Often, dysfunctional behaviors garner greater rewards. Thus, many correctional programs employ operant principles in a variety of ways in order to shape desirable behaviors or suppress undesirable behaviors. Extra recreation time or extra phone call minutes tend to be very effective incentives with this population. They cannot be held or traded, and they are easy to operationalize. Simple daily incentive programs function remarkably well to reduce low-level problem behaviors in the environment which afford staff more time to focus on client skill generalization.

Use of Good Time Many inmates with severe personality disorders have engaged in so many infractions that their segregation days exceed their sentences. Individuals with a bottomless pit of infraction time are more likely to be hopeless, unmotivated for treatment, and dangerous. Programs can use make effective use of "good time." It is possible to hold the segregation time over someone's head; if they graduate from the program, their time may be vacated.

Other programs address great need and increase client motivation by locating programs in segregation areas where inmates are in 23-h lockdown. The most problematic inmates are likely already found there. If they have severe, complex mental illnesses that render them acutely dangerous, creating a unit where the starting point is lockdown can make programming easier and the treatment environment safer. Such an environment in DBT would not look like typical segregation. Rather, a rich thriving treatment would be observable. Treatment participation which involves being removed from one's cell becomes naturally reinforced. As risk decreases and skills are developed, increased freedom can be tied to success working on treatment targets. Programs in general population may be very effective at preventing individuals from moving to a higher level of mental healthcare. However, treatment in general population often competes with television access, socialization, and other leisure time activities. Thus, scheduling with operant principles in mind is extremely important.

Managing Safety Managing safety while providing treatment can be challenging. I have had the experience of leading skills groups where each participant had to be brought in one at a time and handcuffed to a bar around the perimeter of the room. Adjustments often need to be made to ensure safety, and this should not necessarily be seen as incompatible with treatment or even with fostering a therapeutic milieu. Physical space resources can greatly aid in the success of a program. Having observation cells within the program space, the presence of a comfort room with good line of sight (i.e., an empty cell with distress tolerance materials available), having adequate group treatment space with a whiteboard or wall with chalk paint, having an office in the milieu that affords privacy for individual sessions (again with good visual access), having easy access to yards/ recreation areas, and having a visually pleasant space with adequate light can all assist with successful management of the milieu and optimal delivery of treatment.

Culture Change Perhaps the greatest challenge in the successful adaptation of DBT involves shaping correctional settings to be more validating and compassionate. Employing validation is, in many ways, countercultural in corrections. Fear of being "manipulated" or of getting too close to inmates often interferes with implementing DBT. One successful example involved a jail whose practice it was to have inmates face the wall with hands palms facing up behind their backs whenever a civilian walked by. The institution was not willing to change the practice, but it became customary for officers to nod and say "thank you, sir" to those who complied. It was a way to reduce status difference and convey mutual respect to one another.

It is crucial that DBT is not considered a mental health initiative but rather that it is developed, planned, and operated as an integrated custody/mental health program. This entails collaboration of many functions that typically take place in silos.

8.6 Conclusion

In sum, DBT is consistent with RNR, GLM, and TICC approaches. There is a substantial evidence base for DBT in the community and a growing body of studies on the effectiveness of correctional DBT. DBT can be tailored to the level of risk and individual patient needs and learning styles (including those with cognitive limitations). More research is needed on correctional DBT. Studies should clearly describe elements of DBT delivered and mode of delivery. Samples should be described in terms of the level of psychiatric and behavioral severity. Most importantly, measures of fidelity for comprehensive and skills/coaching versions of DBT should be developed and utilized.

For those interested in pursuing the possibility of developing DBT programming in corrections, the first step is to form a multidisciplinary implementation/reading group whose primary task will be to learn more about the treatment, so that a careful decision about adoption can be made. DBT implementation is challenging, particularly in correctional settings. However, the potential for changing the lives of even the most difficult individuals in custody is exciting. Correctional administrators, mental health providers, and officers also stand to benefit significantly from well-designed DBT programs.

References

Andrews, D. A., Zinger, I., Hoge, R. D., Bonta, J., Gendreau, P., & Cullen, F. T. (1990). Does correctional treatment work? A clinically relevant and psychologically informed meta-analysis. *Criminology, 28*(3), 369–404. https://doi.org/10.1111/j.1745-9125.1990.tb01330.x

Asmand, P., Mami, S., & Valizadeh, R. (2015). The effectiveness of dialectical behavior therapy and rational emotive behavior therapy in irrational believes treatment, anxiety among young male prisoners who have antisocial personality disorder in Ilam prison. *International Journal of Health System and Disaster Management, 3*(1), 1–7. https://doi.org/10.4103/2347-9019.147135

Black, D. W., Blum, N., McCormick, B., & Allen, J. (2013). Systems Training for Emotional Predictability and Problem Solving (STEPPS) group treatment for offenders with borderline personality disorder. *The Journal of Nervous and Mental Disease, 201*(2), 124–129. https://doi.org/10.1097/NMD.0b013e31827f6435

Black, D. W., Gunter, T., Allen, J., Blum, N., Arndt, S., Wenman, G., & Silieni, B. (2007). Borderline personality disorder in male and female offenders newly committed to prison. *Comprehensive Psychiatry, 48*(5), 400–405. https://doi.org/10.1016/j.comppsych.2007.04.006

Black, D. W., Gunter, T., Loveless, P., Allen, J., & Sieleni, B. (2010). Antisocial personality disorder in incarcerated offenders: Psychiatric comorbidity and quality of life. *Annals of Clinical Psychiatry, 22*(2), 113–120. Retrieved from https://www.aacp.com/article/buy_now/?id=56

Blanchette, K., Flight, J., Verbrugge, P., Gobeil, R., & Taylor, K. (2011). *Dialectical behaviour therapy within a women's structured living environment.* Ottawa, ON: Correctional Services Canada.

Brown, J. F., Brown, M. Z., & Dibiasio, P. (2013). Treating individuals with intellectual disabilities and challenging behaviors with adapted dialectical behavior therapy. *Journal of Mental Health Research in Intellectual Disabilities, 6*(4), 280–303. https://doi.org/10.1080/19315864.2012.700684

Conn, C., Warden, R., Stuewig, J., Kim, E. H., Harty, L., Hastings, M., & Tangney, J. P. (2010). Borderline personality disorder among jail inmates: How common and how distinct? *Corrections Compendium, 35*(4), 6–13. Retrieved from http://www.aca.org

Dialectic. (2018). In *Merriam-Webster Dictionary*. Retrieved from https://www.merriam-webster.com/dictionary/dialectic

Dimeff, L., & Linehan, M. (2001). Dialectical behavior therapy in a nutshell. *The California Psychologist, 34*(3), 10–13. Retrieved from https://cpapsych.site-ym.com/page/048?

Douglas, K. S., Nicholls, T. L., & Brink, J. (2017). Interventions for the reduction of violence by persons with serious mental illnesses. In P. M. Kleespies (Ed.), *The Oxford handbook of behavioral emergencies and crises* (pp. 466–488). New York, NY: Oxford University Press.

Drake, E., & Barnoski, R. (2006). *Recidivism findings for the juvenile rehabilitation administration's dialectical behavior therapy program: Final report (Document No. 06-07-1202).* Olympia, WA: The Washington State Institute for Public Policy.
Fazel, S., Hayes, A. J., Bartellas, K., Clerici, M., & Trestman, R. (2016). Mental health of prisoners: Prevalence, adverse outcomes, and interventions. *Lancet Psychiatry, 3*(9), 871–881. https://doi.org/10.1016/S2215-0366(16)30142-0
Fazel, S., & Seewald, K. (2012). Severe mental illness in 33,588 prisoners worldwide: Systematic review and meta-regression analysis. *The British Journal of Psychiatry, 200*(5), 364–373. https://doi.org/10.1192/bjp.bp.111.096370
Fellner, J. (2004, February 12). Prisons no place for the mentally ill. *The San Diego Union Tribune*. Retrieved from https://www.hrw.org/news/2004/02/12/prisons-no-place-mentally-ill
Ferreira, C. C. (2012). *The effects of a modified dialectical behavior therapy program on male inmates' coping skills* (Doctoral dissertation, Pacific School of Professional Psychology, Forest Grove, OR).
Ford, M. (2015, June 8). America's largest mental hospital is a jail. *The Atlantic*. Retrieved from https://www.theatlantic.com/politics/archive/2015/06/americas-largest-mental-hospital-is-a-jail/395012/
Frazier, S. N., & Vela, J. (2014). Dialectical behavior therapy for the treatment of anger and aggressive behavior: A review. *Aggression and Violent Behavior, 19*(2), 156–163. https://doi.org/10.1016/j.avb.2014.02.001
Galietta, M., Fineran, V., Fava, J., & Rosenfeld, B. (2010). Antisocial and psychopathic individuals. In D. McKay, J. S. Abramowitz, & S. Taylor (Eds.), *Cognitive-behavioral therapy for refractory cases: Turning failure into success* (pp. 385–405). Washington, DC: American Psychological Association.
Galietta, M., & Rosenfeld, B. (2012). Adapting dialectical behavior therapy (DBT) for the treatment of psychopathy. *International Journal of Forensic Mental Health, 11*(4), 325–335. https://doi.org/10.1080/14999013.2012.746762
Galietta, M., Rosenfeld, B., & Ivanoff, A. (2003, April). *Treating difficult-to-treat forensic patients: Applying DBT to forensic settings.* Symposium presented at the International Association of Forensic Mental Health Services Conference, Miami, FL.
Gee, J., & Reed, S. (2013). The HoST programme: A pilot evaluation of modified dialectical behaviour therapy with female offenders diagnosed with borderline personality disorder. *European Journal of Psychotherapy & Counselling, 15*(3), 233–252. https://doi.org/10.1080/13642537.2013.810659
Goodman, P. R., Page, J., & Phelps, M. (2017). *Breaking the pendulum: The long struggle over criminal justice.* New York, NY: Oxford University Press.
Gunderson, J. G., Weinberg, I., & Choi-Kain, L. (2013). Borderline personality disorder. *Focus, 11*(2), 129–145. https://doi.org/10.1176/appi.focus.11.2.129
Lemmon, G. (2008). *Impact of a modified Dialectical Behavior Therapy treatment on coping methods and impulsiveness in female inmates* (Doctoral dissertation, Pacific University, Forest Grove, OR).
Linehan, M. M. (1993). *Cognitive behavior therapy for borderline personality disorder.* New York, NY: The Guilford Press.
Linehan, M. M. (2013). What psychiatrists should know about dialectical behavior therapy. *Psychiatric Annals, 43*(4), 148. https://doi.org/10.3928/00485713-20130403-02
Linehan, M. M. (2015a). *DBT skills training manual* (2nd ed.). New York, NY: The Guilford Press.
Linehan, M. M. (2015b). *DBT skills training handouts and worksheets* (2nd ed.). New York, NY: The Guilford Press.
Linehan, M. M., Armstrong, H. E., Suarez, A., Allmon, D., & Heard, H. L. (1991). Cognitive-behavioral treatment of chronically parasuicidal borderline patients. *Archives of General Psychiatry, 48*(12), 1060–1064.
Manning, S. Y. (2007). Dialectical behaviour therapy. In C. Freeman & M. Powers (Eds.), *The handbook of evidence based psychotherapies* (pp. 83–92). West Sussex, UK: Wiley.

McCann, R. A., Ball, E. M., & Ivanoff, A. (2000). DBT with an inpatient forensic population: The CMHIP forensic model. *Cognitive and Behavioral Practice, 7*(4), 447–456. https://doi.org/10.1016/S1077-7229(00)80056-5

Miller, N. A., & Najavits, L. M. (2012). Creating trauma-informed correctional care: A balance of goals and environment. *European Journal of Psychotraumatology, 3*(1), 17246. https://doi.org/10.3402/ejpt.v3i0.17246

Moore, K. E., Folk, J. B., Boren, E. A., Tangney, J. P., Fischer, S., & Schrader, S. W. (2018). Pilot study of a brief dialectical behavior therapy skills group for jail inmates. *Psychological Services, 15*(1), 98–108. https://doi.org/10.1037/ser0000105

Raine, A., & Yang, Y. (2006). Neural foundations to moral reasoning and antisocial behavior. *Social Cognitive and Affective Neuroscience, 1*(3), 203–213. https://doi.org/10.1093/scan/nsl033

Rosenfeld, B., Byars, K., & Galietta, M. (2011). Conducting psychotherapy outcome research in forensic settings. In B. Rosenfeld & S. D. Penrod (Eds.), *Research methods in forensic psychology* (pp. 309–324). Hoboken, NJ: Wiley.

Rosenfeld, B., Galietta, M., Ivanoff, A., Garcia-Mansilla, A., Martinez, R., Fava, J., … Green, D. (2007). Dialectical behavior therapy for the treatment of stalking offenders. *International Journal of Forensic Mental Health, 6*(2), 95–103. https://doi.org/10.1080/14999013.2007.10471254

Sakdalan, J. A., Shaw, J., & Collier, V. (2010). Staying in the here-and-now: A pilot study on the use of dialectical behaviour therapy group skills training for forensic clients with intellectual disability. *Journal of Intellectual Disability Research, 54*(6), 568–572. https://doi.org/10.1111/j.1365-2788.2010.01274.x

Sansone, R. A., & Sansone, L. A. (2009). Borderline personality and criminality. *Psychiatry (Edgmont), 6*(10), 16–20. Retrieved from https://www.ncbi.nlm.nih.gov/pmc/articles/PMC2790397/

Shelton, D., Kesten, K., Zhang, W., & Trestman, R. (2011). Impact of a dialectic behavior therapy-corrections modified (DBT-CM) upon behaviorally challenged incarcerated male adolescents. *Journal of Child and Adolescent Psychiatric Nursing, 24*(2), 105–113. https://doi.org/10.1111/j.1744-6171.2011.00275.x

Shelton, D., Sampl, S., Kesten, K. L., Zhang, W., & Trestman, R. L. (2009). Treatment of impulsive aggression in correctional settings. *Behavioral Sciences & the Law, 27*(5), 787–800. https://doi.org/10.1002/bsl.889

Singleton, N., Meltzer, H., & Gatward, R. (1998). *Psychiatric morbidity among prisoners in England and Wales: Summary report*. London, UK: Office for National Statistics.

Skeem, J. L., Polaschek, D. L. L., Patrick, C. J., & Lilienfeld, S. O. (2011). Psychopathic personality: Bridging the gap between scientific evidence and public policy. *Psychological Science in the Public Interest, 12*(3), 95–162. https://doi.org/10.1177/1529100611426706

Stern, S., Galietta, M., Rosenfeld, B., & Curtis, R. (2014, June). *Assessing psychotherapy variables in treatment with psychopathic offenders*. Paper presented at the International Association of Forensic Mental Health Services 2014 Conference, Toronto, Canada.

Swenson, C. R., Sanderson, C., Dulit, R. A., & Linehan, M. M. (2001). The application of dialectical behavior therapy for patients with borderline personality disorder on inpatient units. *Psychiatric Quarterly, 72*(4), 307–324. https://doi.org/10.1023/A:1010337231127

Tomlinson, M. F. (2018). A theoretical and empirical review of dialectical behavior therapy within forensic psychiatric and correctional settings worldwide. *International Journal of Forensic Mental Health, 17*(1), 72–95. https://doi.org/10.1080/14999013.2017.1416003

Trestman, R. (2000). Behind bars: Personality disorders. *The Journal of the American Academy of Psychiatry and the Law, 28*(2), 232–235. Retrieved from http://jaapl.org/content/28/2/232

Wagner, P., & Sawyer, W. (2018, June 14). Mass incarceration: The whole pie 2018. *Prison Policy Initiative*. Retrieved from https://www.prisonpolicy.org/reports/pie2018.html

Wahl, C. T. (2011). *Evaluation of a dialectical behavior therapy skills group for female inmates who voluntarily seek treatment: A pilot study* (Doctoral dissertation). Retrieved from ProQuest Dissertations & Theses Global. (Order No. 3479921).

Ward, T., Melser, J., & Yates, P. M. (2007). Reconstructing the Risk–Need–Responsivity model: A theoretical elaboration and evaluation. *Aggression and Violent Behavior, 12*(2), 208–228. https://doi.org/10.1016/j.avb.2006.07.001

Ward, T., Yates, P. M., & Willis, G. M. (2012). The good lives model and the risk need responsivity model: A critical response to Andrews, Bonta, and Wormith (2011). *Criminal Justice and Behavior, 39*(1), 94–110. https://doi.org/10.1177/0093854811426085

Chapter 9
Incorporating Principles of Trauma-Informed Care Into Evidence-Based Sex Offending Treatment

Jill S. Levenson, Gwenda M. Willis, and David Prescott

9.1 Introduction

Since the 1980s, well-conducted treatment programs for sex offending have been shown to help reduce recidivism by a moderate amount (Hanson et al., 2009; Schmucker & Lösel, 2015). In the USA, however, treatment programs have been very much about control, compliance, containment, and management, driven by presumptions of repetitive patterns, deviant sexual interests, multiple victims, and lifelong risk (see Chap. 2). The advent of strengths-based approaches such as the Good Lives Model (GLM; (Ward & Brown, 2004)) (see Chap. 3) encouraged greater consideration of the *why and how*—why do sexually victimizing behaviors develop, and how can we help our clients recognize the social and emotional needs they are trying to meet through sexual assault? Troubled pasts often pave the way to troubled adulthoods, and many people who have sexually offended are unable to find healthy intimacy and connections to others. Treatment programs, ideally, help clients to address these fundamental problems and learn to meet needs in healthy, non-victimizing ways.

People convicted of sex crimes have high rates of various child maltreatment and family dysfunction as youngsters (Levenson et al., 2015, 2016). Early adversity can create distorted thinking and maladaptive coping mechanisms (including violence).

J. S. Levenson (✉)
Trama-Informed Training Initiative, Barry University School of Social Work, Miami Shores, FL, USA
e-mail: jlevenson@barry.edu

G. M. Willis
School of Psychology, The University of Auckland, Auckland, New Zealand
e-mail: g.willis@auckland.ac.nz

D. Prescott
Becket Family of Services, Falmouth, ME, USA
e-mail: DSP@DavidPrescott.net

E. L. Jeglic, C. Calkins (eds.), *New Frontiers in Offender Treatment*,
https://doi.org/10.1007/978-3-030-01030-0_9

It can interfere with attachment and bonding, especially for children who see little modeling of healthy relationship skills (including empathy) in their families or communities. Criminal offenders have much higher rates of adverse childhood experiences (ACEs) than the general population, and such events change the neurochemistry of the brain, leading to poorer functioning in adulthood.

Knowledge about trauma and about sexual offending have grown, enhancing our understanding of these behaviors. Against a societal backdrop of sexual violence prevention emphasizing offense culpability and punishment, however, it is not surprising that professionals in the field have cautioned that people in treatment might embellish or fabricate stories of childhood abuse to deflect personal responsibility or to generate sympathy. On the other hand, several studies have confirmed that sexual offending treatment (SOTX) samples have higher rates of childhood sexual abuse (CSA) and other early adversities than the general male population (Hanson & Slater, 1988; Jespersen et al., 2009; Levenson et al., 2016; Reavis et al., 2013). With concerns about "abuse excuse," approaches to treatment have been highly risk-focused and confrontational and often neglected the principles of effective correctional rehabilitation and trauma-informed practices.

9.2 What Exactly Is TIC?

It is important to understand that trauma-informed care (TIC) is not the same as trauma resolution therapy, nor is it a specific treatment model or a structured program that is delivered in a standardized way. Likewise, it is not a reframing of clients' lives as victims with no internal locus of control, nor is it an excuse for offending. According to the US Substance Abuse and Mental Health Services Administration (SAMHSA), TIC is an overarching framework that takes a "universal precautions" approach to behavioral health services (SAMHSA, 2014). Trauma-informed practitioners understand that past trauma often manifests as presenting problems, and therefore they must integrate knowledge about the neurobiological, psychological, and social consequences of trauma into policies, procedures, and practices that guide a safe, compassionate, respectful therapy environment (Bloom, 2013; Giller et al., 2006; Miller & Najavits, 2012).

TIC is a way of conceptualizing and responding to problematic behavior and its sequelae through the lens of trauma. By conceptualizing cases through a perspective informed by trauma research, we can understand how past experiences may have contributed to sexually abusive behaviors. Trauma-informed practices guide the therapist to avoid repeating disempowering dynamics in the helping relationship. SOTX programs can use TIC to transform their interventions from primarily content-driven psycho-education to a more collaborative and dynamic, process-oriented approach that utilizes the therapeutic encounter as a corrective emotional experience and helps clients build healthy skills.

TIC is not intended to coddle clients, excuse criminal behavior, or condone victimization. Rarely have we seen clients exploit their "victimhood" to deny accountability or gain sympathy. More likely is that clients do not recognize their own traumatic experiences or think about how those events might have shaped their perceptions and behaviors. The research suggests that men tend to underreport early adversity rather than exaggerate it (Dube et al., 2004; Hardt & Rutter, 2004; Najavits et al., 2009)—because they don't recognize it ("my dad was a raging alcoholic, but that was just normal in our family") and have distorted perceptions about it ("I deserved those beatings") or due to cognitive dissonance ("my mom did the best she could and I love her").

TIC is a strengths-based and empowering framework that can be used within any treatment model or rehabilitation framework such as relapse prevention, risk-needs-responsivity, or Good Lives Model (RP, RNR, GLM) to focus on resilience and personal choice. It requires a professional who can build healing relationships with clients that are safe, respectful, non-shaming, and collaborative—these are the therapeutic alliance qualities that foster human connections, post-traumatic growth, and hope for future possibilities (Bloom, 2013). The key, in trauma-informed care, is to listen to the story from the client's perspective and not to project assumptions onto their narrative; rather, we can provide a safe space for the client to explore the meaning that has become attached to their experiences. TIC helps clients make sense of their lives, acknowledge the circumstances they have lived through, understand their choices and patterns of behavior over time, and identify areas for desired change.

TIC has many Rogerian themes, such as client-centered therapeutic encounters that offer warmth, non-threatening authenticity, and positive regard (Rogers, 1961). In practice it focuses largely on creating an empowering, collaborative, safe milieu in the treatment setting, with an aim to avoid re-creating dynamics that are similar to those in abusive and dysfunctional families. This is something that is often quite challenging for practitioners to do effectively in any nonvoluntary, forensic, correctional, or mandated treatment program. Indeed, treatment approaches that emphasize confrontation, control, and compliance are inconsistent with principles of TIC.

9.3 Why Are Trauma-Informed Practices Important in Treatment for Sexual Offending?

TIC recognizes the prevalence of trauma in contemporary society and especially how impactful a certain set of childhood maltreatments and family dysfunctions called ACEs—adverse childhood experience—can be (Anda et al., 2006; Felitti et al., 1998). There is little doubt scientifically about the neurobiological alterations to the brain that result from chronic toxic stress in childhood and that growing up in an adverse environment can affect behavioral and emotional self-regulation, social interaction, cognitive schemas, and self-efficacy. Early experiences shape expectations and interpretations of self, others, and the world (Creeden, 2009; Grady et al., 2016; Herman, 1992; Marshall, 2010). Not everyone who experiences traumatic events develops post-traumatic stress disorder, and many people flourish with resilience even after dealing with adversity. However, ACEs can contribute to relational and psychosocial problems later in life.

A history of early trauma can set the stage for poorly executed interpersonal skills, which interfere with the capacity to build relationships with others. Sexual scripts resulting from early trauma can further limit opportunities for emotionally intimate relationships. Intimacy deficits have been correlated with sexual offense recidivism (Hanson & Harris, 2001; Hanson & Morton-Bourgon, 2005), but a trauma-informed therapy setting can mitigate the loneliness and alienation often felt by our clients. For some clients, the therapeutic relationship and the treatment group is the most emotionally intimate relationship they have ever had (Marshall & Burton, 2010; Marshall et al., 2013; Sawyer & Jennings, 2016). When SOTX clients engage in human connections with others who validate their experience, opportunities exist for building relational skills relevant to reducing recidivism risk (Levenson et al., 2017a).

The problems of people who have sexually abused manifest in different ways. For some, emotional identification with children protects them against perceived rejection from adults, while for others, hostility toward women is revealed through sexual violence. For some, sex becomes a coping mechanism like self-medication. Sexual abuse can be used as a maladaptive attempt to fulfill a need for attention, affection, or interpersonal connection. Conversely, some use it to avoid the risk and vulnerability of true emotional intimacy. Abusive behavior may not be antisocial per se, but may be learned in a hostile or deprivational environment and adapted as a survival or self-protection strategy. Treatment, then, should facilitate the development of new skills for clients to meet their psychological and social needs in ways that are neither victimizing nor self-destructive (Levenson et al., 2017a).

Dozens of studies document the linear and robust relationship between ACEs and problematic adult outcomes—including medical diseases, mental and behavioral health disorders, substance misuse, school dropout, and interpersonal violence (victimization and perpetration) (Anda et al., 2006). Notably, higher ACE scores are also associated with risky sexual behavior, such as early onset of sexual activity, higher rates of sexually transmitted diseases, unwanted pregnancies, higher numbers of sexual partners, being raped as an adult, and being a victim of sex trafficking (Dietz et al., 1999; Hillis et al., 2000; Levenson et al., 2017b; Naramore et al., 2015). Thus, maltreated children are vulnerable to revictimization, but they may also be at increased risk for engaging in behaviors that violate the sexual boundaries of others.

The goal of TIC is not to excuse abusive behavior or to minimize client resilience. The goal is simply for treatment providers to think about maladaptive behaviors in the context of past trauma and help clients understand how their collective experiences shaped them and contributed to their relationship patterns and coping strategies. TIC encourages an understanding of how maladaptive behavior develops as a survival tool in response to fight-or-flight activation and is maintained over time through triggers and reinforcement. Trauma-informed practitioners respond to clients in non-threatening ways that aim to build adaptive behavior, an internal locus of control, and resilience.

Treatment aimed simply at stopping sexually abusive behavior without considering the past experiences and future well-being of the client may be insufficient. Trauma-informed care can help us in our challenge to develop the most relevant and successful programs and the best methods for delivering them. The principles of effective correctional rehabilitation include individualized assessment and case planning based on risk-needs-responsivity (RNR) (Andrews & Bonta, 2010; Hanson et al., 2009). Not all clients pose the same level of risk for re-offense, and not all possess the same risk factors. As a responsivity factor, trauma requires practitioners to understand how its legacy impacts the client's response to treatment (Giller et al., 2006; Miller & Najavits, 2012). Each client has strengths that can be harnessed in unique ways to build resilience, and these are best cultivated by attending to relational elements in the professional encounter (Giller et al., 2006; Knight, 2015; Levenson, 2017; Miller & Najavits, 2012). Trauma-informed care is a framework and a set of skills that transcends specific models of intervention and can be infused in any type of programming across agency settings and diverse populations. The goal is to create therapeutic spaces that are safe, empowering, collaborative, and corrective.

9.4 Is TIC Evidence-Based?

The role that research plays in designing empirically-informed treatment protocols goes beyond experimental testing in outcome or effectiveness studies (Levenson & Prescott, 2014). It also requires the merger of interdisciplinary and theoretical knowledge as a foundation for understanding client behavior, assessment of client needs, and development of appropriate case plans. It is challenging to "test" TIC in an experimental design, because its application requires an individualized and flexible approach that does not lend itself to the rigid implementation conditions that are required for research replicability. However, TIC rests on an extensive empirical foundation of research about the prevalence and impact of childhood adversity, along with decades of literature about therapeutic alliance, the common factors of psychotherapy, cognitive schemas, self-regulation, and client-centered principles. These areas of knowledge form the evidence base to shape our conceptualization of the importance of trauma-informed care and its application. Evidence-based practices require critical thinking plus an incorporation of research knowledge and best practices designed to address to the unique needs, risks, and strengths of each individual client (Grady et al., 2017).

Advancement in the efficacy of SOTX programs requires an acknowledgment of the role that early adversity plays in the development of sexually abusive behavior. Early trauma lays the groundwork for a range of interpersonal problems, maladaptive coping, relational deficits, and distorted cognitive schema about oneself and others (Adams, 2003; Bloom & Farragher, 2013). Intimacy deficits, which are often related to early adversity and attachment disruptions, have been correlated with sex offense recidivism and are therefore important treatment targets (Hanson & Harris,

2001; Hanson & Morton-Bourgon, 2005). By responding to aggressive and sexualized behavior problems in a more compassionate manner, the trauma-informed therapist creates a corrective emotional experience, fostering resilience and post-traumatic growth. By helping SOTX clients to recognize and change harmful interpersonal patterns, we create opportunities for them to learn new skills, enhance their relationships, and improve their general well-being. This type of personal growth can mitigate future potential to re-offend as the client builds healthy strategies for relating to others and meeting emotional needs in non-victimizing ways (Levenson et al., 2017a).

Our treatment outcome research has produced mixed evidence about the ability of our interventions to reduce recidivism (Hanson et al., 2002; Långström et al., 2013; Marques et al., 2005; Schmucker & Lösel, 2015). We argue that trauma is an important responsivity factor (Bloom, 2013; Miller, 2011; Miller & Najavits, 2012) that SOTX providers should consider when delivering services. It is time to put the therapy back into treatment for sex offending. Though workbooks and treatment manuals can be helpful, any overemphasis on rigidly standardized programming can undermine the principles of psychotherapy, which require flexibility to respond to unique client needs as they present themselves in the therapeutic encounter (see Chap. 5). In this way, approaches that integrate interventions with empirically and theoretically supported principles of change may be most useful for promoting meaningful and successful SOTX practice—ultimately enhancing community safety (Levenson et al., 2017a).

9.5 CARES Model of Trauma-Informed SOTX

Using the acronym CARES (collaboration, autonomy, respect, empathy, safety) will help keep a clinician on track when translating trauma-informed concepts into SOTX practice (Levenson et al., 2017a). TIC moves away from the belief that we must actively restrict and manage client's behavior in order to prevent relapse of sexual assault. Our traditional treatment approaches have moved the locus of control away from the client and undermined the client's investment in change. Instead, TIC shifts from control to collaboration, and does not replace the evidence-based cognitive-behavioral interventions we are familiar with, but provides a framework for delivering those interventions in a way that potentially maximizes client responsivity.

Collaborative approaches allow clients to define their problems and goals and participate in devising strategies through which, together with a caring treatment professional, they can develop internal controls to make the self-improvements they desire.

Autonomy and empowerment honor a client's right to self-determination and allow a client to choose and prioritize his life goals and his pace in treatment in a way that is most meaningful to him.

Respect is crucial; by treating clients in ways that honor their humanity and dignity, we can help restore a sense of value and worth. By treating clients the way we all want to be treated, we reinforce and model the kinds of interactions we want our clients to imitate.

Empathy plays a role in helping clients to appreciate the perspectives of others. When we listen with curiosity and compassion, we model empathy and help our clients to feel connected with others.

Finally, treatment should feel *safe*. Many clients enter treatment with trepidation, shame, defensive denial, fears of judgment, and expectations of rigid authoritarianism. The burden is on treatment providers to create safe spaces for sharing openly and honestly about the sexual behavior problems (Really, safety comes first, but that acronym would be SCARE, which doesn't sound as therapeutic). Safe relationships are consistent, predictable, and non-shaming.

9.6 Translating TIC into SOTX Goals

TIC fits well within RNR, self-regulation, GLM, and RP models of SOTX (ideally, a combination of all). When applied to the common components of sex offending treatment, what becomes important is to utilize the treatment experience to reinforce new skills. In other words, what makes therapy different from a class is that in addition to psychoeducational information, clients have a chance to understand and alter their relational patterns with others in their lives, including group members and therapists. In this section, trauma-informed applications of traditional SOTX goals will be discussed (Levenson et al., 2017a).

9.6.1 Accountability

In our field, we have emphasized admission of offending and full disclosures of sexual history, often before any other treatment goals can be accomplished. While knowing the facts and circumstances around a client's offending behavior is certainly useful in formulating the assessment and treatment plan, the job of the therapist is not to decide whether the client is telling the truth, catch him in a lie, or prove him wrong. Counselors should provide an accepting and safe environment where, perhaps for the first time ever, there is more to be gained than lost by talking about shameful behaviors like sexual abuse. The therapeutic demeanor should say: "I want to listen to you and understand your experience, and I have no need to get into a power struggle or win a debate with you!"

Confrontational approaches to SOTX have historically been popular, and some clinicians fear that without confrontation clients will deceive and manipulate and obfuscate responsibility. However, these tactics may actually disempower and discourage clients from taking responsibility for personal change (Garland & Dougher, 1991;

Kear-Colwell & Pollock, 1997). By challenging and confronting clients in ways that may feel hostile, demeaning, or threatening, therapists may inadvertently reinforce resistance and cause a client to become further entrenched in his own unhelpful ideas (Jenkins, 1990). Negative process can affect group dynamics as well, and persistent, harsh, or adversarial confrontation by group members or therapists can inhibit clients from being forthcoming. On the other hand, respectful challenges from group peers can foster reframing of distorted thinking and lead to increased engagement. Therapeutic confrontation points out inconsistencies and inner conflicts without accusing, blaming, or shaming. It recognizes the fear that goes along with discussing abusive behavior and that people are often ambivalent about change. Utilizing more validating approaches can increase engagement by creating a non-threatening environment, which is less likely to trigger old trauma responses. Decreased defensiveness can lead clients to embrace the possibilities and benefits of change, tolerate emotional distress, and improve patterns of interacting with others (Kear-Colwell & Pollock, 1997; Willemsen et al., 2016).

Accountability should not just be about responsibility for sexually offending behavior. Rather, treatment should offer a more holistic approach to personal accountability in all areas of one's life. It involves a willingness to be honest with oneself and others about weaknesses, mistakes, and character flaws, and to identity the role one plays in contributing to conflict or unhealthy relationship patterns. It requires strength to admit the need for self-improvement in all areas of life, acknowledging truths about oneself that are hard to face. Therapists can model personal responsibility and willingness to admit mistakes and apologize. Therapists can also facilitate the safe and nonjudgmental environment required to recognize one's own human flaws and engage in personal growth. In summary, personal accountability is an important treatment target that goes beyond simply taking responsibility for one's offense. Its goal is to help clients live honestly and with integrity within their value system and be the kind of person they want to be.

9.6.2 Empathy

Empathy is the ability to understand the thoughts and feelings of another, and it seems to be a central reason why we resist harming others—because we can imagine how harm would feel. For our clients, the role of empathy in reducing recidivism is unclear (Fernandez, 2002; Marshall et al., 2001), but its importance may lie in the ability to take the perspective of others. To be able to help our clients with their own self-awareness and perspective-taking, we need to be able to model these skills. This parallel process occurs when the therapist conveys an understanding of the client's experience without judging and recognizes and validates client emotions. It also occurs when we acknowledge trauma and adversity, giving voice and recognition to clients' own inner wounds. Again, this is done not to excuse abusive behavior, but to connect with the feelings and thoughts and meaning attached to victimization experiences.

A lack of a secure attachment to a primary caregiver early in life may hinder empathy development (Adams, 2003; Grady et al., 2016; Marshall, 2010). Abusive or neglectful parenting in childhood fails to model sensitivity to the needs of another, inhibiting the development of skills allowing one to discern the perceptions of those around them. A major ingredient in the parental relationship early in life is a series of "serve and return" encounters between infants and their caregivers, by which parents smile, engage, giggle, coo, and talk, stimulating a reciprocal interaction of social responsiveness (National Scientific Council on the Developing Child, 2012). The absence of early parental responsiveness increases a child's risk for disorganized attachment styles, dependency, detachment, and intimacy deficiencies. Deprivational parenting can lead to narcissistic entitlement and self-centric thinking, with a schema of "get what I can when I can."

An adverse family environment can be a breeding ground for sexually abusive behavior. A lack of nurturing leads to mistrust, hostility, and insecure attachment, which then contribute to social rejection, loneliness, negative peer associations, or delinquent behavior (Hanson & Morton-Bourgon, 2005). "The form of sexuality that develops in the context of pervasive intimacy deficits is likely to be impersonal and selfish, and may even be adversarial... Attitudes allowing non-consenting sex can develop through the individual's effort to understand their own experiences and adopting the attitudes of their significant others (friends, family, abusers)" (Hanson & Morton-Bourgon, 2005, pp. 1154–1155). A trauma-informed therapist modeling empathy provides a new type of encounter and may help shape new awareness about the needs of others. This may in turn reduce criminal attitudes and distorted cognitions about the harmful impact of one's behavior on others. There are many opportunities in treatment groups to engage in trauma-informed responses that model and promote empathy.

In summary, helping clients understand and appreciate victim impact begins with validating their own experiences of being victimized. By giving voice to their own pain, clients can better see abusive actions through the eyes of those they've harmed. By modeling compassion and kindness, we implicitly teach clients to engage with respectful boundaries and non-harmful interactions. By eliminating power struggles, we remove the need for aggression and teach skills of shared power. Facilitating victim empathy is not about shaming, blaming, and confronting clients about how they've hurt people. It is about creating opportunities to practice and rehearse perspective-taking, neutralize power imbalances, and engage in mutual, collaborative decision-making that considers the feelings of others.

9.6.3 Reconstructing Relapse Prevention as Self-Regulation

Traditional relapse prevention approaches emphasize complicated models of cycles and triggers that may not be applicable to all clients. Instead of thinking of relapse prevention as an offense-specific phenomenon, it may be more helpful to focus on self-regulation deficits that create a spectrum of risk factors in clients. Chronic early adversity can alter the architecture of the brain by the overproduction of stress hormones (fight-or-flight responses). The amygdala rules, and the executive functioning of the frontal lobe may be less developed, creating self-regulation deficits in three main areas: *general, sexual, and affect regulation* (Levenson et al., 2017a). These areas are consistent with the items in the Sex Offender Treatment Intervention and Progress Scale (SOTIPS), an empirically designed assessment of improvements in treatment targets (McGrath et al., 2013). Some clients may experience difficulties in multiple categories in all three spheres, while other clients may have problems in very specific areas. It is important for therapists to help each client identify those most applicable to salient behavioral, sexual, or emotional regulation goals.

Children who grow up in chaotic home environments may not get a lot of instruction or modeling in how to be organized, set goals, structure time, or plan ahead. Without a chance to cultivate those skills and practice them early on, their adult lives may mimic the chaos that was so familiar to them in childhood. They may have lacked adult caretakers who created external controls in the environment that restricted the ability to act on impulse. There may have been few chances to learn a decision-making process by which we explore many alternatives and weigh the pros and cons of potential outcomes in order to make a well-reasoned choice. Thus, clients may need help with learning to manage impulsivity, creating routine or structure, becoming organized, managing their time or budget efficiently, and thinking through cause and effect. SOTX counselors should recognize these issues, help clients understand their connection to early life experiences, and coach skills that assist clients to navigate the adult world more successfully.

SOTX programs have typically focused primarily on sexual self-regulation. Obviously this is important, but sexual regulation problems may, for some clients, be representative of other related patterns—in particular, a mechanism to meet emotional or intimacy needs. Some sex offenses occur because a person has a paraphilic interest such as pedophilia, or sexual preoccupation, or an excessive sexual appetite. Sexualized coping may be a way of soothing distress and/or meeting needs for intimacy, affection, attention, power, or control, and this may be especially true for clients with a childhood history of abuse. Molestation in childhood can make a unique contribution to sexually abusive behavior. Sexually abusive behavior may reflect compensation for feelings of powerlessness, social learning by which individuals model their own abuser's behavior and distorted thinking, or the association of sexual arousal with adult-child sexual activity (Seto, 2008). Witnessing violence in the childhood home can contribute to a distorted sense of power dynamics in relationships as well as inaccurate ideas about gender roles, male privilege, respect, and consent. In some cases, sexualized acting out (particularly noncontact offenses like computer-related crimes, exposing, or voyeurism) may be a way of creating distance in interpersonal interactions and avoiding the emotional vulnerability of true intimacy. Clients may have different types of sexual self-regulation issues that differ from paraphilic disorders, such as compulsive masturbation, pornography use, infidelity, sexually harassing behavior, promiscuity, or purchase of sexual services.

Affect regulation is also a prominent theme for many SOTX clients and may manifest in irrational anger, overreaction to environmental stress, "chip on the shoulder," or volatile moods. Interventions can include building skill sets for self-monitoring, de-escalation, distress tolerance, mindfulness, and self-awareness. Addressing conflicts and unhealthy interactions that occur here and now in group therapy sessions are ideal to coach interpersonal skills by creating experiential opportunities for compromise, negotiation, conflict resolution, assertiveness training, and active listening skills. Group therapy is also ideal for helping clients with reality testing, interpersonal competence, and perspective-taking with trusted others. Dialectical behavioral therapy (DBT) can be a helpful supplement for some clients with extreme emotional dysregulation (Linehan, 1993; Stinson, 2016).

Self-regulation skills are crucial in helping people develop a strong sense of self-efficacy, defined as belief in one's own capacity to achieve goals, accomplish tasks, and respond competently to challenges (Bandura, 1977). Emotional competence and self-regulation are important pathways to self-efficacy. Learning how to observe one's own inner experience and become more proficient in managing thoughts, emotions, reactions, relationships, and impulses are essential skills and strategies for preventing re-offense and creating a good life.

9.6.4 Thinking and Cognitions

In most SOTX programs, identifying and restructuring distorted cognitions about offending are common requirements for treatment progress. Offense-related distortions take the form of rationalizing, justifying, and excusing behavior, as well as victim-blaming and denial of the impact of abuse on others. Confrontational approaches are often used in group therapy to address offense-related thinking errors, and clients are often required to "correct" distortions in a cognitive restructuring process. However, trauma-informed approaches suggest that distorted thinking about offending is often tied to larger cognitive schemas about self, others, and the world in general (Levenson et al., 2017a).

Beck defined "cognitive distortions" as "idiosyncratic thought content indicative of distorted or unrealistic conceptualizations" (Beck, 1963, p. 324) that often originate from underlying negative *schemas* or "core beliefs" through which people view themselves, others, the world around them, and the future. Core beliefs reflect "truths" formed in childhood based on experiences that shaped expectations of others and interpretations of events.

Distorted cognitions presented by SOTX clients often reflect entrenched patterns of thinking across many domains of a person's life and relationships. A trauma-informed approach focuses on understanding the origins of maladaptive schemas and exploring the validity of these cognitions in a safe environment. For clients with extensive ACE histories, cognitive treatment targets linked to sexual offending are best conceptualized as symptoms rather than problems, and maladaptive rather than distorted or erroneous (Levenson et al., 2017a).

Offense process work can help clients explore the origins of maladaptive cognitions and identify themes and patterns of expectations about boundaries, adult-child relationships, problem-solving, conflict resolution, sexuality, intimacy, gender roles, power and control, and other relevant relational issues. Often, maladaptive cognitions are connected to early trauma. However, it is important to recognize and acknowledge that other factors, including societal values and cultural norms, can influence the development of offense-related cognitions. These include messages about male privilege, sexualization of youngsters, and the pliable interpersonal boundaries fostered by electronic communication. Rather than simply challenging clients to "correct" their "thinking errors," therapists can promote thoughtful discussions in group that explore harmful social norms as well as individual schemas resulting from personal adversities. In this way, we can empower clients to rethink their own flawed assumptions, enter into a process of self-exploration, and take responsibility for altering their thinking and behavior in healthy ways.

9.6.5 Relationship Skills and the Power of Group Therapy

Relational improvements may be the most important aspect of sex offending treatment, and this begins by modeling within the therapeutic encounter. An important principle of TIC is that respectful language, boundaries, and use of power are crucial to the enactment of safe spaces (Levenson et al., 2017a). Modeling respectful interactions with clients can establish safe and appropriate limits without replicating the oppressive dynamics of other authority figures in their lives (Harris & Fallot, 2001). Safe relationships are consistent, predictable, and non-shaming (Elliott et al., 2005; Marshall 2005; Marshall et al., 2013; Willemsen et al., 2016). The historically confrontational approach of many SOTX programs may inadvertently reproduce disempowering dynamics like those in abusive families (Blagden et al., 2016). This can easily create a parallel process that reactivates trauma and prompts a client's need to respond with old coping skills that were rehearsed over and over in a dysfunctional home. Trauma-informed SOTX can facilitate important changes in relational patterns that might improve self-efficacy and decrease dynamic risk for re-offense.

Erik Erikson proposed that trust in our earliest relationships with caretakers is fundamental to establishing a healthy personality (Erikson, 1993). Maslow's hierarchy advised that all humans have basic needs for survival, physical and psychological safety, social connection, self-esteem, and actualization (Maslow, 1943). Carl Rogers talked about unconditional positive regard, as well as therapist authenticity, as foundational elements of the therapeutic alliance (Rogers, 1961). These core foundations of psychotherapy apply to all clients, including people convicted of sex offenses, and are perhaps even more important in highly dysfunctional patients. When a client's basic need for safety and acceptance in the helping relationship is acknowledged, an atmosphere of trust can be established (Elliott et al., 2005). There are stages of intimacy that all relationships go through, and by allowing the consumer to manage risk-taking at his own pace in the counseling program, the clinician actually models a healthy process of establishing trust based on evidence that another person is listening and responding in a truly reliable and genuine manner.

Most SOTX programs utilize group therapy modalities, and there is growing support for the value of an experiential framework that utilizes interpersonal process in group psychotherapy (Blagden et al., 2016; Gunst, 2012; Levenson, 2014; Marshall & Burton, 2010; Marshall et al., 2013; Sawyer & Jennings, 2016; Willemsen et al., 2016). Relational disturbances can be at the root of sexual offending for many clients, and group allows them to share and process emotions in a safe environment. Being more in touch with feelings can help facilitate emotional and behavioral regulation, as well as deeper intimate connections and improved interactions with others (Blagden et al., 2016; Gunst, 2012; Willemsen et al., 2016). Therapists can foster a group climate in which members establish norms regarding peer support and confrontation, model compassionate interactions, and practice effective communication skills (Macgowan, 2003; Marshall, 2005; Marshall et al., 2013; Marshall et al., 2003; Sawyer & Jennings, 2016). When members see honesty and disclosure being rewarded with support and encouragement, it reduces anxiety and threat, thereby decreasing the need for defensive posturing. A TIC model attempts to employ a respectful and accepting encounter in the group room, maintaining a nonjudgmental atmosphere and avoidance of negative labels (Willis, 2017). Group therapy is an opportunity for strategic process-oriented relational interventions, creating opportunities for clients to relate to others in a meaningful and healthy fashion (Levenson et al., 2009; Levenson & Prescott, 2009).

The power of group cohesion and mutual aid is realized when acceptance and sharing from peers facilitate willingness and ability to interact with others more deeply and honestly (Yalom, 1995). Sexual offending can be a manifestation of having had few opportunities for emotional connection with others (Seidman et al., 1994) due to limited interpersonal skills as well as a desire to hide their sexual interests. Yalom (1995) contended that de-isolation and cohesion results from the discovery that others have similar thoughts and feelings; it is the sharing of one's inner world and subsequent acceptance by others that is a healing force. Group therapy also provides ample opportunities to develop and practice new social skills and constructive conflict resolution in the treatment setting itself (Jennings & Sawyer, 2003). The interactions between group members, and between client and therapist, allow relational patterns to be addressed in a non-threatening way as they present themselves in the therapeutic encounter (Jennings & Sawyer, 2003; Marshall & Burton, 2010; Sawyer & Jennings, 2016; Teyber & McClure, 2011). Therapists can coach clients to engage in effective communication with one another.

9.7 Summary and Conclusions

The success of treatment in reducing recidivism for people who sexually abused remains a subject of controversy (Långström et al., 2013; Levenson & Prescott, 2014), and empirical studies have demonstrated mixed results and small effect sizes.

SOTX treatment exists primarily to prevent future victims. Levenson and Prescott (2014) pointed out, however, that SOTX studies have focused almost exclusively on measuring recidivism rates, while other measures of client improvement have often been ignored. By conceptualizing a broader range of treatment goals, and including various measures of client change, SOTX can foster relational improvements that reduce someone's risk of reoffending (Levenson & Prescott, 2014).

The existing literature in the areas of general psychotherapy, neuroscience, and psychosocial impacts of early adversity have much to offer in our understanding of sexually abusive behavior. TIC brings the therapist back into therapy while incorporating best practice principles of risk-needs-responsivity as well as the strengths-based Good Lives Model of rehabilitation. Areas of focus for trauma-informed SOTX should include the common factors of psychotherapy, attention to the life narratives of clients and the meaning attached to them, awareness of the role of adverse childhood experiences in the development of self-regulation difficulties and maladaptive schema, and use of the therapeutic process to foster a corrective experience and meaningful relational changes.

The definition of evidence-based practice involves using clinical expertise informed by research in the context of unique client strengths and needs. Trauma-informed case conceptualization fosters trauma-informed clinical responses, which creates emotionally safe treatment settings and promotes change through corrective experiences and human connections. TIC empowers clients to define their own goals and make meaningful change that reduces future risk to harm others. Using the acronym CARES (collaboration, autonomy, respect, empathy, safety) will help keep a clinician on track when translating trauma-informed concepts into SOTX practice (Levenson et al., 2017a).

References

Adams, M. J. (2003). Victim issues are key to effective sex offender treatment. *Sexual Addiction & Compulsivity: The Journal of Treatment and Prevention, 10*(1), 79–87. https://doi.org/10.1080/10720160390186330

Anda, R. F., Felitti, V. J., Bremner, J. D., Walker, J. D., Whitfield, C., Perry, B. D., … Giles, W. H. (2006). The enduring effects of abuse and related adverse experiences in childhood. *European Archives of Psychiatry and Clinical Neuroscience, 256*(3), 174–186. https://doi.org/10.1007/s00406-005-0624-4

Andrews, D. A., & Bonta, J. (2010). Rehabilitating criminal justice policy and practice. *Psychology, Public Policy, and Law, 16*(1), 39–55. https://doi.org/10.1037/a0018362

Bandura, A. (1977). Self-efficacy: Toward a unifying theory of behavioral change. *Psychological Review, 84*(2), 191–215. https://doi.org/10.1037/0033-295X.84.2.191

Beck, A. T. (1963). Thinking and depression: I. idiosyncratic content and cognitive distortions. *Archives of General Psychiatry, 9*(4), 324–333. https://doi.org/10.1001/archpsyc.1963.01720160014002

Blagden, N., Winder, B., & Hames, C. (2016). "They treat us like human beings"—Experiencing a therapeutic sex offenders prison: Impact on prisoners and staff and implications for treatment. *International Journal of Offender Therapy and Comparative Criminology, 60*(4), 371–396. https://doi.org/10.1177/0306624x14553227

Bloom, S. L. (2013). *Creating sanctuary: Toward the evolution of sane societies*. New York: Routledge.

Bloom, S. L., & Farragher, B. (2013). *Restoring sanctuary: A new operating system for trauma-informed systems of care*. New York: Oxford University Press.

Creeden, K. (2009). How trauma and attachment can impact neurodevelopment: Informing our understanding and treatment of sexual behaviour problems. *Journal of Sexual Aggression, 15*(3), 261–273. https://doi.org/10.1080/13552600903335844

Dietz, P. M., Spitz, A. M., Anda, R. F., Williamson, D. F., McMahon, P. M., Santelli, J. S., ... Kendrick, J. S. (1999). Unintended pregnancy among adult women exposed to abuse or household dysfunction during their childhood. *JAMA, 282*(14), 1359–1364. https://doi.org/10.1001/jama.282.14.1359

Dube, S. R., Williamson, D. F., Thompson, T., Felitti, V. J., & Anda, R. F. (2004). Assessing the reliability of retrospective reports of adverse childhood experiences among adult HMO members attending a primary care clinic. *Child Abuse & Neglect, 28*(7), 729–737. https://doi.org/10.1016/j.chiabu.2003.08.009

Elliott, D. E., Bjelajac, P., Fallot, R. D., Markoff, L. S., & Reed, B. G. (2005). Trauma-informed or trauma-denied: Principles and implementation of trauma-informed services for women. *Journal of Community Psychology, 33*(4), 461–477. https://doi.org/10.1002/jcop.20063

Erikson, E. H. (1993). *Childhood and society*. New York: W.W. Norton & Company Inc.

Felitti, V. J., Anda, R. F., Nordenberg, D., Williamson, D. F., Spitz, A. M., Edwards, V., ... Marks, J. S. (1998). Relationship of childhood abuse and household dysfunction to many of the leading causes of death in adults: The Adverse Childhood Experiences (ACE) study. *American Journal of Preventive Medicine, 14*(4), 245–258. https://doi.org/10.1016/S0749-3797(98)00017-8

Fernandez, Y. L. (2002). *In their shoes: Examining the issue of empathy and its place in the treatment of offenders*. Oklahoma City, OK: Wood'N'Barnes Publishing.

Garland, R. J., & Dougher, M. J. (1991). Motivational intervention in the treatment of sex offenders. In W. R. Miller & S. Rollnick (Eds.), *Motivational interviewing: Preparing people to change addictive behaviors* (pp. 303–313). New York: The Guilford Press.

Giller, E., Vermilyea, E., & Steele, T. (2006). Risking connection: Helping agencies embrace relational work with trauma survivors. *Journal of Trauma Practice, 5*(1), 65–82. https://doi.org/10.1300/J189v05n01_05

Grady, M. D., Levenson, J. S., & Bolder, T. (2016). Linking adverse childhood effects and attachment: A theory of etiology for sexual offending. *Trauma, Violence, & Abuse, 18*(4), 433–444. https://doi.org/10.1177/1524838015627147

Grady, M. D., Levenson, J. S., & Prescott, D. S. (2017). Empirically informed forensic social work practice. In T. Maschi & G. S. Leibowitz (Eds.), *Forensic social work: Psychosocial and legal issues across diverse populations and settings* (2nd ed., pp. 307–322). New York: Springer.

Gunst, E. (2012). Experiential psychotherapy with sex offenders: Experiencing as a way to change, to live more fulfilling lives, to desist from offending. *Person-Centered & Experiential Psychotherapies, 11*(4), 321–334. https://doi.org/10.1080/14779757.2012.740324

Hanson, R. K., Bourgon, G., Helmus, L., & Hodgson, S. (2009). The principles of effective correctional treatment also apply to sexual offenders: A meta-analysis. *Criminal Justice and Behavior, 36*(9), 865–891. https://doi.org/10.1177/0093854809338545

Hanson, R. K., Gordon, A., Harris, A. J. R., Marques, J. K., Murphy, W., Quinsey, V. L., & Seto, M. C. (2002). First report of the collaborative outcome data project on the effectiveness of treatment for sex offenders. *Sexual Abuse: A Journal of Research and Treatment, 14*(2), 169–194. https://doi.org/10.1023/A:1014624315814

Hanson, R. K., & Harris, A. J. R. (2001). A structured approach to evaluating change among sexual offenders. *Sexual Abuse: A Journal of Research & Treatment, 13*(2), 105–122. https://doi.org/10.1177/107906320101300204

Hanson, R. K., & Morton-Bourgon, K. E. (2005). The characteristics of persistent sexual offenders: A meta-analysis of recidivism studies. *Journal of Consulting and Clinical Psychology, 73*(6), 1154–1163. https://doi.org/10.1037/0022-006X.73.6.1154

Hanson, R. K., & Slater, S. (1988). Sexual victimization in the history of child sexual abusers: A review. *Sexual Abuse: A Journal of Research and Treatment, 1*(4), 485–499. https://doi.org/10.1177/107906328800100402

Hardt, J., & Rutter, M. (2004). Validity of adult retrospective reports of adverse childhood experiences: Review of the evidence. *Journal of Child Psychology and Psychiatry, 45*(2), 260–273. https://doi.org/10.1111/j.1469-7610.2004.00218.x

Harris, M. E., & Fallot, R. D. (2001). *Using trauma theory to design service systems*. San Francisco, CA: Jossey-Bass.

Herman, J. L. (1992). Complex PTSD: A syndrome in survivors of prolonged and repeated trauma. *Journal of Traumatic Stress, 5*(3), 377–391. https://doi.org/10.1002/jts.2490050305

Hillis, S. D., Anda, R. F., Felitti, V. J., Nordenberg, D., & Marchbanks, P. A. (2000). Adverse childhood experiences and sexually transmitted diseases in men and women: a retrospective study. *Pediatrics, 106*(1), 1–6. Retrieved from http://www.pediatrics.org/cgi/content/full/106/1/e11

Jenkins, A. (1990). *Invitations to responsibility*. Richmond, Australia: Dulwich Centre Publications.

Jennings, J. L., & Sawyer, S. (2003). Principles and techniques for maximizing the effectiveness of group therapy with sex offenders. *Sexual Abuse: A Journal of Research & Treatment, 15*(4), 251–267. https://doi.org/10.1177/107906320301500403

Jespersen, A. F., Lalumière, M. L., & Seto, M. C. (2009). Sexual abuse history among adult sex offenders and non-sex offenders: A meta-analysis. *Child Abuse & Neglect, 33*(3), 179–192. https://doi.org/10.1016/j.chiabu.2008.07.004

Kear-Colwell, J., & Pollock, P. (1997). Motivation or confrontation: Which approach to the child sex offender? *Criminal Justice and Behavior, 24*(1), 20–33. https://doi.org/10.1177/0093854897024001002

Knight, C. (2015). Trauma-informed social work practice: Practice considerations and challenges. *Clinical Social Work Journal, 43*(1), 25–37. https://doi.org/10.1007/s10615-014-0481-6

Långström, N., Enebrink, P., Laurén, E.-M., Lindblom, J., Werkö, S., & Hanson, R. K. (2013). Preventing sexual abusers of children from reoffending: Systematic review of medical and psychological interventions. *BMJ: British Medical Journal, 347*(f4630), 1–11. https://doi.org/10.1136/bmj.f4630

Levenson, J. S. (2014). Incorporating trauma-informed care into sex offender treatment. *Journal of Sexual Aggression, 20*(1), 9–22. https://doi.org/10.1080/13552600.2013.861523

Levenson, J. S. (2017). Trauma-informed social work practice. *Social Work, 62*(2), 105–113. https://doi.org/10.1093/sw/swx001

Levenson, J. S., Baglivio, M. T., Wolff, K. T., Epps, N., Royall, W. C., Gomez, K. C., & Kaplan, D. (2017b). You learn what you live: Prevalence of childhood adversity in the lives of juveniles arrested for sexual offenses. *Advances in Social Work, 18*(1), 1–18. https://doi.org/10.18060/21204

Levenson, J. S., Macgowan, M. J., Morin, J. W., & Cotter, L. P. (2009). Perceptions of sex offenders about treatment: Satisfaction and engagement in group therapy. *Sexual Abuse: A Journal of Research & Treatment, 21*(1), 35–56. https://doi.org/10.1177/1079063208326072

Levenson, J. S., & Prescott, D. S. (2009). Treatment experiences of civilly committed sex offenders: A consumer satisfaction survey. *Sexual Abuse: A Journal of Research & Treatment, 21*(1), 6–20. https://doi.org/10.1177/1079063208325205

Levenson, J. S., & Prescott, D. S. (2014). Déjà vu: From Furby to Långström and the evaluation of sex offender treatment effectiveness. *Journal of Sexual Aggression, 20*(3), 257–266. https://doi.org/10.1080/13552600.2013.867078

Levenson, J. S., Willis, G. M., & Prescott, D. S. (2015). Adverse childhood experiences in the lives of female sex offenders. *Sexual Abuse: A Journal of Research & Treatment, 27*(3), 258–283. https://doi.org/10.1177/1079063214544332

Levenson, J. S., Willis, G. M., & Prescott, D. S. (2016). Adverse childhood experiences in the lives of male sex offenders: Implications for trauma-informed care. *Sexual Abuse: A Journal of Research & Treatment, 28*(4), 340–359. https://doi.org/10.1177/1079063214535819

Levenson, J. S., Willis, G. M., & Prescott, D. S. (2017a). *Trauma-informed care: Transforming treatment for people who sexually abuse*. Brandon, VT: Safer Society Press.
Linehan, M. M. (1993). *Cognitive-behavioral treatment of borderline personality disorder*. New York: The Guilford Press.
Macgowan, M. J. (2003). Increasing engagement in groups: A measurement based approach. *Social Work with Groups, 26*(1), 5–28. https://doi.org/10.1300/J009v26n01_02
Marques, J. K., Wiederanders, M., Day, D. M., Nelson, C., & van Ommeren, A. (2005). Effects of a relapse prevention program on sexual recidivism: Final results from California's Sex Offender Treatment and Evaluation Project (SOTEP). *Sexual Abuse: A Journal of Research & Treatment, 17*(1), 79–107. https://doi.org/10.1007/s11194-005-1212-x
Marshall, W. L. (2005). Therapist style in sexual offender treatment: Influence on indices of change. *Sexual Abuse: A Journal of Research & Treatment, 17*(2), 109–116. https://doi.org/10.1177/107906320501700202
Marshall, W. L. (2010). The role of attachments, intimacy, and loneliness in the etiology and maintenance of sexual offending. *Sexual and Relationship Therapy, 25*(1), 73–85. https://doi.org/10.1080/14681990903550191
Marshall, W. L., & Burton, D. L. (2010). The importance of group processes in offender treatment. *Aggression and Violent Behavior, 15*(2), 141–149. https://doi.org/10.1016/j.avb.2009.08.008
Marshall, W. L., Burton, D. L., & Marshall, L. E. (2013). Features of treatment delivery and group processes that maximize the effects of offender programs. In J. L. Wood & T. A. Gannon (Eds.), *Crime and crime reduction: The importance of group processes* (pp. 159–174). New York: Routledge.
Marshall, W. L., Fernandez, Y. M., Serran, G. A., Mulloy, R., Thornton, D., Mann, R. E., & Anderson, D. (2003). Process variables in the treatment of sexual offenders: A review of the relevant literature. *Aggression and Violent Behavior, 8*(2), 205–234. https://doi.org/10.1016/S1359-1789(01)00065-9
Marshall, W. L., Hamilton, K., & Fernandez, Y. (2001). Empathy deficits and cognitive distortions in child molesters. *Sexual Abuse: A Journal of Research & Treatment, 13*(2), 123–130. https://doi.org/10.1177/107906320101300205
Maslow, A. (1943). A theory of human motivation. *Psychological Review, 50*(4), 370–396. https://doi.org/10.1037/h0054346
McGrath, R. J., Cumming, G. F., & Lasher, M. P. (2013). *Sex Offender Treatment Intervention and Progress Scale (SOTIPS) manual*. Middlebury, VT: Author.
Miller, N. A. (2011). *RSAT training tool: Trauma-informed approaches in correctional settings*. Bureau of Justice Assistance. Retrieved from http://www.rsat-tta.com/Training-Curricula/Curricula
Miller, N. A., & Najavits, L. M. (2012). Creating trauma-informed correctional care: A balance of goals and environment. *European Journal of Psychotraumatology, 3*(1), 1–8. https://doi.org/10.3402/ejpt.v3i0.17246
Najavits, L., Schmitz, M., & Johnson, K. M. (2009). Seeking safety therapy for men: Clinical and research experiences. In L. J. Katlin (Ed.), *Men and addictions: New research* (pp. 37–58). Hauppauge, NY: Nova Science Publishers.
Naramore, R., Bright, M. A., Epps, N., & Hardt, N. S. (2015). Youth arrested for trading sex have the highest rates of childhood adversity: A statewide study of juvenile offenders. *Sexual Abuse: A Journal of Research and Treatment, 29*(4), 396–410. https://doi.org/10.1177/1079063215603064
National Scientific Council on the Developing Child. (2012). *The science of neglect: The persistent absence of responsive care disrupts the developing brain: Working paper 12*. Retrieved from http://www.developingchild.harvard.edu
Reavis, J. A., Looman, J., Franco, K. A., & Rojas, B. (2013). Adverse childhood experiences and adult criminality: How long must we live before we possess our own lives? *The Permanente Journal, 17*(2), 44–48. https://doi.org/10.7812/TPP/12-072

Rogers, C. R. (1961). *On becoming a person: A therapist's view of psychotherapy*. New York: Houghton Mifflin Company.
SAMHSA. (2014). *Trauma-informed care in behavioral health services: Treatment Improvement Protocol (TIP) series 57. HHS Publication No. (SMA) 13-4801*. Rockville, MD: Substance Abuse and Mental Health Services Administration. Retrieved from http://store.samhsa.gov/shin/content//SMA14-4816/SMA14-4816.pdf
Sawyer, S., & Jennings, J. L. (2016). *Group therapy with sex offenders: Engaging the full potential of the group experience*. Burlington, VT: Safer Society Press.
Schmucker, M., & Lösel, F. (2015). The effects of sexual offender treatment on recidivism: An international meta-analysis of sound quality evaluations. *Journal of Experimental Criminology, 11*(4), 597–630. https://doi.org/10.1007/s11292-015-9241-z
Seidman, B. T., Marshall, W. L., Hudson, S. M., & Robertson, P. J. (1994). An examination of intimacy and loneliness in sex offenders. *Journal of Interpersonal Violence, 9*(4), 518–534. https://doi.org/10.1177/088626094009004006
Seto, M. C. (2008). *Pedophilia and sexual offending against children: Theory, assessment, and intervention*. Washington, DC: American Psychological Association.
Stinson, J. (2016, April 8). *DBT with sexual offenders*. Paper presented at the Florida Association for the Treatment of Sexual Abusers, Orlando, FL.
Teyber, E., & McClure, F. H. (2011). *Interpersonal process in therapy: An integrative model* (6th ed.). Belmont, CA: Brooks/Cole, Cengage Learning.
Ward, T., & Brown, M. (2004). The good lives model and conceptual issues in offender rehabilitation. *Psychology, Crime & Law, 10*(3), 243–257. https://doi.org/10.1080/10683160410001662744
Willemsen, J., Seys, V., Gunst, E., & Desmet, M. (2016). "Simply speaking your mind, from the depths of your soul": Therapeutic factors in experiential group psychotherapy for sex offenders. *Journal of Forensic Psychology Practice, 16*(3), 151–168. https://doi.org/10.1080/15228932.2016.1172423
Willis, G. M. (2017). Why call someone by what we don't want them to be? The ethics of labeling in forensic/correctional psychology. *Psychology, Crime & Law*, 1–17. https://doi.org/10.1080/1068316X.2017.1421640
Yalom, I. D. (1995). *The theory and practice of group psychotherapy* (4th ed.). New York: Basic Books.

Chapter 10
Can Mindfulness Make Prison a Healthier Place?

Fleet Maull and Kate Crisp

10.1 Introduction and Overview

Mindfulness is a capacity for or state of sustained attention to internal and external stimuli presently arising in conscious awareness moment by moment. The attention aspect of mindfulness, according to its classical roots and the consensus of the majority of clinicians and researchers using contemporary mindfulness-based interventions (MBIs) to prevent or reduce the morbidity related to physical and psychological disorders and enhance physical health and well-being (WB), includes positive attitudinal qualities like nonjudgment, acceptance, friendliness, self-empathy, compassion, kindness, openness, and curiosity. It also includes strategic skills such as attention switching, non-elaboration, letting go, and decentering.

Mindfulness ideally leads to a metacognitive awareness, which includes an awareness that is separate from the contents of awareness (i.e., that one is not one's sensations, thoughts, or feelings) and the possibility of a shift in perspective to a more fluid sense of self or nonself. Mindfulness is also a dispositional trait possessed by everyone to one degree or another, but formal mind training or mindfulness meditation practice increases dispositional mindfulness to sustain the state of mindfulness (Davis & Hayes, 2011; Hussain, 2015; Tang, Hölzel, & Posner, 2015, 2016).

Neuroscientists identified the neural pathways and mechanisms affected by sustained mindfulness, meditation, or mind training and the relation to emotion regulation and well-being (Boccia, Piccardi, & Guariglia, 2015; Davidson & Schuyler, 2015; Grecucci, Pappaianni, Siugzdaite, Theuninck, & Job, 2015; Tang et al., 2015, 2016). Social science and behavioral researchers, as well as neurobiological researchers, suggested a strong potential for mindfulness practice and various MBIs

F. Maull (✉) · K. Crisp
Prison Mindfulness Institute & Center for Mindfulness in Public Safety,
P.O. Box 206, Deerfield 01373, MA, United States
e-mail: fleet@prisonmindfulness.org; kate@prisonmindfulness.org

E. L. Jeglic, C. Calkins (eds.), *New Frontiers in Offender Treatment*,
https://doi.org/10.1007/978-3-030-01030-0_10

to reduce the morbidity associated with physical illness and psychological disorders by promoting improvements in physical health and well-being. In particular, MBIs reduce anxiety and prevent relapse in depressive and addictive disorders (Baer, 2003; Boccia et al., 2015; Brown, Ryan, & Creswell, 2007; Grecucci et al., 2015; Grossman, Neimann, Schmidt, & Walach, 2004; Tang et al., 2015, 2016).

Mindfulness-based interventions (MBIs) like mindfulness-based stress reduction (MBSR), mindfulness-based cognitive therapy (MBCT), acceptance commitment therapy (ACT), dialectical behavioral therapy (DBT), and mindfulness-based relapse prevention (MBRP) have found increasing clinical application in the psychotherapy, counseling, and mental health treatment fields (Brown et al., 2007). Combinations of acceptance-based approaches to cognitive therapy [ACT, DBT, and MBCT] and mindfulness show promise for increasing empathy through greater attentiveness in the present moment to thoughts and feelings experienced by oneself and others and the resulting intimacy and appreciation for the others experience (Block-Lerner, Adair, Plumb, Rhatigan, & Orsillo, 2007). Both a pilot pre-/post study and a follow-up RCT demonstrated gains in self-compassion, mindfulness, and well-being from a mindful self-compassion (MSC) training program sustained at 6-month and 1-year follow-ups (Neff & Germer, 2013).

10.1.1 Mindfulness Programs in Prison Settings

Mindfulness-based programs (MBPs) of varying types, both faith-based and secular, have been offered in the US prison system since at least the 1960s, with mindfulness teachers like Stephen Levine bringing mindfulness practices to death row inmates at San Quentin State Prison in California. A prison dharma movement, disseminating Buddhist mindfulness meditation practices, emerged in the 1980s and grew dramatically over the past three decades. Prison Dharma Network (aka Prison Mindfulness Institute), a nonprofit organization founded in 1989, promotes both faith-based and secular approaches to offering mindfulness to at-risk and incarcerated youth and adults and has over 150 organizations and thousands of individual members in its network supporting meditation programs in jails and prisons all across the United States (Prison Mindfulness Institute, 2018).

During the past two decades, mindfulness-based therapies developed in the 1980s, like DBT (Marsha Linehan) and ACT (Stephen Hays), and have gained traction in forensic psychology and treatment programs with incarcerated youth and adults. More recently, the MBSR model developed by Jon Kabat-Zinn and the MBCT model developed by Zindel Segal and Mark Williams, representing an integration of MBSR and cognitive behavioral therapy (CBT), have found applications with incarcerated populations. Currently, most of the secular and/or clinical mindfulness-based approaches are grouped under the term mindfulness-based interventions or MBIs.

The current landscape of MBPs in US prisons, jails, and juvenile facilities includes both faith-based and secular meditation and yoga programs. Even the faith-based meditation programs offered through prison chapels tend to focus more on mindfulness meditation and physical yoga than on religious teaching. Various clinical MBIs, such as DBT, ACT, MBSR, and MBCT, are gaining traction as therapeutic approaches to offender treatment and rehabilitation. Also, an increasing number of secular mindfulness classes offered by both outside volunteers and to nonclinical offender populations, and several mindfulness-based programs (MBPs) that include a psychoeducational component, like Prison Mindfulness Institute's *Path of Freedom*© and Lionheart Foundation's *Power Source*, are being implemented around the country.

More recently, mindfulness is finding its way into professional development and wellness training for correctional officers and other corrections staff in the form of mindfulness-based wellness programs like Center for Mindfulness in Public Safety's Mindfulness-Based Wellness & Resiliency (MBWR)(c) program. This chapter will focus on reviewing the research on the effectiveness and outcomes of secular MBIs and MBPs employed with both clinical and nonclinical offender populations, as well as mindfulness-based wellness programs for prison staff.

10.1.2 General Research on Mindfulness-Based Interventions (MBIs)

Early research in the behavioral and social science fields included efficacy studies on interventions like MBSR that employ mindfulness techniques and practices to reduce psychological distress and psychopathology. These studies supported the effectiveness of MBIs (MBSR in particular) for ameliorating distressing physical and psychological symptomatology (Anderson, Lau, Segal, & Bishop, 2007; Bishop et al., 2004; Brown et al., 2007; Kabat-Zinn et al., 1992; Shapiro, Carlson, Astin, & Freedman, 2006). A growing body of scientific literature supports the clinical application of MBIs like MBSR, MBCT, DBT, ACT, and MBRT for a variety of psychological disorders including anxiety, depression, addiction, and dual diagnosis (Anderson et al., 2007; Brown et al., 2007; Carmody & Baer, 2008; Grecucci et al., 2015; Gupta, 2014; Hussain, 2015; Lau & Yu, 2009; Tang et al., 2015, 2016).

This chapter will review how new and promising evidence-based MBIs are being employed with both offenders and prison staff. While there has been an increased emphasis on *evidence-based practice* (EBP) within forensic treatment, applications have been limited largely to cognitive behavioral therapy (CBT; see Chap. 4). There remains a disconnect between the growing body of evidence supporting the clinical application of various MBIs and their employment in offender treatment. We seek to bridge that gap by providing an overview of interventions with demonstrated efficacy and how these approaches have been translated into offender treatment. We will highlight how MBIs can be used beyond targeting factors that have traditionally been thought to reduce recidivism and encompass issues related to a more holistic sense of well-being, which more recent research suggests can promote desistance.

Research on treatment approaches including mindfulness will be reviewed. In addition, we will discuss areas where additional research is needed.

10.2 Mindfulness Defined

Kabat-Zinn (1994), a pioneer in the mainstreaming of mindfulness in the healthcare setting, defined mindfulness as "paying attention, on purpose, in the present moment, in a particular way, and nonjudgmentally" (p. 4). Drawing on experiences with Buddhist-derived mindfulness practice, Kabat-Zinn first introduced the MBSR model as a secularized intervention to help patients suffering from chronic pain at the University of Massachusetts Medical Center in 1979 (Kabat-Zinn, 1990, 1994, 2011). MBSR is now the most widely known and popular MBI in clinical settings (Malinowski, 2008).

Mindfulness can be seen both as a set of attention training skills (Carmody, 2009) and a resultant state (Carmody, 2009; Reid, 2011); Kabat-Zinn (2003) described the resultant state of mindfulness as "the awareness that emerges through paying attention on purpose, in the present moment, and nonjudgmentally to the unfolding of experience moment to moment" (p. 145). The type of mindfulness training prominent in mainstream clinical applications has its roots in various Buddhist traditions and training practices aimed at liberating individuals from suffering (Carmody, 2009; Malinowski, 2008).

Current concepts of mindfulness vary along a spectrum, ranging from simple attention training to the proactive cultivation of metacognitive awareness, self-empathy, self-acceptance, and self-compassion (Carmody, 2009; Malinowski, 2008). Carmody (2009) described mindfulness as intentionally paying attention to present moment experiences nonjudgmentally. Bishop et al. (2004), Kabat-Zinn (1994, 2003), Siegel (2006), and others (Anderson et al., 2007; Baldini, Parker, Nelson, & Siegel, 2014; Grecucci et al., 2015; Malinowski, 2008; Reid, 2011) argued for the inclusion of intentional cultivation of openness, curiosity, acceptance, and self-compassion as well as the skill of awareness or metacognition (being aware of being mindful, aware of being aware) in order to realize the full therapeutic potential of mindfulness training to promote healing, enhance overall psychological well-being (PWB), and promote prosocial attitudes and behaviors.

Shapiro et al. (2006) proposed a three-component model (see Fig. 10.1) consisting of (1) intention, (2) attention, and (3) attitude or orientation to experience. Shapiro et al. (2006) also proposed *reperceiving* as a *meta-mechanism of action*, defined as a shift in perspective that allowed a person to "disidentify from the contents of consciousness (i.e., one's thoughts) and view his or her moment-by-moment experiences with greater clarity and objectivity" (p. 3). Others have used terms like meta-awareness, metacognition, or metacognitive awareness to describe this same meta-mechanism, discussing it as *decentering* or a shift in perspective of self (Carmody, 2009; Dorjee, 2016; Hussain, 2015).

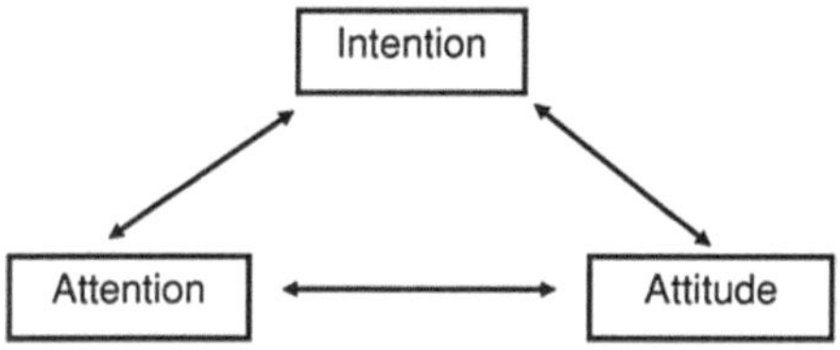

Fig. 10.1 The three axioms of mindfulness—intention, attention, and attitude—are not separate stages but rather interwoven aspects of a single cyclic process occurring simultaneously. Mindfulness is this moment-to-moment process (Shapiro et al., 2006, p. 3)

Shapiro et al. (2006) associated the three core components or *axioms* of their mindfulness model with three of the elements in Kabat-Zinn's (1994) operational definition for mindfulness: intention, *on purpose*; attention, *paying attention*; and attitude, *in a particular way*. Shapiro et al. (2006) further theorized four additional mechanisms of mindfulness that may contribute to the positive outcomes of mindfulness practice: (1) self-regulation and self-management; (2) emotional, cognitive, and behavioral flexibility; (3) values clarification; and (4) exposure.

10.2.1 Benefits of Mindfulness

The benefits of mindfulness meditation practice have been widely shown in the research to date. These benefits include enhancement of individual capacities and other improvements like becoming more accepting, patient, open-hearted, nonreactive, nonjudgmental, and compassionate; attending to moment-to-moment experience; emotional, cognitive, and behavioral flexibility; self-regulation of awareness and attention; emotion regulation and stress reduction; ability to cope with pain and distress; improved working memory; improved physical health and personal well-being; relieving suffering; and increased emotional intelligence, empathy, and prosocial behaviors (Baer, 2003; Bishop et al., 2004; Boccia et al., 2015; Brown et al., 2007; Brown & Ryan, 2003; Carmody, 2009; Carmody & Baer, 2008; Grecucci et al., 2015; Gupta, 2014; Hussain, 2015; Kabat-Zinn, 2003; Mandal, Arya, & Pandey, 2014; Nyklíček, Dijksman, Lenders, Fonteijn, & Koolen, 2014; Shapiro et al., 2006). Further, mindfulness positively correlates with subjective well-being and psychological well-being (Brown et al., 2007; Davidson & Schuyler, 2015; Mathura & Sharma, 2014). In addition, two of the core aspects of mindfulness, awareness and nonjudgmental acceptance of moment-to-moment experience, "are regarded as potentially effective antidotes against common forms of psychological distress, rumination, anxiety, worry, fear, anger and so on …" (Mathura & Sharma, 2014, p. 535). Researchers empirically associated both dispositional mindfulness and enhanced trait mindfulness with positive emotions and an overall positive outlook, optimal mental health, and healthy functioning in life (Boccia et al., 2015; Brown et al., 2007).

Past research supports the positive impact of mindfulness practice and various MBIs and MBPs (MBSR, MBCT, ACT, DBT, and others) on physical and psychological health. Such interventions treat physical illnesses like hypertension, fibromyalgia, heart disease, cancer, and HIV/AIDS and psychological disorders like anxiety, depression, burnout, and PTSD (Anderson et al., 2007; Bishop et al., 2004; Brown et al., 2007; Grecucci et al., 2015; Kabat-Zinn et al., 1992; Khusid & Vythilingam, 2016b; Nyklíček & Kuijpers, 2008; Shapiro et al., 2006).

Various neuroscientific investigations exploring neuroplasticity and the potential for reshaping the brain in support of healthier, more integrated brain functionality have investigated the impact of mindfulness training on neuroplasticity and overall brain health (Baldini et al., 2014; Boccia et al., 2015; Davidson & McEwen, 2012; Davidson & Schuyler, 2015; Garland & Howard, 2009; Rybak, 2013). Functional MRIs and other brain scanning technologies have been combined with psychosocial investigations to demonstrate the salutary impact of various intentional mindfulness practices on the healthy functioning of the human brain and the resulting enhancement of cognitive and emotional function, processing, emotion regulation, well-being, resilience, and inclination toward prosocial and altruistic attitudes and behaviors like caring, compassion, and generosity (Baldini et al., 2014; Boccia et al., 2015; Davidson & McEwen, 2012; Davidson & Schuyler, 2015; Garland & Howard, 2009; Rybak, 2013).

Neurobiological studies using advanced neuroimaging technologies and other neurophysiological markers have produced compelling data in recent years. Studies have demonstrated clear differences in brain structure and function in groups of long-term practitioners of mindfulness when compared to beginning practitioners or non-practitioners (Boccia et al., 2015; Grecucci et al., 2015; Tang et al., 2015, 2016; Tang & Posner, 2013). Longitudinal studies have shown mindfulness training to be a mediator of neuroplasticity, improved brain function, and increases in dispositional mindfulness and well-being (Boccia et al., 2015; Davidson & McEwen, 2012; Davidson & Schuyler, 2015; Grecucci et al., 2015; Tang et al., 2015, 2016; Tang & Posner, 2013).

Davidson and Schuyler (2015) identified four underlying constituents of well-being: (1) positive outlook, (2) resilience, (3) altruistic behaviors (e.g., empathy, compassion, generosity), and (4) attention/mindfulness and have suggested that well-being may be a trainable skill. Davidson and Schuyler (2015) further demonstrated that taking advantage of the neuroplasticity of neural networks involved in experiences of SWB and PWB via various forms of psychotherapy and mindfulness training can enhance the underlying constituents and overall well-being altogether. Sharma and Tomer (2018) found significant correlations between subjective well-being (SWB) and prosocial behaviors. Gesch, Hammond, Hampson, Eves, and Crowder (2002) found correlations between healthy nutrition (intervention involving dietary supplements), SWB, and reduced antisocial behaviors. Thus, given society's interest in reducing antisocial behaviors and promoting prosocial behaviors among incarcerated youth and adults, increasing SWB and PWB through MBIs and MBPs warrants further experimentation and research.

Similarly, there is a growing body of research demonstrating correlations between trait mindfulness, resilience, and various components of resilience as well as increases in resilience associated with mindfulness training (Davidson & Schuyler, 2015; Davies, 2016; Jain & Singh, 2016; Wu et al., 2013). MBIs have preventive and treatment potential for individuals at risk for or suffering from PTSD through the enhancement of resilience (Bernstein, Tanay, & Vujanovic, 2011; Chopko & Schwartz, 2009; Khusid & Vythilingam, 2016a).

What Are the Unique Needs of Incarcerated Individuals That Mindfulness Training Might Address? In addition to helping incarcerated individuals come to terms with the emotional dysregulation and challenges of incarceration, mindfulness meditation also supports those in prison in dealing with the unique systemic effects that prison life has on an individual. Prisons and jails are noisy, stressful, possibly dangerous, and challenging environments. Prisoners experiencing a loss of freedom, family, employment, home, privacy, status, and all familiar reference points and are then thrown into a hostile environment with adversarial relational situations around every corner. These environments do not support the integration of the grief and emotional pain that occurs through this systemic loss. Mindfulness meditation can help prisoners cope with and understand this difficult world they have landed in and provide them with resources that will serve them in the reentry process.

Auty, Cope, and Leibling (2017) performed a systematic review and meta-analysis of research studies on prison yoga and meditation programs prior to December 2014. They found evidence to support the conclusion that prison yoga and meditation programs produce some positive impact on participants' psychological well-being (PWB) and behavioral functioning with a larger effect size for PWB (Cohen's $d = 0.46$) versus behavioral functioning ($d = 0.30$). They theorized that this difference could be attributed to yoga and meditation having a more immediate healthy impact on brain function, as described in other studies (Tang et al., 2007; Zylowska et al., 2008), while effects on behavior might require a study with a longer follow-up period. An earlier systematic review of the research on meditation programs in correctional settings by Himelstein (2011a) also found support for prison meditation programs positively impacting PWB. Himelstein (2011b) in another study also found support for improvements in self-regulation, self-reported drug use, and recidivism.

10.3 The Application of MBIs with Incarcerated Populations

Given that there is a paucity of research, especially studies with rigorous RCT designs, examining outcomes and measuring effectiveness with mindfulness-based interventions (MBIs) and mindfulness-based programs (MBPs) with incarcerated populations, for the purposes of this chapter, we will look at both existing and potential applications of MBIs across three categories of offender issues and needs, including (1) aggression, violence, and antisocial personality disorder (ASPD), (2) substance abuse and addiction, and (3) depression, mental illness, and dual diagnosis. We will address specific applications of MBIs with incarcerated women and juveniles within each of those four categories above where research is available. Finally, we will also address MBIs and MBPs designed to enhance wellness and resiliency among correctional officers and other prison staff as an important component of creating healthier correctional environments.

10.3.1 Aggression, Violence, and Anti-social Personality Disorder (ASPD)

Plambeck (2015) found that ACT showed promise as a treatment for reducing problematic anger-related behaviors in male jail populations. Velotti et al. (2016) found correlations between mindfulness impairment (mentalizing and metacognitive network impairment) and antisocial personality disorder (ASPD) and that mindfulness training may moderate the relationship between aggression and antisocial personality disorder (ASPD) by increasing capacity for awareness of moment-to-moment experiences and behaviors and their underlying personal motives and mental states. Based upon a review of the research literature, Heppner et al. (2008) concluded that higher levels of ego involvement (interpreting daily occurrences as to their self-referenced implications) are associated with greater levels of aggression and hostility and that higher levels of dispositional mindfulness are associated with lower levels of ego involvement. They then theorized that higher levels of trait and state mindfulness would be related to lower levels of aggression and that mindfulness training could reduce aggressive responses. Performing two studies, one examining the relationship between dispositional mindfulness and self-reported aggressiveness and hostility and the other examining the relationship between experimentally induced (state) mindfulness and aggressive responses to social rejection, Heppner et al. (2008) demonstrated that both trait (dispositional) and state (experimentally induced) mindfulness are related to lower levels of aggression in general and specifically in response to social rejection, thus supporting their theory that mindfulness training could reduce aggressive tendencies.

10.3.2 Women at Risk for Anger, Hostility, and Violence

Smith, Tew, and Patel (2015) described a MBP known as CARE, combining mindfulness training (MT) with narrative therapy (NT), that completed a rigorous Correctional Services Accreditation and Advice Panel (CSAAP) accreditation process based on the "what works" literature to become an evidence-based treatment for female offenders at risk for violence in the United Kingdom. Mulay, Kelly, and

Cain (2017) found an 18-month DBT program to be effective in reducing violent behaviors, anger, and hostility in female prisoners.

10.3.3 Juvenile Offenders at Risk for Anger and Hostility

Derezotes (2000) found that an MBP combining yoga and mindfulness meditation led to increased self-control and self-awareness and reduced stress and anger in juvenile sex offenders.

10.3.4 Substance Abuse and Addiction Treatment

Studies strongly suggest that impulse control is a key predictor of criminal behavior and is strongly connected to drug and alcohol addiction (Gottfredson & Hirschi, 1990; Samuelson, Carmody, Kabat-Zinn, & Bratt, 2007). Multiple studies have demonstrated positive effects of mindfulness-based interventions for treating and preventing substance abuse and addiction (Appel & Kim-Appel, 2009; Gelderloos, Walton, Orme-Johnson, & Alexander, 1991; Marlatt & Chawla, 2007; Witkiewitz, Marlatt, & Walker, 2005; Zgierska et al., 2009). In addition, MBCT interventions integrating mindfulness meditation with CBT for substance abuse have been found to positively impact outcome (Alterman, Koppenhaver, Mulholland, Ladden, & Baime, 2004; Amaro et al., 2010; Beitel et al., 2007; Bowen et al., 2009; Brewer et al., 2009; Britton et al., 2010; Garland, Gaylord, Boettiger, & Howard, 2010; Witkiewitz & Bowen, 2010; Zgierska et al., 2008). Khusid and Vythilingam (2016a, 2016b) performed a systematic review of the literature, including high-level studies regarding the effectiveness of MBIs for the treatment of chronic pain, substance abuse, and insomnia, and found a strong support for effectiveness of MBIs like MBSR, MBCT, and MBRP in the treatment of all three conditions.

Mohammadkhani, Khanipour, Azadmehr, Mobramm, and Naseri (2015) explored the relationship between substance abuse, suicidality, and trait mindfulness and found that higher levels of trait mindfulness were strongly correlated with a lower risk of suicidality and other psychiatric symptomatology in prisoners with a history of substance abuse who are at a very high risk for various psychological disturbances and suicidality. They cited research by Chambers, Gullone, and Allen (2009) demonstrating that mindfulness supports healthy adaptive and self-regulation behaviors. Thus, they theorized that mindfulness could act as a protective resilience enhancement lowering the likelihood of maladaptive self-regulation behaviors like suicide attempts. For this reason, they recommended that mindfulness training be included in forensic treatment interventions and programs addressing substance abuse and suicide risk, noting both DBT and MBCT as possible components of an effective treatment strategy (Mohammadkhani et al., 2015).

In another study, Bowen et al. (2006) found preliminary support for the effectiveness of a particular form of mindfulness, known as vipassana meditation (VM), in treating substance abuse disorders among incarcerated populations. They found that participants in a jail-based VM mindfulness course had lower rates of substance abuse across different substances (alcohol, marijuana, and crack cocaine) during a 3-month post-release follow-up, as well as significantly fewer psychiatric symptoms and higher levels of optimism.

10.3.5 Substance Abuse Treatment for Incarcerated Juveniles

Himelstein, Saul, and Garcia-Romeu (2015) employed an RCT design and found that mindfulness training delivered one on one to incarcerated juveniles in a substance abuse treatment program strengthened program outcomes through improvements in participant's behavior regulation. This more rigorous study confirmed preliminary findings from a pilot study that demonstrated improved impulse control and psychological functioning in incarcerated juveniles participating in a mindfulness program (Himelstein, 2011b). Leonard et al. (2013) in an RCT employing a combination of CBT and mindfulness training (MT) found that the CBT/MT combination showed promise as a protective treatment mediating the degradation of attention and cognitive functions due to high stress levels in incarcerated adolescents, factors that could also support effective substance abuse treatment. Evans-Chase (2013) reported preliminary results with new internet-based mindfulness training (MT) intervention with incarcerated juveniles that shows promise for improving self-regulation, an important factor in the success of other treatment interventions.

10.3.6 Depression, Mental Illness, and Dual Diagnosis Treatment

James and Glaze (2006) reported that 74% of state prisoners and 76% of local jail prisoners in the United States meet the criteria of dual diagnosis (substance abuse disorder combined with other depression and/or other psychiatric disorders) and that such complications as major depressive disorder and ASPD increased the probability of reoffending among released prisoners having completed a substance abuse treatment program prior to release. Moyes, Heath, and Dean (2016) recommended improvements to treatment programs for dual diagnosis prisoners including more holistic and integrated approaches and the use of low-level, flexible interventions (possible indication favoring the use of MBIs).

10.3.7 Women Prisoners: Stress, Anxiety, Depression, and Sleep Issues

Incarcerated women in prisons often have histories of trauma and mental health and substance abuse issues. On top of that, considering the stress of incarceration and separation from their children, families, and significant others, it is not surprising that many women experience increased stress, anxiety, depression, and sleep issues. In a study examining the impact of a mindfulness-based emotional intelligence, researchers found promising results. The women exhibited lower scores on stress, anxiety, and depression following the intervention (Ferszt, Miller, Hickey, Maull, & Crisp, 2015).

10.4 Mindfulness-Based Wellness & Resiliency (MBWR) Programs for Prison Staff

The combination of extremely high levels of work stress, lack of healthy stress management knowledge and skills, and the utilization of unhealthy stress coping mechanisms leads to significant physical and mental health risks, including a host of chronic, stress-related illnesses (e.g., obesity, diabetes, hypertension, musculoskeletal disease, cardiovascular disease, and cancer) (Brower, 2013; Keinan & Malach-Pines, 2007; McCraty, Atkinson, Lipsenthal, & Arguelles, 2009). Stress may also lead to anxiety, depression, and suicide (Brower, 2013; Warren, Dussetschleger, Punnet, & Cherniack, 2015). Chronic, stress-related physical and mental illnesses add additional mortality risks to the correctional occupation (Brower, 2013). Suicide risk among correctional officers is also a growing concern; some reports estimated the suicide rate among correctional officers to be twice that of police officers (Brower, 2013).

Wellness programs are a relatively new phenomenon in the corrections field, and there is little data available on the efficacy of such programs (Bezerra, Assis, & Constantino, 2016; Brower, 2013). Page and Vella-Brodrick (2009) explored the "what, how, and why of employee wellbeing" and argued that employee well-being is made up of three sub-constructs: subjective well-being (SWB), workplace well-being, and psychological well-being (PWB). SWB (positive feelings/happiness) includes life satisfaction and dispositional affect. Workplace well-being includes work satisfaction and work-related affect. PWB (positive functioning) includes self-acceptance, positive relations with others, environmental mastery, autonomy, purpose in life, and personal growth (Page & Vella-Brodrick, 2009). Weiss, Westerhof, and Bohlmeijer (2016) conducted a meta-analysis of self-report assessments of various behavioral interventions designed to improve PWB and found that such behavioral interventions significantly enhance PWB.

Researchers reported considerable evidence of correlations between mindfulness as measured by various self-report scales and well-being as measured by various scales measuring either subjective (hedonic) well-being (SWB) or psychological (eudaimonic) well-being (PWB) and correlations between low levels of mindfulness and psychological distress in the general public, meditators and non-meditators, student's critical care unit personnel, public hospital workers, and probation and parole officers (Chang, Huang, & Lin, 2015; Hanley, Warner, & Garland, 2015; Jain & Singh, 2016; Lan, Subramanian, Rahmat, & Kar, 2014; Mitchell & Heads, 2015; Moral, Kumar, & Sharma, 2014; Nyklíček & Kuijpers, 2008; Shonin, Van Gordon, & Griffiths, 2014; Weiss et al., 2016). Jain and Singh (2016) reported on various studies suggesting that low levels of mindfulness, low self-compassion, and low self-efficacy are all predictors of psychological distress. Conversely, high levels of mindfulness, self-compassion, self-efficacy, awareness, and nonjudging are predictors of well-being (Jain & Singh, 2016). Mitchell and Heads (2015) reported increases in self-reported well-being sustained for up to 4 years following the completion of a 5-week adaptation of the normally 8-week MBSR program.

10.5 Implications for Future Research

Past research supports the effectiveness of various MBIs and MBPs to enhance SWB, PWB, and resilience in nonclinical and clinical populations. However, many studies suffered from various weaknesses in design and sample size. More rigorous RCTs are necessary. Researchers shifted from a focus primarily on outcome studies toward identifying, isolating, and investigating the underlying mechanisms and mediating factors of WB, resilience, and mindfulness, but more research is necessary to understand exactly how, why, and to what extent mindfulness prevents or decreases psychological distress while enhancing immunity, physical health, WB, and resilience.

Well-designed, methodologically sound, and robust studies are necessary to further illuminate these various mechanisms, their interactions with each other, and their impact on human health. As stated, the advances in neuroscience research offered a window into the biological and neuronal substrates of SWB, PWB, resilience, and mindfulness and the apparent plasticity of those substrates. However, most studies were cross-sectional in design and subject to selection effects and other problems. More longitudinal studies will determine the impact of mindfulness training on WB, resilience, and overall human health, happiness, and performance over time and to what degree practitioners can sustain that impact. Other areas that require further investigation are the impact of gender, culture, baseline attachment levels, and other individual and group differences regarding how mindfulness functions as a trait or skill in mediating human health.

Corrections research in particular on the use and implementation of various MBIs and MBPs for prisoner treatment and rehabilitation as well as for staff health, wellness, and employee performance is in its infancy. There have been very few empirical studies focused on mindfulness-based prisoner treatment/rehabilitation or staff wellness programs and even fewer have met the rigorous standards for effective

RCTs. Many program evaluations involve insufficient or partially implemented interventions that imply negative results. Rhine, Mawhorr, and Parks (2006) suggested program evaluation reports not be completed until a new intervention or program reaches full operational stability with fidelity to the intervention or program design and that program evaluators focus on helping practitioners improve the quality of the program to its intended operational capacity before writing and delivering reports on effectiveness or ineffectiveness.

10.6 Summary

Overall, there is considerable evidence of mindfulness practice and MBIs and MBPs as effective strategies for the enhancement of well-being and resiliency for prisoners and prison staff—both at risk for chronic stress, primary and secondary trauma exposure, and psychological disorders including substance abuse, depression, PTSD, and suicidality. The evidence thus supports the implementation of MBPs for both prisoners and prisoner workers as an overall strategy for creating healthier correctional environments leading to improved offender outcomes and enhanced public safety.

Creating healthy organizational cultures that enhance well-being and resilience for correctional staff while effectively promoting rehabilitation for offenders are indicated for improving correctional management and outcomes. Training programs for correctional staff and rehabilitation programs for offenders can be effective, as past researchers demonstrated through well-designed, well-implemented, and properly sustained training programs (Bechtel, 2011; Paparozzi & Guy, 2013; Rhine et al., 2006; Trounson & Pfeifer, 2016).

The idea of creating *healthy* prisons is not a new one. The WHO promoted a Health in Prisons model in 1995, suggesting a complete transformation of the punishment-oriented total prison/total institution model into a whole prison model focused on health and sustainability for everyone involved (Ross & Harzke, 2012, p. 16). In the language of this chapter, a *whole prison* is a *mindful prison*. The focus is on promoting health, WB, and resilience for everyone through the application of evidenced-based MBIs and MBPs and sound correctional management practices. Denmark, Finland, Norway, and Sweden developed a very different vision for criminal justice and corrections and developed much more effective policies and correctional facilities that are healthier for everyone involved (Griffin, 2013; Pratt, 2008). There is no particular reason that the United States cannot envision and accomplish the same or at least begin to move in that direction.

References

Alterman, A. I., Koppenhaver, J. M., Mulholland, E., Ladden, L. J., & Baime, M. J. (2004). Pilot trial of effectiveness of mindfulness meditation for substance abuse patients. *Journal of Substance Use, 9*(6), 259–268. https://doi.org/10.1080/14659890410001711698

Amaro, H., Magno-Gatmaytan, C., Meléndez, M., Cortés, D. E., Arevalo, S., & Margolin, A. (2010). Addiction treatment intervention: An uncontrolled prospective pilot study of Spiritual Self-Schema therapy with Latina women. *Substance Abuse, 31*(2), 117–125. https://doi.org/10.1080/08897071003641602

Anderson, N. D., Lau, M. A., Segal, Z. V., & Bishop, S. R. (2007). Mindfulness-based stress reduction and attentional control. *Clinical Psychology and Psychotherapy, 14*(6), 449–463. https://doi.org/10.1002/cpp.544

Appel, J., & Kim-Appel, D. (2009). Mindfulness: Implications for substance abuse and addiction. *International Journal of Mental Health and Addiction, 7*(4), 506–512. https://doi.org/10.1007/s11469-009-9199-z

Auty, K. M., Cope, A., & Leibling, A. (2017). A systematic review and meta-analysis of yoga and mindfulness meditation in prison: Effects on psychological well-being and behavioral functioning. *International Journal of Offender Therapy and Comparative Criminology, 61*(6), 689–710. https://doi.org/10.1177/0306624X15602514

Baer, R. A. (2003). Mindfulness training as a clinical intervention: A conceptual and empirical review. *Clinical Psychology: Science and Practice, 10*(2), 125–143. https://doi.org/10.1093/clipsy.bpg015

Baldini, L. L., Parker, S. C., Nelson, B. W., & Siegel, D. J. (2014). The clinician as neuroarchitect: The importance of mindfulness and presence in clinical practice. *Clinical Social Work Journal, 42*(3), 218–277. https://doi.org/10.1007/s10615-014-0476-3

Bechtel, K. A. (2011). The importance of implementation in corrections. *Corrections Today, 73*, 105–106. Retrieved from http://www.aca.org

Beitel, M., Genova, M., Schuman-Olivier, Z., Arnold, R., Avants, S. K., & Margolin, A. (2007). Reflections by inner-city drug users on a Buddhist-based spirituality-focused therapy: A qualitative study. *American Journal of Orthopsychiatry, 77*(1), 1–9. https://doi.org/10.1037/0002-9432.77.1.1

Bernstein, A., Tanay, G., & Vujanovic, A. A. (2011). Concurrent relations between mindful attention and awareness and psychopathology among trauma-exposed adults: Preliminary evidence of transdiagnostic resilience. *Journal of Cognitive Psychotherapy, 25*(2), 99–113. https://doi.org/10.1891/0889-8391.25.2.99

Bezerra, C. D. M., Assis, S. G., & Constantino, P. (2016). Psychological distress and work stress in correctional officers: A literature review. *Ciência & Saúde Coletiva, 21*(7), 2135–2146. https://doi.org/10.1590/1413-81232015217.00502016

Bishop, S. R., Lau, M., Shapiro, S., Carlson, L., Anderson, N. D., Carmody, J., … Devins, G. (2004). Mindfulness: A proposed operational definition. *Clinical Psychology: Science and Practice, 11*(3), 230–241. https://doi.org/10.1093/clipsy.bph077

Block-Lerner, J., Adair, C., Plumb, J. C., Rhatigan, D. L., & Orsillo, S. M. (2007). The case for mindfulness-based approaches in the cultivation of empathy: Does non-judgmental present-moment awareness increase capacity for perspective-taking and empathic concern? *Journal of Marital and Family Therapy, 33*(4), 501–516. https://doi.org/10.1111/j.1752-0606.2007.00034.x

Boccia, M., Piccardi, L., & Guariglia, P. (2015). The meditative mind: A comprehensive meta-analysis of MRI studies. *BioMed Research International, 2015*, 419808. https://doi.org/10.1155/2015/419808

Bowen, S., Chawla, N., Collins, S. E., Witkiewitz, K., Hsu, S., Grow, J., … Marlatt, A. (2009). Mindfulness-based relapse prevention for substance use disorders: A pilot efficacy trial. *Substance Abuse, 30*(4), 295–305. https://doi.org/10.1080/08897070903250084

Bowen, S., Witkiewitz, K., Dillworth, T. M., Chawla, N., Simpson, T. L., Ostafin, B. D., ... Marlatt, G. A. (2006). Mindfulness meditation and substance use in an incarcerated population. *Psychology of Addictive Behaviors, 20*(3), 343–347. https://doi.org/10.1037/0893-164X.20.3.343

Brewer, J. A., Sinha, R., Chen, J. A., Michalsen, R. N., Babuscio, T. A., Nich, C., ... Rounsaville, B. J. (2009). Mindfulness training and stress reactivity in substance abuse: Results from a randomized, controlled stage I pilot study. *Substance Abuse, 30*(4), 306–317. https://doi.org/10.1080/08897070903250241

Britton, W. B., Bootzin, R. R., Cousins, J. C., Hasler, B. P., Peck, T., & Shapiro, S. L. (2010). The contribution of mindfulness practice to a multicomponent behavioral sleep intervention following substance abuse treatment in adolescents: A treatment-development study. *Substance Abuse, 31*(2), 86–97. https://doi.org/10.1080/08897071003641297

Brower, J. (2013). *Correctional officer wellness and safety literature review*. Washington, DC: OJP Diagnostic Center, Office of Justice Programs. Retrieved from https://www.ojpdiagnosticcenter.org/engagements/publications/correctional-officer-wellness-and-safety-literature-review

Brown, K. W., & Ryan, R. M. (2003). The benefits of being present: Mindfulness and its role in psychological well-being. *Journal of Personality and Social Psychology, 84*(4), 822–848. https://doi.org/10.1037/0022-3514.84.4.822

Brown, K. W., Ryan, R. M., & Creswell, J. D. (2007). Mindfulness: Theoretical foundations and evidence for its salutary effects. *Psychological Inquiry, 18*(4), 211–237. https://doi.org/10.1080/10478400701598298

Carmody, J. (2009). Evolving conceptions of mindfulness in clinical settings. *Journal of Cognitive Psychotherapy, 23*(3), 270–280. https://doi.org/10.1891/0889-8391.23.3.270

Carmody, J., & Baer, R. A. (2008). Relationships between mindfulness practice and levels of mindfulness, medical and psychological symptoms and well-being in a mindfulness-based stress reduction program. *Journal of Behavioral Medicine, 31*(1), 23–33. https://doi.org/10.1007/s10865-007-9130-7

Chambers, R., Gullone, E., & Allen, N. B. (2009). Mindful emotion regulation: An integrative review. *Clinical Psychology, 29*(6), 560–572. https://doi.org/10.1016/j.cpr.2009.06.005

Chang, J.-H., Huang, C.-L., & Lin, Y.-C. (2015). Mindfulness, basic psychological needs fulfillment, and well-being. *Journal of Happiness Studies, 16*(5), 1149–1162. https://doi.org/10.1007/s10902-014-9551-2

Chopko, B. A., & Schwartz, R. C. (2009). The relation between mindfulness and posttraumatic growth: A study of first responders to trauma-inducing incidents. *Journal of Mental Health Counseling, 31*(4), 363–376. https://doi.org/10.17744/mehc.31.4.9w6lhk4v66423385

Davidson, R. J., & McEwen, B. S. (2012). Social influences on neuroplasticity: Stress and interventions to promote well-being. *Nature Neuroscience, 15*(5), 689–695. https://doi.org/10.1038/nn.3093

Davidson, R. J., & Schuyler, B. S. (2015). Neuroscience of happiness. In J. Helliwell, R. Layard, & J. Sachs (Eds.), *World happiness report 2015* (pp. 88–105). New York: Sustainable Development Solutions Network. Retrieved from http://worldhappiness.report/ed/2015/

Davies, N. (2016). Resilience tops bill at psychology conference. *Occupational Health & Wellbeing, 68*(3), 16–17. Retrieved from https://www.personneltoday.com/hr/resilience-workplace-tops-bill-occupational-psychology-conference/

Davis, D. M., & Hayes, J. A. (2011). What are the benefits of mindfulness? A practice review of psychotherapy-related research. *Psychotherapy, 48*(2), 198–208. https://doi.org/10.1037/a0022062

Derezotes, D. (2000). Evaluation of yoga and meditation trainings with adolescent sex offenders. *Child and Adolescent Social Work Journal, 17*(2), 97–113. https://doi.org/10.1023/A:1007506206353

Dorjee, D. (2016). Defining contemplative science: The metacognitive self-regulatory capacity of the mind, context of meditation practice and modes of existential awareness. *Frontiers in Psychology, 7*, 1788. https://doi.org/10.3389/fpsyg.2016.01788

Evans-Chase, M. (2013). Internet-based mindfulness meditation and self-regulation: A randomized trial with juvenile justice involved youth. *Journal of Juvenile Justice, 3*(1), 63–79. Retrieved from http://journalofjuvjustice.org/

Ferszt, G. G., Miller, R. J., Hickey, J. E., Maull, F., & Crisp, K. (2015). The impact of a mindfulness based program on perceived stress, anxiety, depression and sleep of incarcerated women. *International Journal of Environmental Research and Public Health, 12*(9), 11594–11607. https://doi.org/10.3390/ijerph120911594

Garland, E. L., Gaylord, S. A., Boettiger, C. A., & Howard, M. O. (2010). Mindfulness training modifies cognitive, affective, and physiological mechanisms implicated in alcohol dependence: Results of a randomized controlled pilot trial. *Journal of Psychoactive Drugs, 42*(2), 177–192. https://doi.org/10.1080/02791072.2010.10400690

Garland, E. L., & Howard, M. O. (2009). Neuroplasticity, psychosocial genomics, and the biopsychosocial paradigm in the 21st century. *Health & Social Work, 34*(3), 191–199. https://doi.org/10.1093/hsw/34.3.191

Gelderloos, P., Walton, K. G., Orme-Johnson, D. W., & Alexander, C. N. (1991). Effectiveness of the transcendental meditation program in preventing and treating substance misuse: A review. *The International Journal of the Addictions, 26*(3), 293–325. https://doi.org/10.3109/10826089109058887

Gesch, C. B., Hammond, S. M., Hampson, S. E., Eves, A., & Crowder, M. J. (2002). Influence of supplementary vitamins, minerals and essential fatty acids on the antisocial behaviour of young adult prisoners: Randomised, placebo-controlled trial. *The British Journal of Psychiatry, 181*(1), 22–28. https://doi.org/10.1192/bjp.181.1.22

Gottfredson, M. R., & Hirschi, T. (1990). *A general theory of crime*. Stanford, CA: Stanford University Press.

Grecucci, A., Pappaianni, E., Siugzdaite, R., Theuninck, A., & Job, R. (2015). Mindful emotion regulation: Exploring the neurocognitive mechanisms behind mindfulness. *BioMed Research International, 2015*, 670724. https://doi.org/10.1155/2015/670724

Griffin, D. (2013). *Open-minded Finland offers successful alternative to heavy-handed retribution*. Dublin, Ireland: The Irish Times. Retrieved from https://www.irishtimes.com/news/open-minded-finland-offers-successful-alternative-to-heavy-handed-retribution-1.964775

Grossman, P., Neimann, L., Schmidt, S., & Walach, H. (2004). Mindfulness-based stress reduction and health benefits. *Journal of Psychosomatic Research, 57*(1), 34–43. https://doi.org/10.1016/S0022-3999(03)00573-7

Gupta, A. (2014). Methodological analysis of mindfulness and foreign perspective. *Indian Journal of Positive Psychology, 4*(1), 77–80. Retrieved from http://www.iahrw.com/journal.php?numb=2

Hanley, A., Warner, A., & Garland, E. L. (2015). Associations between mindfulness, psychological well-being, and subjective well-being with respect to contemplative practice. *Journal of Happiness Studies, 16*(6), 1423–1436. https://doi.org/10.1007/s10902-014-9569-5

Heppner, W. L., Kernis, M. H., Lakey, C. E., Campbell, W. K., Goldman, B. M., Davis, P. J., & Cascio, E. V. (2008). Mindfulness as a means of reducing aggressive behavior: Dispositional and situational evidence. *Aggressive Behavior, 34*(5), 486–496. https://doi.org/10.1002/ab.20258

Himelstein, S. (2011a). Meditation research: The state of art in correctional settings. *International Journal of Offender Therapy and Comparative Criminology, 55*(4), 646–661. https://doi.org/10.1177/0306624X10364485

Himelstein, S. (2011b). Mindfulness-based substance abuse treatment for incarcerated youth: A mixed method pilot study. *International Journal of Transpersonal Studies, 30*(1–2), 1–10. https://doi.org/10.24972/ijts.2011.30.1-2.1

Himelstein, S., Saul, S., & Garcia-Romeu, A. (2015). Does mindfulness meditation increase effectiveness of substance abuse treatment with incarcerated youth? A pilot randomized controlled trial. *Mindfulness, 6*(6), 1472–1480. https://doi.org/10.1007/s12671-015-0431-6

Hussain, D. (2015). Meta-cognition in mindfulness: A conceptual analysis. *Psychological Thought, 8*(2), 132–141. https://doi.org/10.5964/psyct.v8i2.139

Jain, H., & Singh, R. (2016). Developing psychological capital through mindfulness based stress reduction (MBSR) therapy. *Indian Journal of Health and Wellbeing, 7*(1), 79–84. Retrieved from http://iahrw.com/journal.php?numb=1

James, D. J., & Glaze, L. E. (2006). *Mental health problems of prison and jail inmates*. Washington, DC: Bureau of Justice Statistics, Office of Justice Programs. Retrieved from https://www.bjs.gov/index.cfm?iid=789&ty=pbdetail

Kabat-Zinn, J. (1990). *Full catastrophe living*. New York, NY: Bantam Dell, Random House.

Kabat-Zinn, J. (1994). *Wherever you go, there you are: Mindfulness meditation in everyday life*. New York, NY: Hyperion.

Kabat-Zinn, J. (2003). Mindfulness-based interventions in context: Past, present, and future. *Clinical Psychology: Science and Practice, 10*(2), 144–156. https://doi.org/10.1093/clipsy.bpg016

Kabat-Zinn, J. (2011). Some reflections on the origins of MBSR, skillful means, and the trouble with maps. *Contemporary Buddhism, 12*(1), 281–306. https://doi.org/10.1080/14639947.2011.564844

Kabat-Zinn, J., Massion, A. O., Kristeller, J., Peterson, L. G., Fletcher, K. E., Pbert, L., … Santorelli, S. F. (1992). Effectiveness of a meditation-based stress reduction program in the treatment of anxiety disorders. *The American Journal of Psychiatry, 149*(7), 936–943. https://doi.org/10.1176/ajp.149.7.936

Keinan, G., & Malach-Pines, A. (2007). Stress and burnout among prison personnel: Sources, outcomes, and intervention strategies. *Criminal Justice and Behavior, 34*(3), 380–398. https://doi.org/10.1177/0093854806290007

Khusid, M. A., & Vythilingam, M. (2016a). The emerging role of mindfulness meditation as effective self-management strategy, part 1: Clinical implications for depression, post-traumatic stress disorder, and anxiety. *Military Medicine, 181*(9), 961–968. https://doi.org/10.7205/MILMED-D-14-00677

Khusid, M. A., & Vythilingam, M. (2016b). The emerging role of mindfulness meditation as effective self-management strategy, part 2: Clinical implications for chronic pain, substance misuse, and insomnia. *Military Medicine, 181*(9), 969–975. https://doi.org/10.7205/MILMED-D-14-00678

Lan, H. K., Subramanian, P., Rahmat, N., & Kar, P. C. (2014). The effects of mindfulness training program on reducing stress and promoting well-being among nurses in critical care units. *Australian Journal of Advanced Nursing (Online), 31*(3), 22–31. Retrieved from http://www.ajan.com.au/

Lau, M. A., & Yu, A. R. (2009). New developments in research on mindfulness-based treatments: Introduction to the special issue. *Journal of Cognitive Psychotherapy, 23*(3), 179–184. https://doi.org/10.1891/0889-8391.23.3.179

Leonard, N. R., Jha, A. P., Casarjian, B., Goolsarran, M., Garcia, C., Cleland, C. M., … Massey, Z. (2013). Mindfulness training improves attentional task performance in incarcerated youth: A group randomized controlled intervention trial. *Frontiers in Psychology, 4*, 792. https://doi.org/10.3389/fpsyg.2013.00792

Malinowski, P. (2008). Mindfulness as psychological dimension: Concepts and applications. *The Irish Journal of Psychology, 29*(1–2), 155–166. https://doi.org/10.1080/03033910.2008.10446281

Mandal, S. P., Arya, Y. K., & Pandey, R. (2014). Understanding emotion regulatory effect of mindfulness: Role of differentiation and range of emotional experiences. *Indian Journal of Positive Psychology, 4*(3), 356–362. Retrieved from http://www.iahrw.com/journal.php?numb=2

Marlatt, G. A., & Chawla, N. (2007). Meditation and alcohol use. *The Southern Medical Journal, 100*(4), 451–453. https://doi.org/10.1097/SMJ.0b013e3180381416

Mathura, R., & Sharma, S. (2014). A study of well-being and its positive concomitants. *Indian Journal of Positive Psychology, 4*(4), 534–539. Retrieved from http://www.iahrw.com/journal.php?numb=2
McCraty, R., Atkinson, M., Lipsenthal, L., & Arguelles, L. (2009). New hope for correctional officers: An innovative program for reducing stress and health risks. *Applied Psychophysiology and Biofeedback, 34*(4), 251–272. https://doi.org/10.1007/s10484-009-9087-0
Mitchell, M., & Heads, G. (2015). Staying well: A follow up of a 5-week mindfulness based stress reduction programme for a range of psychological issues. *Community Mental Health Journal, 51*(8), 897–902. https://doi.org/10.1007/s10597-014-9825-5
Mohammadkhani, P., Khanipour, H., Azadmehr, H., Mobramm, A., & Naseri, E. (2015). Trait mindfulness, reasons for living and general symptom severity as predictors of suicide probability in males with substance abuse or dependence. *Iranian Journal of Psychiatry, 10*(1), 56–63. Retrieved from http://ijps.tums.ac.ir/index.php/ijps
Moral, A., Kumar, R., & Sharma, M. (2014). A study of well-being in meditators. *Indian Journal of Health and Wellbeing, 5*(10), 1229–1231. Retrieved from http://iahrw.com/journal.php?numb=1
Moyes, H. C. A., Heath, J. J., & Dean, L. V. (2016). What can be done to improve outcomes for prisoners with a dual diagnosis? *Advances in Dual Diagnosis, 9*(1), 14–25. https://doi.org/10.1108/ADD-07-2015-0016
Mulay, A. L., Kelly, E., & Cain, N. M. (2017). Psychodynamic treatment of the criminal offender: Making the case for longer-term treatment in a longer-term setting. *Psychodynamic Psychiatry, 45*(2), 143–173. https://doi.org/10.1521/pdps.2017.45.2.143
Neff, K. D., & Germer, C. K. (2013). A pilot study and randomized controlled trial of the mindful self-compassion program. *Journal of Clinical Psychology, 69*(1), 28–44. https://doi.org/10.1002/jclp.21923
Nyklíček, I., Dijksman, S. C., Lenders, P. J., Fonteijn, W. A., & Koolen, J. J. (2014). A brief mindfulness based intervention for increase in emotional well-being and quality of life in percutaneous coronary intervention (PCI) patients: The MindfulHeart randomized controlled trial. *Journal of Behavioral Medicine, 37*(1), 135–144. https://doi.org/10.1007/s10865-012-9475-4
Nyklíček, I., & Kuijpers, K. F. (2008). Effects of mindfulness-based stress reduction intervention on psychological well-being and quality of life: Is increased mindfulness indeed the mechanism? *Annals of Behavioral Medicine, 35*(3), 331–340. https://doi.org/10.1007/s12160-008-9030-2
Page, K. M., & Vella-Brodrick, D. A. (2009). The 'what,' 'why' and 'how' of employee well-being: A new model. *Social Indicators Research, 90*(3), 441–458. https://doi.org/10.1007/s11205-008-9270-3
Paparozzi, M. A., & Guy, R. (2013). The trials and tribulations of implementing what works: Training rarely trumps values. *Federal Probation Journal, 77*(2), 36–42. Retrieved from http://www.uscourts.gov/statistics-reports/publications/federal-probation-journal
Plambeck, K. L. (2015). *Acceptance and commitment therapy (ACT) treatment groups targeting the reduction of problematic anger-related behaviors and psychological inflexibility in incarcerated men: A pilot study* (Doctoral dissertation) (Order No. 3664509). Retrieved from ProQuest Dissertations and Theses Global. (Order No. 3664509).
Pratt, J. (2008). Scandinavian exceptionalism in an era of penal excess: Part I: The nature and roots of Scandinavian exceptionalism. *The British Journal of Criminology, 48*(2), 119–137. https://doi.org/10.1093/bjc/azm072
Prison Mindfulness Institute. (2018). Retrieved from https://www.prisonmindfulness.org/
Reid, D. (2011). Mindfulness and flow in occupational engagement: Presence in doing. *Canadian Journal of Occupational Therapy, 78*(1), 50–56. https://doi.org/10.2182/cjot.2011.78.1.7
Rhine, E. E., Mawhorr, T. L., & Parks, E. C. (2006). Implementation: The bane of effective correctional programs. *Criminology & Public Policy, 5*(2), 347–358. https://doi.org/10.1111/j.1745-9133.2006.00382.x

Ross, M. W., & Harzke, A. J. (2012). Toward healthy prisoners: The TECH model and its applications. *International Journal of Prisoner Health, 8*(1), 16–26. https://doi.org/10.1108/17449201211268255
Rybak, C. (2013). Nurturing positive mental health: Mindfulness for wellbeing in counseling. *International Journal for the Advancement of Counseling, 35*(2), 110–119. https://doi.org/10.1007/s10447-012-9171-7
Samuelson, M., Carmody, J., Kabat-Zinn, J., & Bratt, M. A. (2007). Mindfulness-based stress reduction in Massachusetts correctional facilities. *The Prison Journal, 87*(2), 254–268. https://doi.org/10.1177/0032885507303753
Shapiro, S. L., Carlson, L. E., Astin, J. A., & Freedman, B. (2006). Mechanisms of mindfulness. *Journal of Clinical Psychology, 62*(3), 373–386. https://doi.org/10.1002/jclp.20237
Sharma, S., & Tomer, S. (2018). Psychosocial antecedents of prosocial behavior and its relationship with subjective well-being in adolescents. *Indian Journal of Positive Psychology, 8*(1), 14–21. Retrieved from http://www.iahrw.com/journal.php?numb=2
Shonin, E., Van Gordon, W., & Griffiths, M. D. (2014). Meditation awareness training (MAT) for improved psychological well-being: A qualitative examination of participant experiences. *Journal of Religion and Health, 53*(3), 849–863. https://doi.org/10.1007/s10943-013-9679-0
Siegel, D. J. (2006). An interpersonal neurobiology approach to psychotherapy. *Psychiatric Annals, 36*(4), 248–256. Retrieved from https://www.healio.com/psychiatry/journals/psycann
Smith, N., Tew, J., & Patel, P. (2015). The CARE programme: An accredited offending behaviour programme specifically for female offenders at risk of violence. *Journal of Aggression, Conflict and Peace Research, 7*(4), 275–286. https://doi.org/10.1108/JACPR-02-2015-0164
Tang, Y., Hölzel, B. K., & Posner, M. I. (2015). The neuroscience of mindfulness meditation. *Nature Reviews Neuroscience, 16*(4), 213–225. https://doi.org/10.1038/nrn3916
Tang, Y.-Y., Hölzel, B. K., & Posner, M. I. (2016). Traits and states in mindfulness meditation. *Nature Reviews Neuroscience, 17*(1), 59. https://doi.org/10.1038/nrn.2015.7
Tang, Y.-Y., Ma, Y., Wang, J., Fan, Y., Feng, S., Lu, Q., … Posner, M. I. (2007). Short-term meditation training improves attention and self-regulation. *Proceedings of National Academy of Sciences of the United States, 104*(43), 17152–17156. https://doi.org/10.1073/pnas.0707678104
Tang, Y.-Y., & Posner, M. I. (2013). Tools of the trade: Theory and method in mindfulness neuroscience. *Social Cognitive and Affective Neuroscience, 8*(1), 118–120. https://doi.org/10.1093/scan/nss112
Trounson, J. S., & Pfeifer, J. E. (2016). Promoting correctional officer wellbeing: Guidelines and suggestions for developing psychological training programs. *Advancing Corrections Journal, 1*, 57–64. Retrieved from https://icpa.ca/advancing-corrections-journal/
Velotti, P., Garofalo, C., D'Aguanno, M., Petrocchi, C., Popolo, R., Salvatore, G., & Dimaggio, G. (2016). Mindfulness moderates the relationship between aggression and antisocial personality disorder traits: Preliminary investigation with an offender sample. *Comprehensive Psychiatry, 64*, 38–45. https://doi.org/10.1016/j.comppsych.2015.08.004
Warren, N., Dussetschleger, J., Punnet, L., & Cherniack, M. G. (2015). Musculoskeletal disorder symptoms in correctional officers: Why do they increase rapidly with job tenure? *Human Factors: The Journal of the Human Factors and Ergonomics Society, 57*(2), 262–275. https://doi.org/10.1177/0018720814547569
Weiss, L. A., Westerhof, G. J., & Bohlmeijer, E. T. (2016). Can we increase psychological well-being? The effects of interventions on psychological well-being: A meta-analysis of randomized controlled trials. *PLoS One, 11*(6), e0158092. https://doi.org/10.1371/journal.pone.0158092
Witkiewitz, K., & Bowen, S. (2010). Depression, craving, and substance use following a randomized trial of mindfulness-based relapse prevention. *Journal of Consulting and Clinical Psychology, 78*(3), 362–374. https://doi.org/10.1037/a0019172
Witkiewitz, K., Marlatt, G. A., & Walker, D. (2005). Mindfulness-based relapse prevention for alcohol and substance abuse disorders. *Journal of Cognitive Psychotherapy, 19*(3), 211–228. https://doi.org/10.1891/jcop.2005.19.3.211

Wu, G., Feder, A., Cohen, H., Kim, J. J., Calderon, S., Charney, D. S., & Mathé, A. A. (2013). Understanding resilience. *Frontiers in Behavioral Neuroscience, 7*, 10. https://doi.org/10.3389/fnbeh.2013.00010

Zgierska, A., Rabago, D., Chawla, N., Kushner, K., Koehler, R., & Marlatt, A. (2009). Mindfulness meditation for substance use disorders: A systematic review. *Substance Abuse, 30*(4), 266–294. https://doi.org/10.1080/08897070903250019

Zgierska, A., Rabago, D., Zuelsdorff, M., Coe, C., Miller, M., & Fleming, M. (2008). Mindfulness meditation for alcohol relapse prevention: A feasibility pilot study. *Journal of Addiction Medicine, 2*(3), 165–173. https://doi.org/10.1097/ADM.0b013e31816f8546

Zylowska, L., Ackerman, D. L., Yang, M. H., Futrell, J. L., Horton, N. L., Hale, T. S., … Smalley, S. L. (2008). Mindfulness meditation training in adults and adolescents with ADHD: A feasibility study. *Journal of Attention Disorders, 11*(6), 737–746. https://doi.org/10.1177/1087054707308502

Chapter 11
Motivational Interviewing with Court-Ordered Populations

Jill D. Stinson

11.1 Introduction

Motivational interviewing originated as an approach to assist those with problems related to smoking and substance abuse in making a commitment to pursue healthier life choices (Miller & Rollnick, 1991, 2002). Based upon a client-centered counseling style, motivational interviewing prioritizes a strengths-based approach to behavioral change as well as respect for individual autonomy. Since its introduction in the early 1980s, motivational interviewing has thrived, with empirical evidence demonstrating effectiveness for not only those who struggle with substance abuse but also as a means of promoting effective healthcare practices (e.g., diabetes management, medication compliance, chronic pain; McCracken & Corrigan, 2008; Rau, Ehlebracht-König, & Petermann, 2008; Steinberg & Miller, 2015), enhanced educational programming (e.g., Rollnick, Kaplan, & Rutschman, 2016), and improved outcomes in mental health treatment (e.g., Arkowitz, Miller, & Rollnick, 2015).

Predicated on the recognition that people who face important decisions about life change are often ambivalent about such change, motivational interviewing is an approach that lends particularly well to working with clients mandated to treatment, including those who have been court-ordered to complete a treatment program. The mere act of requiring a legal order to engage in treatment implies substantial ambivalence on the part of the client. In this chapter, a broad overview of the purpose and effectiveness of motivational interviewing with court-ordered populations will include a discussion of important elements of motivational interviewing, factors that make it particularly suitable for this client population, evidence of its effectiveness, and important considerations and future steps with regard to implementing and evaluating the use of motivational interviewing with this population.

J. D. Stinson (✉)
Department of Psychology, East Tennessee State University, Johnson City, TN, USA
e-mail: STINSON@mail.etsu.edu

E. L. Jeglic, C. Calkins (eds.), *New Frontiers in Offender Treatment*,
https://doi.org/10.1007/978-3-030-01030-0_11

11.2 Motivational Interviewing: What Is It?

Motivational interviewing is a unique approach to navigating ambivalence about change. When a person feels more than one way about a potential decision, they are ambivalent, and this ambivalence can sometimes prevent them from making a choice and moving forward. Ambivalence, however, is idiosyncratic to the individual and can present a substantial challenge for clinicians and others who wish to facilitate decision-making. An important goal of motivational interviewing is to resolve this ambivalence through the use of a guiding, rather than directive, conversational style. Miller and Rollnick (2013) define motivational interviewing thusly:

> Motivational interviewing is a collaborative conversation style for strengthening a person's own motivation and commitment to change. (p. 12)

Within this approach is a fundamental respect for autonomy and choice, an emphasis on evoking a person's own strengths to help them accomplish important goals, and the call for compassion, acceptance, empathy, and recognition of absolute worth when working with even the most challenging of clients. These aspects of the spirit of motivational interviewing, coupled with the four fundamental processes of this approach—engaging, focusing, evoking, and planning—set the stage for the important work of growth and change (Miller & Rollnick, 2013).

Motivational interviewing involves movement through the four processes noted above. The first of these, *engaging*, establishes a collaborative partnership and orients the listener to the client's experience. Use of open-ended questions, affirmations, simple and complex reflections, and summaries aids the listener in moving the conversation forward while also giving the speaker room to develop his or her narrative. The next process is *focusing*, which allows the client to explore competing goals with the ultimate aim of establishing a direction. The listener aids in this process through agenda mapping and orienting so that the client has a clearer sense of where he or she would like to go with regard to continuing the conversation. The third process, *evoking*, is intended to facilitate the client's recognition of inherent strengths, generate change talk, and elicit increased hope and confidence in the ability to effect successful life changes. It is here that ambivalence is most salient, with the listener guiding the client toward increased talk in favor of change, rather than dwelling on talk that sustains the status quo. Again, open-ended questions, reflections, affirmations, and summaries, along with other strategies meant to elicit values and visions of a changed future, assist with this process. The final step is *planning*, in which the client develops a plan and is assisted by the listener in troubleshooting and fine-tuning details of the plan so as to improve the chance of success. Additional tasks here include evoking intention and strengthening commitment.

Motivational interviewing is often viewed as a necessary step in guiding clients through the process of change. Early work identifying the stages of change (Prochaska & DiClemente, 1982, 1992) described five nonlinear processes through which a person moves as they consider a potential change. The first of these, *pre-contemplation*, applies to persons who deny the need to change. They may be unaware of the effects of their behavior, or they lack the ability to appreciate negative consequences that arise. The second stage is *contemplation*, or when the individual first begins thinking about the need for change. It is at this point that the problem has perhaps become more real or that the individual feels some ambivalence about continuing their behavior as usual. This may be followed by *preparation*, a time during which the person is more actively contemplating change and seeking information or taking some small measures to plan potential behavioral change. The *action* phase is the point at which the person is more engaged in making relevant changes and showing some observable success in doing so. The final step is *maintenance*, when the individual has successfully made changes and maintained them, planning in advance for challenges or potential setbacks. Court-ordered clients may present with a range of willingness to change, though motivational interviewing is perhaps best indicated for those in the pre-contemplation or contemplation stages. Still, even individuals in planning or action stages may still benefit from discussion to evoke strengths and solidify commitment.

Despite a clear set of processes and associated tools associated with the practice of motivational interviewing, this approach is not merely a set of techniques or strategies meant to push a person in a given direction (i.e., toward making a change). In fact, such directive effort will likely only result in the person advocating for the very behavior one wishes to address. Instead, this is, at its core, a method of participating in a conversation in a mindful way, with the goal of helping the client call forth his or her own motivation for self-improvement. The four processes are not linear, as a disruption in the conversation or loss of a sense of collaborative partnership may call for further engaging. And with regard to integration with other treatment efforts, the planning stage may be preempted by an existing plan that has been designed by a court or other outside agency. With court-ordered clients, this is often the case—a primary aim is to develop sufficient motivation and commitment to the plan that has been identified by the court. The stated goal is to comply with court orders. But the real goal is to promote behavioral change that will result in reduced recidivism and safer communities. Increased motivation and genuine, self-driven commitment to change will achieve both.

11.3 Why Use Motivational Interviewing with Court-Ordered Clients?

For persons who have been mandated by the court for evaluation or treatment, the use of motivational interviewing is rooted in the science of evidence-based approaches for offender populations. For the past 30 years, the criminal justice literature has endorsed the risk-needs-responsivity (RNR) model, noting the need to match level of service provision with the offender's level of risk, to attend to empirically derived criminogenic needs, and to deliver treatment in such a way as to incorporate the client's motivation, learning style, and strengths (Andrews, Bonta, & Hoge, 1990; Bonta & Andrews, 2007). The responsivity principle, in particular, calls for us to not only administer treatment in a way that fosters motivation and potential for growth but also to incorporate motivation as an important aspect of the treatment itself.

Motivational interviewing is uniquely ideal for working with court-ordered clients. First, such clients often present with specific characteristics that impair their motivation or offer the potential to impede treatment. As noted above, the presence of a legal order to initiate treatment communicates a lack of voluntariness on the part of the client. The client did not decide to independently pursue treatment, and this may connote significant ambivalence, a desire to maintain current behaviors, or even lack of awareness, minimization, or denial of the problem. Relatedly, court-mandated clients are often those with poor motivation (e.g., Begun et al., 2003; Chamberlain, Patterson, Reid, Kavanaugh, & Forgatch, 1984; Hartford, Ungerer, & Kinsella, 1976; Miller & Rollnick, 1991), given that they may enter treatment with multiple failed attempts to rectify the problem in the past, increased resistance to intervention, and lack of insight regarding the seriousness of the problem. Further, by nature, court-ordered treatment implies some degree of illegality of behavior, and the stigma associated with such intervention may negatively impact the client's motivation to openly pursue needed change. Moreover, with regard to individual characteristics, court-ordered populations often present with a greater likelihood of interfering mental health symptoms and personality psychopathology (e.g., Black, Gunter, Loveless, Allen, & Sieleni, 2010; Evans, Li, & Hser, 2009), as well as histories of maltreatment and trauma (e.g., Cima, Smeets, & Jelicic, 2008; Harlow, 1999; Ireland & Widom, 1994; Wang et al., 2012; Wolff & Shi, 2010), marginalization in treatment, and difficulty with developing positive therapeutic bonds (e.g., Connors et al., 2000; Honea-Boles & Griffin, 2001; Satterfield, Buelow, Lyddon, & Johnson, 1995) that further diminish their motivation and ability to fully benefit from available treatment opportunities.

A second relevant consideration is that motivational interviewing is intended to enhance motivation, confidence, and commitment to change in the service of improving treatment outcomes. With persons referred by the court for intervention or treatment, the outcomes are presumably quite important, with lack of commitment to change, poor motivation, and treatment failure implying negative legal sanctions for the individual and potential risk to the public. Poor engagement in court-ordered populations may precipitate any number of additional consequences, including increased community supervision or incarceration for the individual, additional financial costs to the public to cover court-related or criminal justice expenses, and the potential for future victimization of others.

Third, motivational interviewing is not itself a treatment approach. It is a manner of facilitating a conversation that evokes motivation for change. Thus, it does not inherently conflict with court-preferred or other statutorily defined mechanisms for addressing specific behaviors in treatment. Motivational interviewing can be integrated with other treatment approaches as a method of improving treatment commitment, maintaining treatment motivation, and developing a plan for sustaining treatment benefit after active intervention is complete. Further, a distinct advantage is that motivational interviewing can be administered by a range of individuals. While it can certainly be practiced by clinical professionals from varying backgrounds (e.g., psychology, counseling, social work, or medicine), this method is also approachable for direct care service staff, including correctional officers, psychiatric technicians, probation and parole officers, and frontline case managers. Given the crucial and nuanced roles that many of these individuals play in the successful risk management of court-ordered clients, their familiarity with and use of motivational interviewing can be vital in promoting positive outcomes for this population.

Finally, a crucial reason for considering motivational interviewing as an approach for court-ordered clients is that it *works*. Motivational interviewing has been demonstrated as an effective practice with a variety of offender and other court-ordered populations, as will be described further below, and has been identified as an evidence-based practice within the "Evidence-Based Policy and Practice" initiative promoted by the National Institute of Corrections (Bogue et al., 2004; Crime and Justice Institute at Community Resources for Justice, 2009). Further, adherence to the principles of motivational interviewing facilitates effectiveness of treatment at multiple stages, including treatment engagement and retention, enhancing intrinsic motivation to change, and actual behavioral change over time (see further McMurran, 2009). Thus, it works with diverse populations of court-ordered clients, it aligns with the RNR framework and best practices with court-ordered and offender populations, and it promotes effective treatment outcomes at differing points of contact.

11.4 What's the Evidence?

As previously noted, motivational interviewing has been extensively examined within the context of treatment motivation, engagement, and effectiveness for substance abuse intervention and smoking cessation. While many persons may voluntarily seek treatment for such concerns, they may have already demonstrated sufficient motivation to initiate and sustain treatment without further motivational enhancement. Many persons, however, find themselves court-ordered or otherwise compelled to seek such treatment to maintain employment, avoid legal sanction, or prevent other negative consequences. Similarly, other involuntary or court-ordered populations in need of treatment have benefitted from motivational interviewing as well. Empirical study of this approach with court-ordered populations can be divided into several categories. The first includes a review of the effectiveness of motivational interviewing by population, noting its success with varying groups or presenting problems. This is primarily helpful for those who seek a quick summary of how motivational interviewing has been implemented with their target population. Another is to examine the impact of motivational interviewing on differing components of treatment involvement, including initial and sustained motivation, actual treatment engagement, and treatment outcome results (e.g., McMurran, 2009). Finally, some examinations of motivational interviewing emphasize dissemination and training for providers, as well as how a given provider's approach impacts treatment engagement, retention, and successful completion. Within this section, I will present evidence in each of these categories for ease of access for the interested reader.

Effectiveness by Population The earliest evidence for the effectiveness of motivational interviewing involved original empirical studies and extensive reviews and meta-analyses of this approach with persons with problems with smoking, alcohol consumption, and substance abuse. While not explicitly intended to address court-ordered clients, it is also true that many persons with substance-related disorders or difficulties have had court involvement or may be seeking treatment following a directive from others. Meta-analyses of motivational interviewing have supplied evidence for its effectiveness with smoking cessation (e.g., Heckman, Egleston, & Hofmann, 2010; Hettema & Hendricks, 2010; Lai, Cahill, Qin, & Tang, 2010), alcohol abuse (e.g., Kohler & Hofmann, 2015; Vasilaki, Hosier, & Cox, 2006), and substance-related problems (e.g., Lenz, Rosenbaum, & Sheperis, 2016; Li, Zhu, Tse, Tse, & Wong, 2016; Sayegh, Huey, Zara, & Jhaveri, 2017). Importantly, other literature has explored the impact of motivational interviewing and associated motivational enhancement approaches with offender populations who also engage in problematic alcohol and substance abuse. Such research has highlighted motivational interviewing's contribution to success in alcohol and substance abuse treatment for adolescent offenders (Battjes et al., 2004; D'Amico, Osilla, & Hunter, 2010; Stein et al., 2006), offenders in co-occurring treatment for domestic violence (Crane, Eckhardt, & Schlauch, 2015; Easton, Swan, & Sinha, 2000; Roffman, Edleson, Neighbors, Mbilinyi, & Walker, 2008), probationers mandated to alcohol or substance abuse treatment (Carroll et al., 2006; Harper & Hardy, 2000; Sinha, Easton, Renee-Aubin, & Carroll, 2003), offenders referred for substance abuse treatment who presented with comorbid mental health concerns (Miles, Dutheil, Welsby, & Haider, 2007), and offenders with intellectual disability (Mendel & Hipkins, 2002). Collectively, these studies have underscored the importance of addressing motivation and treatment engagement for substance abusers who are offenders engaged in other forms of therapy and the positive impact of motivational interviewing on treatment attendance, completion, and recidivism.

Other examinations have emphasized the use of motivational interviewing with violent offender populations, including those with sexual offenses, histories of domestic violence, and varied forms of violent criminal activity. Examinations of motivational interviewing with violent or general offenders have primarily explored the impact of motivational approaches on treatment engagement and readiness to change (Anstiss, Polaschek, & Wilson, 2011; Austin, Williams, & Kilgour, 2011; Chambers, Eccleston, Day, Ward, & Howells, 2008). Case examples of the effectiveness of motivational interviewing with men in sex offender treatment were provided by Miller and Rollnick (1991) and Mann and Rollnick (1996). Later publications included an examination of motivational interviewing with youth who had engaged in sexual violence (Patel, Lambie, & Glover, 2008) and texts devoted to using this approach with sex offense-specific populations (Prescott, 2009, 2013).

More extensive research exists describing the impact of motivational interviewing on the treatment of men referred for domestic violence intervention (e.g., Crane et al., 2015; Easton et al., 2000; Kistenmacher & Weiss, 2008; Murphy & Baxter, 1997; Musser & Murphy, 2009; Musser, Semiatin, Taft, & Murphy, 2008; Roffman et al., 2008; Zalmanowitz, Babins-Wagner, Rodger, Corbett, & Leschied, 2013). Additionally, some research has explored the ability of motivational approaches to reduce vulnerability to domestic and intimate partner violence victimization in female offenders (Weir et al., 2009). Collectively, this research does indicate that motivational interviewing has improved readiness for change and treatment completion, though researchers frequently note a number of particular challenges specific to treatment of perpetrators of domestic violence, including stigma, interfering alcohol and substance abuse problems, traditionally high rates of treatment non-completion, and comorbid mental health problems and interpersonal skills deficits, often requiring a multimodal treatment approach.

Finally, limited research includes the impact of motivational interviewing on women who are involved in the criminal justice system (e.g., Weir et al., 2009) and families of adolescents who have committed offenses (Slavet et al., 2005). In the former, the emphasis was less on the women's participation in offense-related interventions but instead on safety behaviors and reducing risk of victimization and HIV-related risks.

Effectiveness by Stage of Treatment Research describing the application of motivational interviewing with offender and other court-ordered populations includes recognition of distinct stages or desired outcomes associated with treatment and court-ordered supervision: readiness to change or initial treatment engagement, continuing treatment engagement, treatment completion, positive treatment outcome, and reduction in recidivism post-intervention. Here, research regarding the effectiveness of motivational approaches is decidedly mixed, recognizing the complex factors associated with court-ordered treatment for diverse offenders and in diverse settings.

A number of researchers have focused on readiness to change and enhancing early treatment engagement in mandated treatment populations. Findings from their studies indicate that even brief (typically ranging from one to three sessions pretreatment) motivational interviewing or motivational enhancement therapy (MET; Miller, Zweben, DiClemente, & Rychtarik, 1992) sessions result in measurable improvements in readiness to change or stage of change (Anstiss et al., 2011; Austin et al., 2011; Easton et al., 2000; Kistenmacher & Weiss, 2008; Mendel & Hipkins, 2002). Case study evidence additionally supports the use of motivational interviewing to improve initial treatment interest and engagement in court-ordered clients (Mann & Rollnick, 1996; Musser & Murphy, 2009; Patel et al., 2008). Mechanisms of measuring treatment engagement in these studies have ranged from self-reported stage of change, self-reported improvements in confidence and self-efficacy to make change (e.g., D'Amico et al., 2010; Mendel & Hipkins, 2002; Slavet et al., 2005), facilitator-evaluated readiness to change, and rates of treatment attendance versus refusal.

Engagement has also been operationalized as a fluid and continuing construct, with some research measuring not only initial treatment interest and engagement but continuing participation and progress throughout a term of intervention. This also includes a focus on rates of successful treatment completion, which rely on continuous attendance and compliance. Here, research application of motivational interviewing and MET or other brief engagement interventions varies more widely, with some utilizing a time-limited motivational intervention prior to treatment initiation, while others incorporate the spirit of or techniques associated with motivational interviewing throughout a period of treatment for the experimental group. Overall, the majority of these studies demonstrate that motivational interviewing is effective in enhancing treatment participation, compliance, and completion in diverse populations (Carroll et al., 2006; Crane et al., 2015; Lincourt, Kuettel, & Bombardier, 2002; Sinha et al., 2003). However, highlighting the complexity of treatment engagement and completion in court-ordered clients, given the complexity of their individualized needs, Stein et al. (2006) found that while participation in an initial motivational interviewing session (as opposed to a control group relaxation training) did mitigate negative treatment engagement for substance abuse-referred adolescents, other measured features of treatment engagement did not reach significance.

The next form of evaluation includes measurement of behavioral change associated with the use of motivational interviewing to enhance change outcomes as well as consideration of recidivism or relapse. These outcomes are typically more salient with regard to treatment with court-ordered clients, as a return to prior behavior may result in legal sanction, loss of additional freedoms, or harm to others. Conservatively, some researchers have used rearrest and reconviction rates to measure the impact of motivational interviewing on sustaining posttreatment change. Such studies have found significant reductions in formally detected recidivism for general offenders (Anstiss et al., 2011) and persons with histories of illegal substance use (Letizia & Keaton, 2014; Sinha et al., 2003), though this was not the case in a specific comparison between the impact of motivational interviewing with psychoeducation while incarcerated for alcohol-related driving offenses and mere incarceration, as there were no post-incarceration differences in alcohol-related driving offense recidivism (Woodall, Delaney, Kunitz, Westerberg, & Zhao, 2007).

More commonly, researchers have relied on self-reported accounts of post-intervention behavioral change. Again, results vary depending on type of court-ordered treatment, population studied, and the presence of comorbidities or other factors that may make treatment more complex. For example, an examination of motivational interviewing with a group of adolescents in substance abuse treatment yielded marked reductions in marijuana use 6 and 12 months posttreatment, though there were no differences between groups with regard to alcohol abuse or criminal activity (Battjes et al., 2004). Similarly, a sample of females involved in the criminal justice system and who were additionally diagnosed as HIV positive were involved in a randomized control trial to use motivational interviewing to reduce HIV-related risks and exposure to potential intimate partner violence; results indicated that those who received the brief motivational intervention demonstrated significant reductions in risky sexual behaviors and needle sharing, but no differences with regard to their involvement in relationship violence (Weir et al., 2009). Here, then, the challenges of working with court-ordered populations may more strongly impact treatment outcomes. Still, motivational interviewing has shown improvements in self-reported outcomes such as reduced marijuana use (Battjes et al., 2004; Carroll et al., 2006; Sinha et al., 2003), substance abuse (Harper & Hardy, 2000; Miles et al., 2007) and problematic alcohol use (Harper & Hardy, 2000; Woodall et al., 2007) among offenders and others court-ordered to treatment.

Effectiveness Within a System Finally, numerous authors have noted the importance of involving members of the criminal justice, correctional, and forensic mental health systems in motivational interviewing training efforts (e.g., Clark, 2005; Clark, Walters, Gingerich, & Meltzer, 2006; Farbring & Johnson, 2008; Stinson & Clark, 2017; Walters, Clark, Gingerich, & Meltzer, 2007). In a recent study surveying persons who routinely train a variety of professionals in the practice and implementation of motivational interviewing, it was notable that more barriers to implementation and use of motivational interviewing were apparent among corrections staff than was true for other groups (Schumacher, Madson, & Nilsen, 2014). Specifically, trainers felt that corrections staff were markedly less interested in hearing what the clients felt or thought, had significantly less respect for their clients, were more likely to struggle with taking the client's perspective, held a more negative opinion toward motivational interviewing and its components, and were more likely to require training to "undo" what they had previously learned about interacting with clients. These barriers, along with historical values and attitudes associated with many agencies who serve court-ordered clients (Stinson & Clark, 2017), make it all the more important that professionals and staff who work with court-ordered populations see motivational interviewing as an approach that can improve outcomes for their clients and enhance their ability to effectively perform their jobs.

With regard to the effect of training members of a system or agency in motivational interviewing, results are promising, though mixed with regard to outcome. In one randomized control trial of motivational interviewing training for probation officers, it was noted that while the training did significantly improve the skills of individual officers, there were no differences in outcomes for offenders, nor did the rated level of competence in motivational interviewing by officer relate to probationers' outcomes (Walters, Vader, Nguyen, Harris, & Eells, 2010). Similarly, in a study of corrections staff who either had or had not received training in motivational interviewing, there were no significant differences in recidivism among a sample of offenders with substance abuse histories, though it was noted that the recidivism rates between groups were different by as high as 10% (30% for the group who worked with staff who had received motivational interviewing training, as opposed to 40% in the other group; Letizia & Keaton, 2014). Though small, reductions in recidivism still indicate reduced victimization, improved safety, and decreased cost to the system. Finally, although the goal was not to measure the impact of motivational interviewing training on outcomes for court-ordered probationers, Harper and Hardy (2000) found that probationers whose probation officers had received motivational interviewing training showed significantly improved attitudes and relationships with the probation office, which may contribute to improved compliance with court orders and improved treatment outcomes.

11.5 What Does It Look Like in Practice?

The challenges of working with court-ordered clients are certainly real. As noted previously within this chapter, such clients present with complex histories and symptoms of psychopathology, may fail to recognize the extent of their problems, or lack confidence in their ability to successfully make and sustain meaningful behavioral change. There may be multiple issues to address, and it simply becomes overwhelming for providers and clients alike to know where or how to start. Here let us consider the example of Mike, a hypothetical client who may be familiar to many who work with court-ordered populations.

Mike presents with a referral from the court for substance abuse treatment and counseling as a condition of intensive probation. Mike is a 35-year-old, unemployed man who dropped out of high school in the 11th grade due to poor grades. Mike has a history of physical abuse from his stepfather and often ran away from home to live with his grandmother. He has held a number of jobs doing roofing and landscaping work, though he has difficulty maintaining a job due to his substance abuse problems. He abuses opioid pain medication and alcohol, and he has been arrested for possession of prescription medication that is not his and alcohol-related offenses on numerous occasions. He has additionally been arrested for theft, as he sometimes steals small sums of money in order to support his drug habit. He has very little social support, and his previous efforts to engage in treatment, all court-ordered, have resulted in relapses and short-term jail stays.

Initially, Mike presents to his case manager in the probation office as disengaged and only minimally interested in treatment. He feels as though the judge didn't really listen to him when he said treatment had never worked before, and he expresses that it's just a "set up for failure." The case manager proceeds with *engaging*, listening carefully to Mike's story and drawing from him his perceptions of his past, his most recent encounter with the judge, and his past experiences with treatment. Consistent with the spirit of motivational interviewing, the case manager is striving to understand the situation from Mike's perspective, maintaining accurate empathy and reflecting back important elements of Mike's experience. Once a strong and collaborative relationship has been established, the case manager begins *focusing*, talking with Mike about what aspects of his life he would most like to address. He is able to identify several treatment targets, including his lasting depression, which he also feels contributes to his drug and alcohol abuse, as well as how substance abuse treatment could be different from his previous attempts to change. It becomes apparent that his depression likely contributes to his relapses, and his lack of confidence in himself and frequent self-criticism interfere with his engagement in treatment efforts. Moving into the *evoking* phase, the case manager and Mike discuss his ambivalence further, focusing primarily on Mike's statements that evidence willingness and reasons for change. His desire for greater stability, to feel satisfied with himself and his life, and to avoid further repercussions from the court are cited as crucial reasons for pursuing change. He and his case manager additionally discuss factors that can facilitate his success, including his perseverance (e.g., surviving years of violent abuse in his home), his insight into his symptoms of depression, and his willingness to make radical changes when necessary (e.g., leaving to live with his grandmother to escape an abusive and chaotic home). Toward the end of this phase, Mike exhibits substantially greater change talk and acknowledges a noticeable increase in his level of confidence to improve his mental health and work on his substance abuse problems. With regard to *planning*, the case manager is able to offer him a range of treatment options that will satisfy his probation requirements, reviewing the pros and cons of each option with Mike's worldview and expectations under consideration.

Mike concludes his intake meeting with his case manager with a renewed sense of confidence and a commitment to make important changes in his life. Moreover, he has a strong, collaborative relationship with his case manager and feels as though she listens to and understands him. He believes it will be easier to talk with her about any obstacles he encounters as he initiates treatment, potentially preventing future relapses or treatment failure. From the perspective of the case manager, her work with Mike during this initial session provided valuable and "real" information about Mike and his approach to satisfying the judge's orders, and the conversation moved far more smoothly than the typical confrontational approach she has seen used by others in their work with similar clients. She also believes Mike will be more open about his progress in treatment, as well as any problems with which he continues to struggle.

11.6 What Happens Now?

From this review, it is evident that motivational interviewing is appropriate and useful with court-ordered clients, and that it may offer a unique contribution to treatment by enhancing motivation, evoking self-initiated change and treatment participation, and maintaining treatment effects over time. Further, it may improve relationships between clients and the persons who work most closely with them, mitigating the suspicion and mistrust that court-ordered clients may feel toward their providers. Empirical findings suggest effectiveness for a number of commonly court-ordered populations, including juveniles and adults, violent and nonviolent offenders, and persons with substance abuse concerns, among others. However, as is evident from the discussion here, there are clear needs for future evaluation.

A primary need is for replication and controlled research trials. Though a handful of studies suggest effectiveness with varying court-ordered populations, these are limited in that they involve small samples (a frequent concern with court-ordered treatment research), inconsistent goals, implementation, follow-up across studies, and interwoven confounds (e.g., comorbidities, differential availability of resources across jurisdictions) that are characteristic of working with court-ordered populations. Additionally, the ethics of conducting controlled research trials with court-ordered populations prohibit random exclusionary access to what is known to be a best practice, intentional harm to a vulnerable population, and the requirement of participation in research to those who are legally involved. It is important, therefore, for future research to be as deliberate as possible in acknowledging and controlling (where ethically and scientifically reasonable) variables that limit our ability to more broadly study the impact of motivational interviewing on diverse samples. Additionally, future research should address the broader aims of using motivational interviewing with court-ordered samples at different stages of the legal process.

A secondary need is for additional research on systems implementation of motivational interviewing with professionals who work with court-ordered clients. Though there are a number of empirical studies on the success of correctional and other criminal justice system staff in learning and using motivational interviewing (Bogue et al., 2004; Bogue, Diebel, & O'Connor, 2008; Bogue, Pampel, & Pasini-Hill, 2013; Walters et al., 2010), there remains a need to link these training and implementation efforts to outcomes for clients, as well as how such changes have impacted treatment participation and completion among differing groups. Systems are slow to change and may be reluctant to change course with regard to infused treatment approaches. However, the overwhelming evidence for motivational interviewing's effectiveness in dealing with complex problems in the area of substance abuse treatment, healthcare systems, and schools speaks to a broad applicability across systems, settings, and agencies. It is likely, given the available research, that implementation and dissemination of motivational interviewing would have a salient and measurable effect on multiple outcomes, though more research is needed to ensure that this is true and to provide a stronger evidence base within agencies and systems that serve court-ordered clients.

Finally, in order for motivational interviewing to be successfully implemented with court-ordered clients, we must continue to foster an emerging paradigm shift in how such clients are viewed by society, the courts, and the systems involved in their care. A long era of being "tough on crime" and punitive approaches to illegal use of alcohol and other substances have fostered negative attitudes toward those with court involvement and the belief that confrontational approaches are superior to a rehabilitative philosophy (Stinson & Clark, 2017). Confrontational and hostile attitudes toward clients are ineffective in motivating lasting behavioral change (Hubble, Duncan, & Miller, 1999; Miller & Rollnick, 2003) and are in fact a barrier to implementing motivational interviewing (Schumacher et al., 2014). A gradual shift in recent decades, prompted first by consideration of the responsivity principle (Andrews et al., 1990; Bonta & Andrews, 2007) and then bolstered by the introduction of strengths-based approaches to offender work (e.g., Ward & Maruna, 2007), has led to a growing realization that more effective service for court-ordered clients involves empathy, collaboration, and building strengths and self-efficacy. This shift in the approach to treating clients with legal or other court involvement aligns well with the spirit of motivational interviewing and can facilitate its effectiveness in a variety of service settings.

11.7 Concluding Thoughts

Clients who seek assessment or treatment services at the behest of the court are a particular challenge for providers. They may present with varying levels of motivation or commitment to change, past failures in making significant behavioral change, mental health comorbidities, greater deficits in skills and available resources, and potential serious consequences for non-completion of services. However, it can be very rewarding when one is able to promote growth and meaningful change for even one client. Motivational interviewing presents us with an evidence-based approach for accomplishing this. Emerging empirical literature suggests that motivational interviewing can be effective in improving motivation, treatment engagement, retention, and completion, as well as reduced rates of recidivism and greater compliance with community or agency supervision efforts. Such effects are seen across offender or court-ordered groups, including alcohol and substance abusers, perpetrators of domestic violence, offenders who have committed sexual and violent offenses, and adults, adolescents, and families. Further, it can promote more effective practices among providers and community supervision agents, which may in turn enhance outcomes for court-ordered clients. Though additional research is needed, motivational interviewing is a translatable and sustainable approach that aligns with evidence-based practice and offers the promise of greater treatment effectiveness with a challenging client population.

References

Andrews, D. A., Bonta, J., & Hoge, R. D. (1990). Classification for effective rehabilitation: Rediscovering psychology. *Criminal Justice and Behavior, 17*(1), 19–52. https://doi.org/10.1177/0093854890017001004

Anstiss, B., Polaschek, D. L. L., & Wilson, M. (2011). A brief motivational interviewing intervention with prisoners: When you lead a horse to water, can it drink for itself? *Psychology, Crime & Law, 17*(8), 689–710. https://doi.org/10.1080/10683160903524325

Arkowitz, H., Miller, W. R., & Rollnick, S. (Eds.). (2015). *Motivational interviewing in the treatment of psychological problems*. New York, NY: The Guilford Press.

Austin, K. P., Williams, M. W. M., & Kilgour, G. (2011). The effectiveness of motivational interviewing with offenders: An outcome evaluation. *New Zealand Journal of Psychology, 40*(1), 55–67. Retrieved from http://www.psychology.org.nz/publications-media/new-zealand-journal-of-psychology/

Battjes, R. J., Gordon, M. S., O'Grady, K. E., Kinlock, T. W., Katz, E. C., & Sears, E. A. (2004). Evaluation of a group-based substance abuse treatment program for adolescents. *Journal of Substance Abuse Treatment, 27*(2), 123–134. https://doi.org/10.1016/j.jsat.2004.06.002

Begun, A. L., Murphy, C. M., Bolt, D., Weinstein, B., Strodthoff, T., Short, L., & Shelley, G. (2003). Characteristics of the safe at home instrument for assessing readiness to change intimate partner violence. *Research on Social Work Practice, 13*(1), 80–107. https://doi.org/10.1177/1049731502238758

Black, D. W., Gunter, T., Loveless, P., Allen, J., & Sieleni, B. (2010). Antisocial personality disorder in incarcerated offenders: Psychiatric comorbidity and quality of life. *Annals of Clinical Psychiatry, 22*(2), 113–120. Retrieved from https://www.aacp.com/article/buy_now/?id=56

Bogue, B., Campbell, N., Carey, M., Clawson, E., Faust, D., Florio, K., … Woodward, W. (2004). *Implementing evidence-based practice in community corrections: The principles of effective intervention*. Washington, DC: National Institute of Corrections.

Bogue, B., Diebel, J., & O'Connor, T. (2008) Combining officer supervision skills: A new model for increasing success in community corrections. *Perspectives: The Journal of the American Probation and Parole Association, 32*(2), 30–45. Retrieved from https://www.appa-net.org/eweb/DynamicPage.aspx?Site=APPA_2&WebCode=VC_PubsReports

Bogue, B., Pampel, F., & Pasini-Hill, D. (2013). Progress toward motivational interviewing proficiency in corrections: Results of a Colorado staff development program. *Justice Research and Policy, 15*(1), 37–66. https://doi.org/10.3818/JRP.15.1.2013.37

Bonta, J., & Andrews, D. A. (2007). Risk-need-responsivity model for offender assessment and rehabilitation. *Rehabilitation, 6*, 1–22. Retrieved from https://www.publicsafety.gc.ca/cnt/rsrcs/pblctns/rsk-nd-rspnsvty/index-en.aspx

Carroll, K. M., Easton, C. J., Nich, C., Hunkele, K. A., Neavins, T. M., Sinha, R., … Rounsaville, B. J. (2006). The use of contingency management and motivational/skills-building therapy to treat young adults with marijuana dependence. *Journal of Consulting and Clinical Psychology, 74*(5), 955–966. https://doi.org/10.1037/0022-006X.74.5.955

Chamberlain, P., Patterson, G., Reid, J., Kavanaugh, K., & Forgatch, M. (1984). Observation of client resistance. *Behavior Therapy, 15*(2), 144–155. https://doi.org/10.1016/S0005-7894(84)80016-7

Chambers, J. C., Eccleston, L., Day, A., Ward, T., & Howells, K. (2008). Treatment readiness in violent offenders: The influence of cognitive factors on engagement in violence programs. *Aggression and Violent Behavior, 13*(4), 276–284. https://doi.org/10.1016/j.avb.2008.04.003

Cima, M., Smeets, T., & Jelicic, M. (2008). Self-reported trauma, cortisol levels, and aggression in psychopathic and non-psychopathic prison inmates. *Biological Psychology, 78*(1), 75–86. https://doi.org/10.1016/j.biopsycho.2007.12.011

Clark, M. D. (2005). Motivational interviewing for probation staff: Increasing the readiness to change. *Federal Probation, 69*(2), 22–28. Retrieved from http://www.uscourts.gov/federal-probation-journal/2005/12/motivational-interviewing-probation-staff-increasing-readiness

Clark, M. D., Walters, S., Gingerich, R., & Meltzer, M. (2006). Motivational interviewing for probation officers: Tipping the balance toward change. *Federal Probation, 70*(1), 38–44. Retrieved from http://www.uscourts.gov/federal-probation-journal/2006/06/motivational-interviewing-probation-officers-tipping-balance

Connors, G. J., DiClemente, C. C., Dermen, K. H., Kadden, R., Carroll, K. M., & Frone, M. R. (2000). Predicting the therapeutic alliance in alcoholism treatment. *Journal of Studies on Alcohol and Drugs, 61*(1), 139–149. https://doi.org/10.15288/jsa.2000.61.139

Crane, C. A., Eckhardt, C. I., & Schlauch, R. C. (2015). Motivational enhancement mitigates the effects of problematic alcohol use on treatment compliance among partner violent offenders: Results of a randomized clinical trial. *Journal of Consulting and Clinical Psychology, 83*(4), 689–695. https://doi.org/10.1037/a0039345

Crime and Justice Institute at Community Resources for Justice. (2009). *Implementing evidence-based policy and practice in community corrections* (2nd ed.). Washington, DC: National Institute of Corrections.

D'Amico, E. J., Osilla, K. C., & Hunter, S. B. (2010). Developing a group motivational interviewing intervention for first-time adolescent offenders at-risk for an alcohol or drug use disorder. *Alcoholism Treatment Quarterly, 28*(4), 417–436. https://doi.org/10.1080/07347324.2010.511076

Easton, C., Swan, S., & Sinha, R. (2000). Motivation to change substance use among offenders of domestic violence. *Journal of Substance Abuse Treatment, 19*(1), 1–5. https://doi.org/10.1016/S0740-5472(99)00098-7

Evans, E., Li, L., & Hser, Y. (2009). Client and program factors associated with dropout from court mandated drug treatment. *Evaluation and Program Planning, 32*(3), 204–212. https://doi.org/10.1016/j.evalprogplan.2008.12.003

Farbring, C. Å., & Johnson, W. R. (2008). Motivational interviewing in the correctional system: An attempt to implement motivational interviewing in criminal justice. In H. Arkowitz, H. A. Westra, W. R. Miller, & S. Rollnick (Eds.), *Motivational interviewing in the treatment of psychological problems* (pp. 304–323). New York, NY: The Guilford Press.

Harlow, C. W. (1999). *Prior abuses reported by inmates and probationers (Publication No. NCJ 172879)*. Washington, DC: U.S. Department of Justice, Bureau of Justice Statistics. Retrieved from https://www.bjs.gov/index.cfm?ty=pbdetail&iid=837

Harper, R., & Hardy, S. (2000). Research note. An evaluation of motivational interviewing as a method of intervention with clients in a probation setting. *The British Journal of Social Work, 30*(3), 393–400. https://doi.org/10.1093/bjsw/30.3.393

Hartford, R. J., Ungerer, J. C., & Kinsella, J. K. (1976). Effects of legal pressure on prognosis for treatment of drug dependence. *The American Journal of Psychiatry, 133*(12), 1399–1404. https://doi.org/10.1176/ajp.133.12.1399

Heckman, C. J., Egleston, B. L., & Hofmann, M. T. (2010). Efficacy of motivational interviewing for smoking cessation: A systematic review and meta-analysis. *Tobacco Control, 19*(5), 410–416. https://doi.org/10.1136/tc.2009.033175

Hettema, J. E., & Hendricks, P. S. (2010). Motivational interviewing for smoking cessation: A meta-analytic review. *Journal of Consulting and Clinical Psychology, 78*(6), 868–884. https://doi.org/10.1037/a0021498

Honea-Boles, P., & Griffin, J. E. (2001). The court-mandated client: Does limiting confidentiality preclude a therapeutic encounter? *Journal of Professional Counseling, Practice, Theory, & Research, 29*(2), 149–160. Retrieved from https://www.txca.org/tca/TCA_Publications.asp

Hubble, M. A., Duncan, B. L., & Miller, S. D. (1999). *The heart and soul of change: What works in therapy*. Washington, DC: American Psychological Association.

Ireland, T., & Widom, C. S. (1994). Childhood victimization and risk for alcohol and drug arrests. *International Journal of the Addictions, 29*(2), 235–274. https://doi.org/10.3109/10826089409047380

Kistenmacher, B. R., & Weiss, R. L. (2008). Motivational interviewing as a mechanism for change in men who batter: A randomized controlled trial. *Violence and Victims, 23*(5), 558–570. https://doi.org/10.1891/0886-6708.23.5.558

Kohler, S., & Hofmann, A. (2015). Can motivational interviewing in emergency care reduce alcohol consumption in young people? A systematic review and meta-analysis. *Alcohol and Alcoholism, 50*(2), 107–117. https://doi.org/10.1093/alcalc/agu098

Lai, D. T., Cahill, K., Qin, Y., & Tang, J.-L. (2010). Motivational interviewing for smoking cessation. *Cochrane Database of Systematic Reviews*, 1, CD006936. https://doi.org/10.1002/14651858.CD006936.pub2

Lenz, A. S., Rosenbaum, L., & Sheperis, D. (2016). Meta-analysis of randomized controlled trials of motivational enhancement therapy for reducing substance use. *Journal of Addictions & Offender Counseling, 37*(2), 66–86. https://doi.org/10.1002/jaoc.12017

Letizia, D., & Keaton, M. A. (2014). The impact of motivational interviewing training with corrections staff on recidivism rates for substance abusing offenders. *American Journal of Forensic Psychology, 32*(3), 45–56. Retrieved from http://www.forensicpsychology.org/journal.htm

Li, L., Zhu, S., Tse, N., Tse, S., & Wong, P. (2016). Effectiveness of motivational interviewing to reduce illicit drug use in adolescents: A systematic review and meta-analysis. *Addiction, 111*(5), 795–805. https://doi.org/10.1111/add.13285

Lincourt, P., Kuettel, T. J., & Bombardier, C. H. (2002). Motivational interviewing in a group setting with mandated clients: A pilot study. *Addictive Behaviors, 27*(3), 381–391. https://doi.org/10.1016/S0306-4603(01)00179-4

Mann, R. E., & Rollnick, S. (1996). Motivational interviewing with a sex offender who believed he was innocent. *Behavioural and Cognitive Psychotherapy, 24*(2), 127–134. https://doi.org/10.1017/S1352465800017392

McCracken, S. G., & Corrigan, P. W. (2008). Motivational interviewing for medication adherence in individuals with schizophrenia. In H. Arkowitz, H. A. Westra, W. R. Miller, & S. Rollnick (Eds.), *Applications of motivational interviewing. Motivational interviewing in the treatment of psychological problems* (pp. 249–276). New York, NY: The Guilford Press.

McMurran, M. (2009). Motivational interviewing with offenders: A systematic review. *Legal and Criminological Psychology, 14*(1), 83–100. https://doi.org/10.1348/135532508X278326

Mendel, E., & Hipkins, J. (2002). Motivating learning disabled offenders with alcohol-related problems: A pilot study. *British Journal of Learning Disabilities, 30*(4), 153–158. https://doi.org/10.1046/j.1468-3156.2002.00209.x

Miles, H., Dutheil, L., Welsby, I., & Haider, D. (2007). 'Just say no': A preliminary evaluation of a three-stage model of integrated treatment for substance use problems in conditions of medium security. *The Journal of Forensic Psychiatry & Psychology, 18*(2), 141–159. https://doi.org/10.1080/14789940601101897

Miller, W. R., & Rollnick, S. (2013). *Motivational interviewing: Helping people change* (3rd ed.). New York, NY: The Guilford Press.

Miller, W. R., & Rollnick, S. (1991). *Motivational interviewing: Preparing people to change addictive behavior*. New York, NY: The Guilford Press.

Miller, W. R., & Rollnick, S. (2002). *Motivational interviewing: Preparing people for change* (2nd ed.). New York, NY: The Guilford Press.

Miller, W. R., & Rollnick, S. (2003). Motivational interviewing: Preparing people for change. *Journal for Healthcare Quality, 25*(3), 46. Retrieved from https://journals.lww.com/jhqonline/Citation/2003/05000/Motivational_Interviewing__Preparing_People_for.13.aspx

Miller, W. R., Zweben, A., DiClemente, C. D., & Rychtarik, R. G. (1992). *Motivational enhancement therapy training manual: A clinical research guide for therapists treating individuals with alcohol abuse and dependence*. Rockville, MD: National Institute on Alcohol Abuse and Alcoholism.

Murphy, C. M., & Baxter, V. A. (1997). Motivating batterers to change in the treatment context. *Journal of Interpersonal Violence, 12*(4), 607–619. https://doi.org/10.1177/088626097012004009

Musser, P. H., & Murphy, C. M. (2009). Motivational interviewing with perpetrators of intimate partner abuse. *Journal of Clinical Psychology, 65*(11), 1218–1231. https://doi.org/10.1002/jclp.20642

Musser, P. H., Semiatin, J. N., Taft, C. T., & Murphy, C. M. (2008). Motivational interviewing as a pregroup intervention for partner-violent men. In C. M. Murphy & R. D. Maiuro (Eds.), *Motivational interviewing and stages of change in intimate partner violence* (pp. 61–88). New York, NY: Springer Publishing Company.

Patel, S. H., Lambie, G. W., & Glover, M. M. (2008). Motivational counseling: Implications for counseling male juvenile sex offenders. *Journal of Addictions & Offender Counseling, 28*(2), 86–100. https://doi.org/10.1002/j.2161-1874.2008.tb00035.x

Prescott, D. S. (2009). *Building motivation for change in sexual offenders*. Brandon, VT: Safer Society Press.
Prescott, D. S. (2013). *Enhancing motivation in treatment: A case study and professional development planning method*. Fitchburg, MA: NEARI Press.
Prochaska, J. O., & DiClemente, C. C. (1982). Transtheoretical therapy: Toward a more integrative model of change. *Psychotherapy: Theory, Research, and Practice, 19*(3), 276–288. https://doi.org/10.1037/h0088437
Prochaska, J. O., & DiClemente, C. C. (1992). Stages of change in the modification of problem behaviors. In M. Hersen, R. M. Eisler, & P. M. Miller (Eds.), *Progress in behavior modification* (pp. 184–214). Sycamore, IL: Sycamore Press.
Rau, J., Ehlebracht-König, I., & Petermann, F. (2008). Impact of a motivational intervention on coping with chronic pain: Results of a controlled efficacy study. *Schmerz, 22*(5), 575–578. https://doi.org/10.1007/s00482-008-0658-4
Roffman, R. A., Edleson, J. L., Neighbors, C., Mbilinyi, L., & Walker, D. (2008). The men's domestic abuse check-up: A protocol for reaching the nonadjudicated and untreated man who batters and who abuses substances. *Violence Against Women, 14*(5), 589–605. https://doi.org/10.1177/1077801208315526
Rollnick, S., Kaplan, S. G., & Rutschman, R. (2016). *Motivational interviewing in schools: Conversations to improve behavior and learning*. New York, NY: The Guilford Press.
Satterfield, W. A., Buelow, S. A., Lyddon, W. J., & Johnson, J. T. (1995). Client stages of change and expectations about counseling. *Journal of Counseling Psychology, 42*(4), 476–478. Retrieved from http://www.apa.org/pubs/journals/cou/index.aspx
Sayegh, C. S., Huey, S. J., Jr., Zara, E. J., & Jhaveri, K. (2017). Follow-up treatment effects of contingency management and motivational interviewing on substance use: A meta-analysis. *Psychology of Addictive Behaviors, 31*(4), 403–414. https://doi.org/10.1037/adb0000277
Schumacher, J. A., Madson, M. B., & Nilsen, P. (2014). Barriers to learning motivational interviewing: A survey of motivational interviewing trainers' perceptions. *Journal of Addictions & Offender Counseling, 35*(2), 81–96. https://doi.org/10.1002/j.2161-1874.2014.00028.x
Sinha, R., Easton, C., Renee-Aubin, L., & Carroll, K. M. (2003). Engaging young probation-referred marijuana-abusing individuals in treatment: A pilot trial. *The American Journal on Addictions, 12*(4), 314–323. https://doi.org/10.1111/j.1521-0391.2003.tb00546.x
Slavet, J. D., Stein, L. A. R., Klein, J. L., Colby, S. M., Barnett, N. P., & Monti, P. M. (2005). Piloting the family check-up with incarcerated adolescents and their parents. *Psychological Services, 2*(2), 123–132. https://doi.org/10.1037/1541-1559.2.2.123
Stein, L. A. R., Colby, S. M., Barnett, N. P., Monti, P. M., Golembeske, C., Lebeau-Craven, R., & Miranda, R. (2006). Enhancing substance abuse treatment engagement in incarcerated adolescents. *Psychological Services, 3*(1), 25–34. https://doi.org/10.1037/1541-1559.3.1.0
Steinberg, M. P., & Miller, W. R. (2015). *Motivational interviewing in diabetes care*. New York, NY: The Guilford Press.
Stinson, J. D., & Clark, M. D. (2017). *Motivational interviewing with offenders: Engagement, rehabilitation, and reentry*. New York, NY: The Guilford Press.
Vasilaki, E. I., Hosier, S. G., & Cox, W. M. (2006). The efficacy of motivational interviewing as a brief intervention for excessive drinking: A meta-analytic review. *Alcohol and Alcoholism, 41*(3), 328–335. https://doi.org/10.1093/alcalc/agl016
Walters, S. T., Clark, M. D., Gingerich, R., & Meltzer, M. L. (2007). *Motivating offenders to change: A guide for probation and parole*. Washington, DC: National Institute of Corrections.
Walters, S. T., Vader, A. M., Nguyen, N., Harris, T. R., & Eells, J. (2010). Motivational interviewing as a supervision strategy in probation: A randomized effectiveness trial. *Journal of Offender Rehabilitation, 49*(5), 309–323. https://doi.org/10.1080/10509674.2010.489455
Wang, Y., Xu, K., Cao, G., Qian, M., Shook, J., & Ai, A. L. (2012). Child maltreatment in an incarcerated sample in China: Prediction for crime types in adulthood. *Children and Youth Services Review, 34*(8), 1553–1559. https://doi.org/10.1016/j.childyouth.2012.04.015
Ward, T., & Maruna, S. (2007). *Rehabilitation*. London, UK: Routledge.

Weir, B. W., O'Brien, K., Bard, R. S., Casciato, C. J., Maher, J. E., Dent, C. W., … Stark, M. J. (2009). Reducing HIV and partner violence risk among women with criminal justice system involvement: A randomized controlled trial of two motivational interviewing-based interventions. *AIDS and Behavior, 13*(3), 509–522. https://doi.org/10.1007/s10461-008-9422-0

Wolff, N. L., & Shi, J. (2010). Trauma and incarcerated persons. In C. L. Scott (Ed.), *Handbook of correctional mental health* (2nd ed., pp. 277–320). Washington, DC: American Psychiatric Publishing.

Woodall, W. G., Delaney, H. D., Kunitz, S. J., Westerberg, V. S., & Zhao, H. (2007). A randomized trial of a DWI intervention program for first offenders: Intervention outcomes and interactions with antisocial personality disorder among a primarily American-Indian sample. *Alcoholism: Clinical and Experimental Research, 31*(6), 974–987. https://doi.org/10.1111/j.1530-0277.2007.00380.x

Zalmanowitz, S. J., Babins-Wagner, R., Rodger, S., Corbett, B. A., & Leschied, A. (2013). The association of readiness to change and motivational interviewing with treatment outcomes in males involved in domestic violence group therapy. *Journal of Interpersonal Violence, 28*(5), 956–974. https://doi.org/10.1177/0886260512459381

Chapter 12
Assertive Community Treatment with People with Combined Mental Illness and Criminal Justice Involvement

Joseph S. DeLuca, Lauren K. O'Connor, and Philip T. Yanos

12.1 Introduction

Studies in the United States estimate that over 50% of state prisoners, nearly 50% of all federal prisoners and approximately 65% of jail inmates, meet criteria for a mental disorder (James & Glaze, 2006). It is further estimated that between 10 and 30% of incarcerated adults in the United States have a diagnosable severe mental illness (SMI) (generally defined as including schizophrenia-spectrum disorders, bipolar disorder, and treatment-resistant major depressive disorder) (Fontanarosa, Uhl, Oyesanmi, & Schoelles, 2013; Prins, 2014; Steadman, Osher, Clark Robbins, Case, & Samuels, 2009). Given that roughly 25% of the general US population meets criteria for mental illness (Kessler, Chiu, Demler, & Walters, 2005) and 6% meet criteria for SMI (Substance Abuse and Mental Health Services Administration, 2010), these estimates suggest that mental disorders and SMI are overrepresented in the criminal justice system.

The overrepresentation of persons diagnosed with SMI in the US criminal justice system can be traced back several decades ago. In the late 1950s and early 1960s, *deinstitutionalization* occurred amidst a host of cultural changes (e.g., civil rights movements), treatment developments (e.g., antipsychotics), and sociopolitical shifts in society (e.g., shifting spending from state budgets to the federal budget). Deinstitutionalization called for a gradual reduction of available state psychiatric hospital beds, with the goal of discharged patients being transitioned into newly created community-based treatment centers (Anthony, 1993). Simultaneously, the United States' federally initiated *war on drugs* and subsequent *mass incarceration*

J. S. DeLuca (✉) · L. K. O'Connor · P. T. Yanos
John Jay College of Criminal Justice and the Graduate Center, City University of New York, New York, NY, USA
e-mail: jdeluca@gradcenter.cuny.edu; loconnor@jjay.cuny.edu; pyanos@jjay.cuny.edu

E. L. Jeglic, C. Calkins (eds.), *New Frontiers in Offender Treatment*,
https://doi.org/10.1007/978-3-030-01030-0_12

movements created conditions in which there was a threefold increase in the overall incarceration rate between 1970 and 2005, with low-income persons and persons of color at a significantly greater risk of arrest and incarceration (Kearney, Harris, Jacome, & Parker, 2014). Although many endorse the perspective that deinstitutionalization was the primary driver for the overrepresentation of people with SMI in the criminal justice system (Lamb, Weinberger, & Gross, 2004; Talbott, 2004; Torrey, 2012), others (Fisher, Silver, & Wolff, 2006) attribute it, at least partially, to the effects of criminological risk factors that affect all persons of low socioeconomic status.

Few individuals diagnosed with a mental health problem receive treatment while incarcerated (James & Glaze, 2006), and those that do often receive subpar care that is not evidence-based (Baillargeon, Hoge, & Penn, 2010). It appears that significant shortcomings in recommended practices for intake screening and assessment for mental illness, related to shrinking public funding for correctional mental health services, are partially to blame for this. Thus, such deficiencies in mental health care must be taken into account when formulating discharge plans for such inmates. To this end, studies have also indicated that offenders diagnosed with mental illness tend to have higher rates of recidivism than offenders without mental illness (e.g., Messina, Burdon, Hagopian, & Prendergast, 2004; Skeem, Winter, Kennealy, Louden, & Tatar, 2014).

Since most incarcerated individuals are eventually released back into society, evidence-based interventions and systems to prevent recidivism and enhance community integration are imperative. In this chapter, we first describe a well-established, intensive community treatment for individuals diagnosed with SMI—assertive community treatment (ACT). We then describe the forensic adaptation of this treatment—forensic assertive community treatment (FACT)—along with a case example of how ACT can be used with forensically involved clients (and how FACT can further meet forensic needs of clients). We conclude with future directions for the field.

12.2 History and Origins of Assertive Community Treatment

ACT is a comprehensive approach to treating people with SMI in the community. Unlike many other approaches to treatment for this population, it is characterized as a system of care or framework for organizing services, rather than a clinical intervention in itself (DeLuca, Moser, & Bond, 2008). Nevertheless, ACT is distinguished by a set of key approaches to offering treatment that set it apart from many of methods of providing psychiatric treatment to people with SMI.

ACT has its origins in the pioneering work of Leonard Stein, Mary Ann Test, and Arnold J. Marx, who established the *Training in Community Living* program (later *Program for Assertive Community Treatment*) in Madison, Wisconsin in 1972 (see Stein & Test, 1985; Thompson, Griffith, & Leaf, 1990). The originators of ACT had worked in Wisconsin's Mendota State Hospital and sought to establish a model that could allow persons who had been discharged from Mendota to be "successfully treated in the community" without the need for extended state rehospitalization (Gold Award: A Community Treatment Program, 2000, p. 755). Stein, Test, and Marx strongly believed that hospitalization promoted dependency that interfered with successful adaptation to community life, leading to high rates of "treatment failure" (Gold Award: A Community Treatment Program, 2000, p. 755) among those discharged from state hospitals. Focusing specifically on addressing the needs of these "treatment failures," they developed a model that focused on providing services in the community, with an emphasis on teaching skills to cope with the challenges of community living. Some of the original features of the *Training in Community Living* approach that its originators established are still key parts of the ACT model: services provided predominantly in the community by a multidisciplinary team, 24-h staff availability (through an on-call phone system), and low client-to-staff ratio (Drake, 1998). The principle that ACT services are provided predominantly in the community (including clients' residences and workplaces) represented a radical departure from traditional office-based service models and is still the most distinguishing feature of the ACT model.

An interesting window into the service environment of the original *Training in Community Living* team is provided by Estroff (1981), who conducted a landmark ethnographic study of the lives of "psychiatric clients" (p. xv) receiving services from that program in the 1970s. Estroff described a committed team of staff who were "community converts" (p. 49), highly focused on practical issues such as employment and housing and often believing more strongly in the potential for clients to live in the community than the clients themselves. For example, when asked about "the biggest obstacles to curing people," a staff member stated "I don't believe in curing," and then stated "employment," explaining that a lack of opportunity keeps many clients from reaching their full potential (p. 123). This indicates that the prototypical ACT team was in some ways ahead of its time in conceiving of what would later be known as "recovery" as a social phenomenon that occurs independently from symptomatic improvement. Mental health *recovery* has been defined as a deeply personal, subjective, and unique process of living a hopeful, satisfying, and meaningful life, even when one is experiencing mental health symptoms (Anthony, 1993). At the same time, however, Estroff described an atmosphere of service provision that was at times paternalistic, with staff attempting to "re-parent" clients and occasionally engaging in a "testing of wills" (p. 48). The tension between these dimensions of ACT (both person-centered and paternalistic) has been an ongoing theme in the evolution of ACT that will be discussed further below.

12.3 Principles of ACT and their Evolution

Following reports of the success of the "Program for Assertive Community Treatment," ACT services were implemented in a variety of locations, such that programs existed in 14 US states by the early 1990s (Gold et al., 2003). However, a barrier to the dissemination of ACT programs was a lack of clearly delineated criteria for what constituted ACT. This changed with the development of the Dartmouth Assertive Community Treatment Scale (Teague, Bond, & Drake, 1998) in the mid-1990s. The DACTS was developed after a series of practices were derived from multiple sources, including Test, Stein, and Marx's original writings and key informant interviews. It was intended to be used as a tool for evaluating the "fidelity" of ACT programs to prevent "program drift" away from core ACT principles. The DACTS eventually included 28 items addressing three aspects of ACT service practice: Human Resources–Structure and Composition (e.g., "Small Caseload," "ACT Team Size"), Organizational Boundaries (e.g., "Responsibility for Crisis Services," "Responsibility for Hospital Discharge Planning"), and Nature of Services (e.g., "Community Based Services," "Assertive Engagement Mechanisms").

The DACTS facilitated the further implementation of ACT, such that, by 2014, it was estimated that 40 US states and much of Canada had ACT teams. However, an area of particular controversy concerned the "Assertive Engagement Mechanisms" item of the DACTS Fidelity Scale (Teague et al., 1998, p. 218; "[ACT team] uses street outreach, plus legal mechanisms (e.g., representative payees, probation/parole, OP commitment) as indicated"), which many interpreted to mean that it was appropriate for ACT teams to use "coercive" methods, such as threats of hospitalization, to maintain treatment engagement (see Gomory, 2002, for an extensive discussion of this perspective). To address this concern, Salyers and Tsemberis (2007) made an explicit call for a modernization of ACT fidelity criteria so that they were more clearly aligned with "recovery-oriented" principles of consumer choice, self-determination, and belief in the possibility of recovery (for a discussion of principles of recovery-oriented services, see O'Connell, Tondora, Croog, Evans, & Davidson, 2005). Although Salyers and Tsemberis (2007) did not explicitly recommend that fidelity criteria should be revised, they recommended that ACT teams simultaneously train staff in recovery-oriented practices and monitor the use of these practices in addition to ACT fidelity.

Subsequent research on the nature of "engagement strategies" used by ACT teams has suggested that teams primarily use person-centered strategies that are consistent with principles of recovery-oriented care, but that coercive strategies are also sometimes used. For example, while Kidd et al. (2010) found that ACT teams generally scored fairly high on measures of recovery-orientation, Manuel et al. (2013) noted significant variation in team practices, finding evidence that some ACT teams routinely used "conditional involvement" strategies, such as telling a client that they would only be assisted if they complied with treatment requirements.

Partly in response to controversies about the types of "engagement strategies" that might most appropriately be used by ACT teams, researchers eventually moved to develop a new fidelity rating scale, called the Tool for Measurement of Assertive Community Treatment (TMACT; Monroe-DeVita, Teague, & Moser, 2011). The TMACT revised and expanded upon DACTS items, dividing 47 items into 6 subscales: Operations and Structure, Core Team, Specialist Team, Core Practices, Evidence-Based Practices, and Person-Centered Planning and Practices. The "Person-Centered Planning and Practices" subscale is composed of four completely new items and makes explicit recommendations for the use of recovery-oriented practices and de-emphasizes the use of coercive strategies that the DACTS appeared to sanction. The TMACT's increased focus on the use of evidence-based practices represents another modernization of ACT fidelity, as it explicitly recognized a need to integrate practices such as illness self-management and integrated dual disorder treatment into ACT services. Research on the impact of the TMACT is still in its infancy, but many locations are now adopting TMACT fidelity criteria, suggesting that they will replace the DACTS as the primary guiding force for ACT services.

Given the above focus on fidelity criteria and the possibility that one might not be able to distinguish the "forest from the trees" in ACT services, we will describe what we believe to be the "essence" of ACT services based on our experience working within ACT teams. In our experience, the essence of this model is contained in the act of going out into the field to meet with clients in their own environments (their home, school, or other locations in their neighborhood) and in the relaxed "human-to-human" nature of interactions that often occur in this context. Although interactions with clients inevitably revolve around clinical topics such as life goals and the impact of psychiatric symptoms on them, it is also perfectly appropriate to discuss common interests such as music and sports with clients as a way of building trust and rapport. These types of interactions are often experienced as less artificial and inherently stigmatizing by clients than office-based interactions, and, as a result, many clients find it difficult to transition to more traditional services when they are considered to be no longer in need of ACT services.

12.4 Evidence Supporting ACT

ACT is considered an evidence-based practice for the treatment of schizophrenia (Kreyenbuhl, Buchanan, Dickerson, & Dixon, 2009). Since its inception, numerous meta-analyses and systematic reviews have been conducted on the effectiveness of ACT for individuals with SMI. These reviews are comprised of studies from the United States, Canada, Australia, and the United Kingdom and include myriad adaptations of the ACT model (e.g., for individuals with co-occurring substance use disorders, experiences of homelessness, and/or justice involvement). While some reviews synthesize findings across a broad range of ACT interventions and subpopulations (e.g., Bond, McGrew, & Fekete, 1995; Mueser, Bond, Drake, & Resnick, 1998; Ziguras & Stuart, 2000), more recent reviews have focused specifically on particular adaptations (e.g., Coldwell & Bender, 2007; De Vet et al., 2013; Fries & Rosen, 2011).

A significant reduction in psychiatric hospitalizations (both frequency and duration) has been the strongest and most consistently reported outcome of ACT (Bond, Drake, Mueser, & Latimer, 2001; Burns, 2001; Mueser et al., 1998). One analysis estimated that ACT reduced hospitalizations by 78% compared with standard care and 58% compared with low-intensity case management (Latimer, 1999). In addition to this consistent finding, ACT has been found to increase community housing stability, independent living, and patient satisfaction (Burns, 2001; Latimer, 1999; Mueser et al., 1998; Ziguras & Stuart, 2000). Additionally, ACT has been found to moderately reduce symptom severity, improve subjective quality of life (Bond et al., 2001), and significantly decrease family burden and increase family satisfaction (Ziguras & Stuart, 2000). These varying outcomes are particularly pronounced for interventions with higher implementation fidelity (Burns, 2001; Latimer, 1999). For instance, higher-fidelity programs (using the DACTS) have been found to reduce inpatient days by about 23% more than lower-fidelity programs (Latimer, 1999).

Mixed or weaker findings for traditional ACT demonstrate that it has little impact on social functioning, arrests and incarcerations, vocational functioning, substance use, and medication compliance (Burns, 2001; Mueser et al., 1998). Specific to substance use, Fries and Rosen (2011) conducted a review of four randomized controlled trials (RCTs) that looked at the efficacy of traditional ACT in treating individuals with co-occurring alcohol and/or drug use disorders. With consistency, these RCTs showed that compared to treatment-as-usual, ACT showed small to no significant difference in substance abuse, though both conditions showed improvements in substance abuse over time. Based on these findings, Fries and Rosen (2011) suggested that the substance abuse treatment provided within these interventions may not be sufficient and that the addition of an evidence-based substance abuse treatment may be indicated. Similarly, other weak outcome findings have been used to inform additional developments and adaptations of the ACT model over time, including Forensic ACT (FACT) (see following discussion).

In addition to the presence of weaker findings, more recent studies (many coming out of the UK) with strong comparison conditions have found that intensive case management programs may be just as effective as ACT (Essock et al., 2006; King, 2006). Despite the presence of some weaker findings, the literature on ACT is notable for its relative absence of negative outcomes; ACT has rarely been shown to worsen outcomes, and clients appear to be generally satisfied with the services (McGrew, Wilson, & Bond, 1996; McGrew, Wilson, & Bond, 2002). Criticisms suggesting that ACT may be paternalistic or coercive notwithstanding (e.g., Levine, Toro, & Perkins, 1993), a research study exploring which features of ACT were least liked by clients found that only 6% stated they felt the program was too intrusive and 1% felt it fostered dependence, while 44% either stated that there was nothing they disliked about the program or voluntarily made a positive statement about ACT in place of a critique (McGrew et al., 2002).

In addition to its clinical benefits, ACT treatment has been found to reduce mental health costs for high-frequency inpatient users within the United States and Canada. Through offsetting the costs of inpatient hospitalizations, ACT has been found to be cost-effective for those with high levels of hospitalizations (about 4 days/month over the past 2 years) while less cost-effective for infrequently hospitalized clients (Dieterich, Irving, Park, & Marshall, 2010; Latimer, 1999). With that, more recent cost analyses of ACT in the United Kingdom have shown less promising results (McCrone et al., 2009), suggesting that these findings may be context and system specific.

Given the structure and flexibility of the ACT model, research has also focused on the effectiveness of specific adaptations, many of which incorporate supported housing for individuals with histories of homelessness or co-occurring substance use disorders. Three reviews have been conducted to synthesize research on ACT for homeless adults with SMI (Coldwell & Bender, 2007; De Vet et al., 2013; Nelson, Aubry, & Lafrance, 2007). In addition to standard benefits of ACT, compared to those in standard care, ACT clients had significantly fewer days of homelessness and more stable days of housing, especially when treatment was integrated with evidence-based housing models (Tsemberis, Gulcur, & Nakae, 2004). In addition to adaptations for individuals with co-occurring substance use disorders and experiences of homelessness, ACT has also been adapted for use with forensically involved clients (FACT). The following sections will review this specific treatment adaptation and provide a review of initial research findings supporting its implementation.

12.5 Adapting ACT with Forensically Involved Clients

Given the relative success of ACT, forensic ACT (FACT) was created in order to help transition criminal justice-involved individuals diagnosed with SMI into community treatment. While traditional ACT teams have served—and continue to serve—individuals involved in the criminal justice system (or otherwise forensically involved, such as Assisted/Mandatory Outpatient Treatment), studies suggest that the traditional ACT model may not meet the specific needs of forensic clients (e.g., individuals with a history of arrest or incarceration, currently on parole, etc.). For example, in one longitudinal study of nearly 5000 ACT clients in New York State (Beach et al., 2013), forensic clients (v. non-forensic clients) had significantly higher arrest and incarceration rates, risk of homelessness, and risk of early discharge from ACT. In particular, 33% of ACT clients with recent forensic histories (i.e., criminal justice involvement <6 months before enrollment), and 14% of clients with past forensic histories (i.e., criminal justice involvement >6 months before enrollment), were rearrested or incarcerated within 1 year of enrollment (compared to 5% of non-forensic ACT clients). Beach et al. (2013) concluded that the poor outcomes for ACT clients with forensic histories highlight the failure of traditional ACT models in improving criminal justice outcomes and "underscores the need for ACT teams to incorporate interventions targeted at improving forensic outcomes in this population" (p. 443). Such goals can be achieved via FACT principles and programming, discussed below.

12.5.1 Inception of FACT

With the proliferation of individuals diagnosed with mental health problems in the criminal justice system, programs to meet the needs of such individuals have similarly proliferated. FACT began to gain momentum as a potentially structured, intensive treatment program for justice-involved individuals in the early 2000s. Lamberti, Weisman, and Faden (2004) conducted a national survey of members of the National Association of County Behavioral Health Directors (NACBHD) in order to identify existing ACT programs in the United States that had been modified to prevent the rearrest and incarceration of justice-involved adults diagnosed with SMI. Lamberti et al. (2004) identified three criteria for inclusion in their study: (1) client history of involvement with the criminal justice system was an admission requirement; (2) a criminal justice agency was the primary source of referrals; and (3) the program had a close partnership with a criminal justice agency to perform jail diversion. Using this definition, Project Link, developed in 1999 in Rochester, New York, is said to be the first recognized FACT program, followed by Chicago's Thresholds Jail Linkage Project in 2001 (Lamberti & Weisman, 2010)—both of which have won Gold Achievement Awards from the American Psychiatric Association.

Sixteen programs in 9 states ended up meeting Lamberti et al. (2004) critesria (it should be noted that the NACBHD only comprised 28 US states at the time, so this was likely an underestimate, as the authors noted). All programs received funding through Medicaid, in addition to further funding through grants and various local, state, and federal resources. Eighty-one percent of these programs primarily received clients from local jails, 50% of the programs accepted clients under involuntary outpatient treatment statutes, 81% of programs accepted clients who had recently committed a violent crime, and 69% incorporated probation officers as members of their ACT teams. Program capacities ranged from 25 to 108, with a mean level enrollment of 53 clients; approximately 50% of clients were from a racial or ethnic minority group, and 32% of staff members were from a racial or ethnic minority group (Lamberti and colleagues highlighted the importance of maintaining a diverse group of service providers to meet the needs of diverse clients involved in the legal system). Most clients had a schizophrenia-spectrum diagnosis (56%) or bipolar diagnosis (21%), and 89% had a co-occurring substance use disorder. Based on this initial survey, Lamberti et al. (2004) concluded that FACT was an emerging and important model and that more research was needed to establish its structure and core elements. They further added that, "… we suggest that the primary distinction between FACT and standard assertive community treatment programs lies in the extent to which the goals of preventing arrest and incarceration determine program structure and function" (p. 1289).

Overall, while traditional ACT teams serve justice-involved individuals, this is not the program's main purpose, and arrests or incarceration are often not key outcomes variable for ACT teams. FACT, on the other hand, is designed to meet the needs of justice-involved individuals and integrates mental health and criminal justice service systems. Criminal justice system employees may be embedded within FACT teams, for example, which can promote effective interdisciplinary communication and legal leverage when needed and appropriate. Lamberti et al. (2004) have also noted that another distinction between FACT and ACT is the type of housing provided, with many FACT programs using supervised residential components, compared to ACT's focus on supportive community housing or independent living. Lastly, Lamberti et al. (2004) noted the importance of considering various social-environmental variables in predicting recidivism (e.g., Bonta, Law, & Hanson, 1998) and, hence, the importance of multidimensional treatment goals, including cognitive-behavioral therapy (CBT) and interventions that target trauma, antisocial attitudes, and substance abuse. Thus, the conceptual framework for FACT generally aligns with the *risk, needs, and responsivity* (RNR) [see Chap. 2] model (Andrews & Bonta, 2010; Lamberti & Weisman, 2010), wherein modifiable general risk factors are targeted in order to prevent recidivism and improve quality of life.

12.5.2 Evolution of FACT

To track the evolution of FACT programs after the landmark 2004 national survey study, a follow-up national survey was conducted several years later (see Lamberti, Deem, Weisman, & LaDuke, 2011; Lamberti & Weisman, 2010), and a chapter was written on FACT in order to describe its origins, current practice, and future directions (Lamberti & Weisman, 2010). Using the same methodology as the 2004 study, Lamberti and Weisman (2010) surveyed NACBHD members again (now representing 30 US states and the District of Columbia) and identified 28 programs meeting FACT study criteria, a 75% increase from the 16 programs identified in the original survey (all 12 programs were initiated after the publication of the 2004 survey). While new programs appeared to maintain similar ingredients (e.g., probation officers and residential components), the authors noted that FACT continued "... to show a significant degree of variability in terms of structure and function. For example, programs continue to show variable fidelity to the ACT model, different admission criteria, and differences in collaboration between the clinicians and the criminal justice system representatives" (p. 9). Thus, calls were made again for the standardization and experimental study of FACT. Lamberti and Weisman (2010) also specifically took this opportunity to describe the guiding principles of FACT model development, ostensibly to promote standardization.

12.5.3 Guiding Principles and Key Components of FACT

As stated, the FACT model is heavily based on Andrews and Bonta's (2010) *RNR* theory, which calls for the targeting of various general and specific risk factors for recidivism (e.g., substance abuse, low levels of satisfaction with work/school, family conflict, lack of healthy recreational pursuits, antisocial traits). This model seems particularly applicable to offenders diagnosed with mental illness (Skeem, Steadman, & Manchak, 2015), especially since <8% of crimes committed by those with SMI are directly related to symptoms (Peterson, Skeem, Kennealy, Bray, & Zvonkovic, 2014). Instead, the majority of crimes committed by those with SMI are related to common factors for criminal behavior, such as antisocial cognitions (Peterson et al., 2014). For crimes that *do* directly relate to psychiatric symptoms, most relate to symptoms of mania rather than depression or psychosis (Peterson et al., 2014). Further, when looking at this specific subset of crimes, about 40% are classified as crimes against another person, while the remaining crimes are either property-related or minor offenses, such as trespassing (Peterson et al., 2014). In addition to targeting such modifiable risk factors and other relevant risk factors in ACT models (e.g., mental illness, homelessness), Lamberti and Weisman (2010) argued that interventions in FACT must also be *accessible* and should incorporate the use of *legal leverage* (e.g., using the legal authority of a probation officer to enhance commitment to treatment).

Lack of access to care remains a widespread issue for individuals living with mental health problems, especially for those living with SMI. FACT ensures access to a wide variety of services (e.g., mental health and addictions, vocational, residential) and delivers these services through outreach. ACT is already an evidence-based model that targets many of these modifiable risk factors; FACT takes this evidence-based model further by targeting additional factors and building connections to the criminal justice system. For example, partnerships with criminal justice staff (e.g., probation officers) bridge additional gaps between systems (that can be challenging to navigate and are critical for clients who may be frequently cycling between systems). To this end, many FACT teams also provide "inreach" in correctional facilities in order to begin discharge and service planning prior to release (Lamberti & Weisman, 2010).

In regard to legal leverage, Lamberti et al. (2004) have stated that FACT's use of such leverage (e.g., for treatment adherence) could seem to be at odds with ACT's client-centered philosophy. However, Lamberti et al. (2004) argued that such leverage can be understood "on a continuum of interventions that may be necessary to promote engagement" (p. 1290), and that such leverage could still remain client-centered if guided by individual clients' needs/strengths and the least restrictive alternative. Similarly, Lamberti and Weisman (2010) argued that FACT teams first utilize legal leverage by establishing partnerships with judges, probation, parole, and police officers (depending on clients' needs and system involvement), and then extend such leverage as needed. Overall, the FACT model emphasizes prevention and intervention (e.g., problem-solving) rather than punishment in addressing behavioral problems that arise. With these shared goals and values in mind (partially accomplished via cross-training), in addition to comprehensive services and outreach offered to clients, maximized outcomes can be had for both clients and communities (Lamberti & Weisman, 2010; Swartz & Swanson, 2004). However, FACT and other programs must contend with the risk that over-involvement by criminal justice staff in mental health diversion programs can also lead to negative outcomes, if not implemented carefully (e.g., Solomon, Draine, & Marcus, 2002).

Dual Agency

It should be noted that these same "dual agency roles" are seen in other intensive treatment and diversion programs for justice-involved individuals (e.g., mental health courts; see Castellano, 2011), and the tension between "community protection" and "individual healing" has been discussed elsewhere (e.g., Yanos, Knight, Vayshenker, Gonzales, & DeLuca, 2017). Nonetheless, Lamberti et al. (2011) have found that, while the most common barrier to collaboration among FACT team clinicians and probation officers tends to be differences in philosophy (e.g., health concerns v. public safety), such collaborations remain common and are viewed by the majority of FACT program leaders as helpful in reducing rearrests (87% agreed). Additionally, 60% of programs had a full-time probation officer on staff, 73% of probation officers on FACT teams received some type of mental health training, and 75% of probation officers on FACT teams performed community outreach with team clinicians. Lamberti et al. (2011) concluded that probation officers are generally reported to be positive features of FACT teams.

Several years later, Lamberti et al. (2014) conducted a qualitative study with 31 adult FACT clients across the United States in order to understand clients' experiences of legal leverage and coercion. Results indicated that the experience of legal leverage varied widely, with some clients perceiving consistent coercion and others perceiving less coercion and more autonomy over time.

Unsurprisingly, clients were more motivated to participate in FACT (and felt more autonomous) if they liked the "structure" FACT gave them and/or perceived the judge and other FACT staff members as caring, supportive, and knowledgeable. Similar to Lamberti et al. (2004) earlier views on emphasizing prevention and shared values, Lamberti et al. (2014) concluded that legal leverage can likely be used effectively and humanely within FACT if it is applied in a supportive manner and used "in ways that support patients' basic psychological needs: to be one's own person, to feel able to accomplish one's goals, and to have positive relationships" (p. 8).

12.6 Evidence Supporting FACT

While the evidence base for ACT is extensive and well-documented, FACT remains a relatively underutilized and understudied program (Landess & Holoyda, 2017), in part due to the heterogeneity and nascence of programs in the United States (Marquant, Sabbe, Van Nuffel, & Goethals, 2016; Morrissey, 2013). For example, many FACT programs continue to differ in regard to standardized admission criteria, diagnoses and demographics of clients, and methods to incorporate clinicians and criminal justice staff—thus making comparisons of programs difficult. Nonetheless, Marquant et al. (2016) review of the FACT literature concluded that, while limited evidence for its effectiveness exists, FACT appears to be a promising model. Based on available data from three RCTs of FACT interventions (and seven non-controlled studies), these authors found that FACT had generally positive effects on forensic outcomes (e.g., reduced recidivism in the form of arrests, incarceration, and/or length of stay in jail/prison). However, much of this evidence came from the non-controlled studies included in the review. Further, it should be noted that the one RCT that did demonstrate a significant effect on arrests (Cusack, Morrissey, Cuddeback, Prins, & Williams, 2010) also had a high model adherence to ACT (measured using the DACTS), suggesting that model adherence may be a crucial factor for success. In regard to non-forensic outcomes (e.g., quality of life, substance use, hospitalization, community functioning), it was found that the evidence for FACT was largely limited in this regard and generally produced nonsignificant results. It should be noted that some FACT clients see benefits in well-being and on clinical variables, but more research is needed in this area.

Two additional studies have been published since Marquant et al. (2016) review of FACT. Lamberti et al. (2017) recently conducted a RCT of the Rochester FACT team in New York. Participants included 70 adults who were diagnosed with SMI and arrested for misdemeanor crimes. Clients who received the FACT intervention had fewer convictions for new crimes, fewer days in jail and the hospital, and more days spent in outpatient mental health treatment (compared to TAU at a 1-year follow-up). The Rochester program showed high fidelity to the ACT model. Additionally, FACT clients in Rochester received active judicial monitoring (including weekly meetings between a FACT team liaison, the presiding judge, public defenders—all who worked to actively problem solve issues that arose for clients), support from staff highly trained in mental health-criminal justice collaboration, and service planning that incorporated modifiable risk factors for criminal recidivism. To this end, FACT team clinicians in this study received training in CBT for antisocial cognitions/behaviors—known risk factors for recidivism and part of the RNR model. To date, this study provides the strongest evidence for FACT and guidance for how such programs should be structured.

In one other recent study, the FACT model was utilized in Belgium for patients being released from a forensic hospital, and outcomes were tracked over a 33-month period (Marquant, Sabbe, Van Nuffel, Verelst, & Goethals, 2018). Marquant et al. (2018) analyzed retrospective data on 70 FACT clients (who were receiving FACT embedded in a continuum of discharge care) and found significantly better forensic outcomes for such clients (v. discharged patients receiving general community-based care), including lower arrest rates (3% v. 14% in the control group) and incarceration rates (4% v. 58% in the control group) at a nearly 3-year follow-up. Rehospitalization rates, however, were significantly higher in the FACT group; nonetheless, FACT still appeared to help clients remain in the community for more days, compared to the control group, which was largely due to the number of days spent in detention/jail for control group participants.

12.6.1 Factors Related to Outcomes in FACT

Regarding other factors related to outcomes in FACT, Marquant et al. (2016) summarized data from multiple studies, finding that a history of violent offending, the presence of antisocial personality traits, previously failed residential care, and substance abuse may all impede progress in FACT—consistent with the RNR model. Substance abuse, residential instability, and criminological needs also emerged as factors that impeded FACT progress in a recent multi-method, non-controlled study of a US FACT program (Kelly, Barrenger, Watson, & Angell, 2017). Marquant et al. (2016) also noted that there appears to be a small percentage of "revolving door patients" who account for a large amount of rearrests and therefore may not be benefitting from FACT. However, Lamberti et al. (2017) found that their sample appeared to be at a higher risk of recidivism than individuals in other jail diversion studies but still demonstrated positive effects on forensic outcomes, suggesting that strong and standardized FACT programs may be effective for a wide range of high-risk clients. Nevertheless, Lamberti et al. (2017) also found that clients with higher scores on an assessment tool used to measure reoffending, as well as clients with more severe psychiatric symptoms, were significantly more likely to fail a conditional discharge (e.g., failure to comply with the judge's legal conditions).

In regard to promotive factors, as stated, high fidelity to the ACT model appears to be an important factor in producing positive outcomes in FACT, as evidenced by two RCTs. Moreover, one of the key ingredients in FACT appears to be collaboration and communication with the courts; for example, Lamberti et al. (2017) reported that although there were similar arrests among participants in the study, FACT clients had fewer convictions. This was likely due to judges issuing bench warrants for arrests for clients who missed court dates, in order to reengage and problem solve rather than punish. Similarly, Marquant et al. (2018) findings suggest that FACT teams may have been better able to direct at-risk clients into treatment (hospitalization) when necessary, rather than involve authorities and increase the chances of incarceration. Further, in one qualitative study of FACT (Lamberti et al., 2014), clients noted the importance of their relationships with FACT program judges and clinicians, as is evident from the following client's quote:

> "What really shocked me is that the judge knew about me. I thought he don't know what's going on, he don't know about my doctors, my suicide attempts, my hepatitis, but he knew everything. I wasn't just another number in there. He knew about me and talked to me in a way that made me feel like I wanted to make this change; I want to work this program" (Lamberti et al., 2014, p. 5).

Overall, more research is needed to explore other factors related to FACT program success. Further randomized research is also needed to establish a solid evidence base for FACT; mixed-methods research would also supplement this evidence base by integrating clients' experiences, likes, and dislikes of FACT. In addition to forensic outcomes, outcomes related to service utilization, clinical and well-being outcomes, and cost-effectiveness, among a diverse group of clients and practitioners, are of interest.

12.7 Case Example

Chris[1] is a 28-year-old Hispanic male, living in a large metropolitan city. He is diagnosed with schizophrenia and has been involved with a local ACT team for the last few months. He reports periodically using marijuana but denies other drug use. Prior to joining ACT, Chris was hospitalized four times over a period of 3 months

[1] Name changed and other identifying information masked or changed.

due to deteriorating mental health and concurrent behavioral problems in the community (e.g., exhibitionism, which culminated in Chris exposing his genitals to females and masturbating in public). After his last hospital discharge, Chris was referred to an outpatient treatment program for adults with SMI and substance use problems, but these services were quickly terminated after similar behavioral problems in the local community occurred, in addition to a continued lack of adherence to treatment. Chris was subsequently referred to the ACT team to better meet his treatment needs.

When Chris first joined the ACT team, he had an unstable housing situation, was unemployed, and had a poor social network and support system. In fact, many of Chris' friends were engaged in illegal activities in the community. Chris was also working to manage his fluctuating psychotic symptoms and depressed mood.

Chris grew up in a community marked by violence and chaos. In high school, Chris joined a local gang and participated in numerous illegal activities, ranging from drug sales to assaults. As a result, he served some time in a juvenile detention facility as an adolescent. Shortly after being released into the community as a young adult, Chris resumed his gang involvement, was subsequently arrested for a burglary, and served time at the local jail. Since being released from jail several years ago, Chris severed his ties with his gang and old peers but continued to cycle through the criminal justice and mental health systems. When arrested by police for illegal activity (including trespassing and recent sexual behaviors in the community), he is generally hospitalized for brief periods of time, rather than incarcerated (due to often presenting to law enforcement with co-occurring psychotic symptoms).

Over the last few months, the ACT team helped Chris to improve his quality of life. For instance, early on, the treatment team helped Chris to apply for, and successfully obtain, supportive housing in the community. Additionally, Chris was provided with information for local food banks and signed up for social services via case management services. The flexible ACT model also seemed to keep Chris engaged in the treatment process. Chris historically had difficulties making his appointments, which often precipitated psychiatric relapse. On ACT, the treatment team would meet Chris in the community, sometimes at his residence and sometimes in the community, such as at his favorite coffee shop. During these visits, Chris might be visited by a nurse or psychiatrist to provide medication, by a substance abuse specialist to work on his substance use, by a vocational rehabilitation specialist to work on employment goals, and also by a social worker or psychologist who provided individual therapy and additional case management. Chris' connection to the team and engagement in his treatment process became clear as he gradually began to visit the ACT office just to check in or to receive additional services (including a substance abuse support group). Chris even attended a holiday party for ACT clients and became friendly with other clients. The informality of ACT services was an important part of the process of keeping him engaged, as ACT team members asked Chris about his various interests, including the type of music that he listened to, religious interests, family relationships, and a stated interest in writing a book. Discussion of clinical concerns within the context of these interests and goals helped Chris to identify a *reason* to want to reduce his interactions with the police and stay out of the hospital.

By all accounts, Chris was making strides in improving his quality of life and meeting many of ACT's traditional outcomes, such as reduced hospitalizations, increased treatment adherence and reduced psychiatric symptoms, increased vocational abilities, and somewhat reduced substance abuse. However, Chris continued to engage in exhibitionistic behaviors in the community. As a result of these behaviors, he had consistent contact with the local police. Chris was arrested twice during his early months on the ACT team but never charged (due to victims who did not wish to press criminal charges or insufficient evidence). Chris was also never hospitalized during this period, ostensibly due to psychiatric symptom management. Nevertheless, the local police became familiar with Chris and kept an eye on him. Chris' housing supervisor also became worried about this behavior after seeing Chris masturbating in public in the local community. Several joint meetings were set up between Chris' housing provider and the ACT team, and it became clear that Chris might be at risk of losing his housing.

Chris' inappropriate behaviors never extended to ACT staff, but he did sometimes exhibit personal boundary issues (e.g., hugging female staff members, holding on to handshakes too long with female staff). Nonetheless, Chris continued to engage in such behavior in the community and was at a high chance of recidivating. Chris' behavior was subsequently conceptualized via the RNR model by the team. First, in regard to risk, it appeared that Chris might not be receiving the necessary type of services to meet his risk for reoffending, given his continued sexual behaviors. Second, in regard to needs, it appeared that Chris maintained many antisocial and criminogenic thinking patterns that needed to be targeted, in addition to other modifiable risk factors. For instance, when asked about his sexual behavior, Chris might say that the women "deserved it," "wanted it," or were "asking for it." It should also be noted that there did not appear to be a strong link between Chris' mental health symptoms and sexual behavior in the community (he also denied past trauma or abuse). However, occasionally preceding inappropriate sexual behavior, Chris might state that other women were giving him "the eyes," which may have been the product of both delusional symptoms and poor social skills. In addition to the aforementioned boundary issues, Chris also appeared to have some deficits in social interaction. He frequently misread cues and social situations, which sometimes lead to inappropriate sexual behavior. For instance, if a woman complimented Chris on his shirt, he might interpret this as a sexual advance or interest. If he perceived a woman to be giving him "the eyes," this might lead to him exposing himself. Chris was also struggling to maintain prosocial contacts and had yet to find a significant other—one of his main goals. Further, Chris did not have many recreational or leisure activities and was still trying to find employment; thus, his days had little routine or scheduled activities. Lastly, in regard to responsivity, it appeared that Chris might benefit the most from a CBT treatment tailored to his learning style and criminogenic cognitions. While traditional CBT had been implemented already via traditional ACT services, it appeared that a more specific approach was needed.

Drawing from the literature on CBT for forensic populations, the ACT team first had to educate themselves on evidence-based practices for forensic populations: Chris was having frequent contact with law enforcement, and it was necessary to incorporate these additional needs and services into his treatment plan. It should be noted that many team members had little knowledge or comfort working with individuals involved in the criminal justice system. Given the sexual nature of the offenses, and the stigma that is attached to this particular group of offenders, it was also not surprising that some team members were frankly appalled and perplexed by Chris' behavior. During one team meeting, one team member incredulously asked, "How do you even treat this?"

The team gradually became familiar with the RNR model and tailored CBT practices for forensic populations (i.e., to target Chris' antisocial and criminogenic cognitions) through personal literature reviews and research and also via psychoeducation from social work and psychology staff. Further, the team's social work and psychology staff helped the team conceptualize Chris' problems in a multifaceted fashion. For instance, Chris' problems were explained in light of his early antisocial peer group and offending experiences, which culminated in a lack of prosocial socialization and community involvement, as well as basic skill deficits. To this end, Chris did not have many fulfilling relationships in his life, especially romantic relationships. On top of this, he appeared to have some baseline impulse control issues. In terms of the modifiable risk factors as described in the RNR, Chris had a low level of satisfaction and performance with work and school and a long history of family conflict (his family largely distanced themselves after his early gang involvement). He also did not have many healthy recreational pursuits. This conceptualization helped both to humanize Chris' problems, and to provide a tangible framework for reducing Chris' inappropriate behaviors. This work was supplemented by specific treatments to target exhibitionistic behaviors (see Marshall & Marshall, 2015). Thus, some of these additional targets included a focus on lack of intimacy, emotional loneliness, poor self-regulation, sexual preoccupation, and attitudes supportive of sexual offending (e.g., aforementioned hostility toward women). Broadly, the team was also encouraged to help Chris develop prosocial skills and facilitate meaningful life goals while keeping their biases in check and treating Chris warmly, empathically, and without judgment (Chris was insightful about stigma and worried the team would judge him).

12.7.1 FACT for Chris

As discussed, one main barrier to meeting Chris' needs in traditional ACT services was the staff's lack of experience and knowledge of forensic populations, specifically sexual offenders. In this case, the team adjusted, but there was a learning curve. As Lamberti and Weisman (2010) note, competent care is a necessary component to FACT teams. FACT staff must be comfortable working with forensic populations and should also be knowledgeable about the criminal justice system and how to partner with this system. To this end, Chris may have benefitted from some form of "legal leverage." Chris would have met the criteria for many FACT programs just for his arrest history and may have even entered FACT programs in other communities after being arrested and transferred to mental health court, for example. Whatever the criteria or mechanism, Chris' involvement on a FACT team would have put him under some sort of supervision from the criminal justice system. This leverage may have helped Chris remain more adherent to treatment; it may have also allowed Chris to engage in early problem-solving and other alternatives to arrest. Overall, while Chris benefitted in some ways from traditional ACT services, he may have benefitted more from specific FACT services. Ideally, Chris would have learned about FACT while incarcerated (inreach) and would have joined the team once released from jail or another hospitalization.

12.8 Challenges and Future Directions

ACT and FACT are intensive and innovative treatment models that meet the needs of many individuals diagnosed with SMI. While ACT demonstrates good outcomes regarding housing and independent living, hospitalizations and symptom severity, quality of life and client satisfaction, subjective perceptions of recovery, and cost-effectiveness, outcomes are less clear in regard to social functioning, arrests and incarcerations, vocational functioning, substance use, and medication compliance. The advent and evolution of FACT have partially addressed this gap by showing promising results as they pertain to forensic outcomes. FACT appears to be a particularly promising evidence-based practice that implements many RNR principles. A common denominator of success for both ACT and FACT programs appears to be a high implementation fidelity to the ACT model.

Several challenges lie ahead for both ACT and FACT programs. First, ACT is traditionally and historically known as a client-centered model, yet some implementations run the risk of being too paternalistic. Although many clients report liking the ACT model and appear to be satisfied with the program, those who oversee the implementation of ACT programs should be mindful of the risk of paternalism in ACT services and should evaluate fidelity using the TMACT if possible. FACT programs may be even more vulnerable to this risk, given their close connection to criminal justice agencies and the aforementioned issues related to dual agency and legal leverage, and it is unclear whether FACT programs have been able to demonstrate fidelity to TMACT principles. More research is needed to better understand FACT clients' perceptions of coercion. In Lamberti et al. (2017) recent RCT, a measure of perceived autonomy related to taking antipsychotic medications was used, but this showed no significant relationship to outcomes. Overall, FACT clients reported above-average autonomy related to medication use in this study. Future studies (on ACT and FACT) may employ additional measures related to working alliance with staff, perceived coercion experienced at entering treatment, and perceived procedural justice. ACT and FACT staff may also be surveyed in regard to balancing different roles and treatment principles, and how staff burnout and turnover may impact teams and services provided.

Second, diversity issues must also be taken into account in future research and implementations of ACT and FACT. FACT is particularly understudied and largely limited to a few North American and some European samples. Moreover, while ACT has been well-studied among North American and some European samples, few studies have examined its effectiveness with underserved and diverse groups (e.g., recent immigrants, refugees, individuals from racial and ethnic minority groups, and individuals with cultural or language barriers). Such individuals not only have the stigma of a severe mental illness but also additional stigmas and stressors related to acculturation, language difficulties, lack of family support (or family members living in the same country), financial disadvantages, and lack of access to services (Yang et al., 2005). Yang et al. (2005) described one best practice approach for ACT clients from ethnic minority groups (primarily East and South Asian clients), based on the work of an ACT team in Toronto, Canada. This team included an acculturation assessment, culturally meaningful group activities and links to local community agencies, and psychoeducational multifamily groups (see also Chow et al., 2010, for more research on such groups). All staff were also bilingual, and cultural matches between staff and clients were also attempted. Using this culturally adapted model, Yang et al. (2005) found significant reductions in hospitalizations, improvements in psychiatric symptoms, and a high satisfaction rate (91%).

Diversity issues are particularly salient in forensic settings, given the mass incarceration of ethnic minority individuals worldwide. In fact, nearly three-quarters of the sample in a recent FACT RCT were African-American (Lamberti et al., 2017). Further, in their review of FACT, Lamberti and Weisman (2010) highlighted the importance of recognizing cultural and language barriers to engage and treat clients and attempting to match staff members' cultural expertise and clients' needs whenever possible. An additional consideration in forensic settings is the threat of internalized stigma from various sources, which can further impede treatment. For instance, ACT and FACT clients may internalize stigma about mental illness (e.g., inability to recover, dangerousness) into their own identity, which is known to predict poor treatment outcomes. The self-stigma process may be even more pernicious for clients contending with "double" or "triple" stigmas (e.g., mental illness, race/ethnicity, and/or criminal offense history; see West, Yanos, & Mulay, 2014). Treatment needs related to various other intersectionalities, such as gender and sexuality (e.g., transgender or gender-nonconforming individuals and the larger LGBTQ community), should also be considered in future ACT and FACT adaptations.

Lastly, several challenges lie ahead specifically for FACT implementation and operation. Lamberti and Weisman (2010, p. 16) highlight some of these common challenges, including establishing admission and discharge criteria with key stakeholders and referral sources (see Landess & Holoyda, 2017, for perspective on how FACT can be a diversion program for mental health courts); addressing incomplete staffing and the need for specialty training; identifying and managing communication and collaboration barriers between clinical teams and criminal justice partners; managing staff issues, including safety, burnout, and turnover; obtaining residential services and developing partnerships with local residential service providers; obtaining primary care services and developing partnerships with local primary care clinics; achieving continuity of care and developing intermediate step-down services; and managing dual agency role confusion. Sustainability also can be a problem for FACT programs, which are often dependent on grants and temporary contracts (Lamberti et al., 2004). More broadly, the core components of FACT need to be refined, including how best to adapt the RNR model to individuals diagnosed with SMI (see Lamberti, 2016; Skeem et al., 2015). Future FACT studies can also shed light on various outcomes, ranging from recidivism to subjective perceptions of recovery, in addition to cost-effectiveness.

References

Andrews, D. A., & Bonta, J. (2010). *The psychology of criminal conduct*. London, UK: Routledge.

Anthony, W. A. (1993). Recovery from mental illness: The guiding vision of the mental health service system in the 1990s. *Psychosocial Rehabilitation Journal, 16*(4), 11–23. https://doi.org/10.1037/h0095655

Baillargeon, J., Hoge, S. K., & Penn, J. V. (2010). Addressing the challenge of community reentry among released inmates with serious mental illness. *American Journal of Community Psychology, 46*(3–4), 361–375. https://doi.org/10.1007/s10464-010-9345-6

Beach, C., Dykema, L.-R., Appelbaum, P. S., Deng, L., Leckman-Westin, E., Manuel, J. I., … Finnerty, M. T. (2013). Forensic and nonforensic clients in assertive community treatment: A longitudinal study. *Psychiatric Services, 64*(5), 437–444. https://doi.org/10.1176/appi.ps.201200170

Bond, G. R., Drake, R. E., Mueser, K. T., & Latimer, E. (2001). Assertive community treatment for people with severe mental illness. *Disease Management and Health Outcomes, 9*(3), 141–159. https://doi.org/10.2165/00115677-200109030-00003

Bond, G. R., McGrew, J. H., & Fekete, D. M. (1995). Assertive outreach for frequent users of psychiatric hospitals: A meta-analysis. *The Journal of Mental Health Administration, 22*(1), 4–16. https://doi.org/10.1007/BF02519193

Bonta, J., Law, M., & Hanson, K. (1998). The prediction of criminal and violent recidivism among mentally disordered offenders: A meta-analysis. *Psychological Bulletin, 123*(2), 123–142. https://doi.org/10.1037/0033-2909.123.2.123

Burns, B. J. (2001). A critique of the effectiveness of assertive community treatment. *Psychiatric Services, 52*(10), 1394–a–1395. https://doi.org/10.1176/appi.ps.52.10.1394-a

Castellano, U. (2011). Courting compliance: Case managers as "double agents" in the mental health court. *Law & Social Inquiry, 36*(2), 484–514. https://doi.org/10.1111/j.1747-4469.2011.01239.x

Chow, W., Law, S., Andermann, L., Yang, J., Leszcz, M., Wong, J., & Sadavoy, J. (2010). Multi-family psycho-education group for assertive community treatment clients and families of culturally diverse background: A pilot study. *Community Mental Health Journal, 46*(4), 364–371. https://doi.org/10.1007/s10597-010-9305-5

Coldwell, C. M., & Bender, W. S. (2007). The effectiveness of assertive community treatment for homeless populations with severe mental illness: A meta-analysis. *American Journal of Psychiatry, 164*(3), 393–399. https://doi.org/10.1176/ajp.2007.164.3.393

Cusack, K. J., Morrissey, J. P., Cuddeback, G. S., Prins, A., & Williams, D. M. (2010). Criminal justice involvement, behavioral health service use, and costs of forensic assertive community treatment: A randomized trial. *Community Mental Health Journal, 46*(4), 356–363. https://doi.org/10.1007/s10597-010-9299-z

De Vet, R., Van Luijtelaar, M. J. A., Brilleslijper-Kater, S. N., Vanderplasschen, W., Beijersbergen, M. D., & Wolf, J. R. L. M. (2013). Effectiveness of case management for homeless persons: A systematic review. *American Journal of Public Health, 103*(10), E13–E26. https://doi.org/10.2105/AJPH.2013.301491

DeLuca, N. L., Moser, L. N., & Bond, G. R. (2008). Assertive community treatment. In K. T. Mueser & D. V. Jeste (Eds.), *Clinical handbook of schizophrenia* (pp. 329–338). New York, NY: The Guilford Press.

Dieterich, M., Irving, C. B., Park, B., & Marshall, M. (2010). Intensive case management for severe mental illness. *Cochrane Database of Systematic Reviews, 2010*(10), CD007906. https://doi.org/10.1002/14651858.CD007906.pub2

Drake, R. E. (1998). Brief history, current status, and future place of assertive community treatment. *American Journal of Orthopsychiatry, 68*(2), 172–175. https://doi.org/10.1037/h0085086

Essock, S. M., Mueser, K. T., Drake, R. E., Covell, N. H., McHugo, G. J., Frisman, L. K., … Swain, K. (2006). Comparison of ACT and standard case management for delivering integrated treatment for co-occurring disorders. *Psychiatric Services, 57*(2), 185–196. https://doi.org/10.1176/appi.ps.57.2.185

Estroff, S. E. (1981). *Making it crazy: An ethnography of psychiatric clients in an American community*. Berkeley, CA: University of California Press.

Fisher, W. H., Silver, E., & Wolff, N. (2006). Beyond criminalization: Toward a criminologically informed framework for mental health policy and services research. *Administration and Policy in Mental Health and Mental Health Services Research, 33*(5), 544–557. https://doi.org/10.1007/s10488-006-0072-0

Fontanarosa, J., Uhl, S., Oyesanmi, O., & Schoelles, K. M. (2013). *Interventions for adult offenders with serious mental illness: Executive summary, Comparative Effectiveness Review, 121*. Rockville, MD: Agency for Healthcare Research and Quality. Retrieved from https://www.ncbi.nlm.nih.gov/books/NBK158915/

Fries, H. P., & Rosen, M. I. (2011). The efficacy of assertive community treatment to treat substance use. *Journal of the American Psychiatric Nurses Association, 17*(1), 45–50. https://doi.org/10.1177/1078390310393509

Gold Award: A Community Treatment Program. (2000). *Psychiatric Services, 51*(6), 755–758. https://doi.org/10.1176/appi.ps.51.6.755

Gold, P. B., Meisler, N., Santos, A. B., Keleher, J., Becker, D. B., Knoedler, W. H., … Stormer, G. (2003). The program of assertive community treatment: Implementation and dissemination of an evidence-based model of community-based care for persons with severe and persistent mental illness. *Cognitive and Behavioral Practice, 10*(4), 290–303. https://doi.org/10.1016/S1077-7229(03)80047-0

Gomory, T. (2002). The origins of coercion in assertive community treatment: A review of early publications from the special treatment unit of Mendota state hospital. *Ethical Human Sciences and Services, 4*(1), 3–16. https://doi.org/10.1891/1523-150X.4.1.3

James, D. J., & Glaze, L. E. (2006). *Mental health problems of prison and jail inmates*. Washington, DC: U.S. Department of Justice, Office of Justice Programs. Retrieved from https://www.bjs.gov/index.cfm?iid=789&ty=pbdetail

Kearney, M. S., Harris, B. J., Jacome, E., & Parker, L. (2014). *Ten economic facts about crime and incarceration in the United States*. Washington, DC: The Hamilton Project. Retrieved from http://www.hamiltonproject.org/papers/ten_economic_facts_about_crime_and_incarceration_in_the_united_states

Kelly, B. L., Barrenger, S. L., Watson, A. C., & Angell, B. (2017). Forensic assertive community treatment: Recidivism, hospitalization, and the role of housing and support. *Social Work in Mental Health, 15*(5), 567–587. https://doi.org/10.1080/15332985.2016.1261754

Kessler, R. C., Chiu, W. C., Demler, O., & Walters, E. E. (2005). Prevalence, severity, and comorbidity of 12-month DSM-IV disorders in the National Comorbidity Survey Replication. *Archives of General Psychiatry, 62*(6), 617–627. https://doi.org/10.1001/archpsyc.62.6.617

Kidd, S. A., George, L., O'Connell, M., Sylvestre, J., Kirkpatrick, H., Browne, G., & Thabane, L. (2010). Fidelity and recovery-orientation in assertive community treatment. *Community Mental Health Journal, 46*(4), 342–350. https://doi.org/10.1007/s10597-009-9275-7

King, R. (2006). Intensive case management: A critical re-appraisal of the scientific evidence for effectiveness. *Administration and Policy in Mental Health and Mental Health Services Research, 33*(5), 529–535. https://doi.org/10.1007/s10488-006-0051-5

Kreyenbuhl, J., Buchanan, R. W., Dickerson, F. B., & Dixon, L. B. (2009). The schizophrenia patient outcomes research team (PORT): Updated treatment recommendations 2009. *Schizophrenia Bulletin, 36*(1), 94–103. https://doi.org/10.1093/schbul/sbp130

Lamb, H. R., Weinberger, L. E., & Gross, B. H. (2004). Mentally ill persons in the criminal justice system: Some perspectives. *Psychiatric Quarterly, 75*(2), 107–126. https://doi.org/10.1023/B:PSAQ.0000019753.63627.2c

Lamberti, J. S. (2016). Preventing criminal recidivism through mental health and criminal justice collaboration. *Psychiatric Services, 67*(11), 1206–1212. https://doi.org/10.1176/appi.ps.201500384

Lamberti, J. S., Deem, A., Weisman, R. L., & LaDuke, C. (2011). The role of probation in forensic assertive community treatment. *Psychiatric Services, 62*(4), 418–421. https://doi.org/10.1176/ps.62.4.pss6204_0418

Lamberti, J. S., Russ, A., Cerulli, C., Weisman, R. L., Jacobowitz, D., & Williams, G. C. (2014). Patient experiences of autonomy and coercion while receiving legal leverage in forensic assertive community treatment. *Harvard Review of Psychiatry, 22*(4), 222–230. https://doi.org/10.1097/01.HRP.0000450448.48563.c1

Lamberti, J. S., Weisman, R., & Faden, D. I. (2004). Forensic assertive community treatment: Preventing incarceration of adults with severe mental illness. *Psychiatric Services, 55*(11), 1285–1293. https://doi.org/10.1176/appi.ps.55.11.1285

Lamberti, J. S., & Weisman, R. L. (2010). Forensic assertive community treatment: Origins, current practice and future directions. In H. A. Dlugacz (Ed.), *Reentry planning for offenders with mental disorders: Policy and practice* (pp. 7-1–7-27). Kingston, NJ: Civic Research Institute.

Lamberti, J. S., Weisman, R. L., Cerulli, C., Williams, G. C., Jacobowitz, D. B., Mueser, K. T., ... Caine, E. D. (2017). A randomized controlled trial of the Rochester forensic assertive community treatment model. *Psychiatric Services, 68*(10), 1016–1024. https://doi.org/10.1176/appi.ps.201600329

Landess, J., & Holoyda, B. (2017). Mental health courts and forensic assertive community treatment teams as correctional diversion programs. *Behavioral Sciences and the Law, 35*(5–6), 501–511. https://doi.org/10.1002/bsl.2307

Latimer, E. A. (1999). Economic impacts of assertive community treatment: A review of the literature. *The Canadian Journal of Psychiatry, 44*(5), 443–454. https://doi.org/10.1177/070674379904400504

Levine, M., Toro, P. A., & Perkins, D. V. (1993). Social and community interventions. *Annual Review of Psychology, 44*(1), 525–558. https://doi.org/10.1146/annurev.ps.44.020193.002521

Manuel, J. I., Appelbaum, P. S., Le Melle, S. M., Mancini, A. D., Huz, S., Stellato, C. B., & Finnerty, M. T. (2013). Use of intervention strategies by assertive community treatment teams to promote patients' engagement. *Psychiatric Services, 64*(6), 579–585. https://doi.org/10.1176/appi.ps.201200151

Marquant, T., Sabbe, B., Van Nuffel, M., & Goethals, K. (2016). Forensic assertive community treatment: A review of the literature. *Community Mental Health Journal, 52*(8), 873–881. https://doi.org/10.1007/s10597-016-0044-0

Marquant, T., Sabbe, B., Van Nuffel, M., Verelst, R., & Goethals, K. (2018). Forensic assertive community treatment in a continuum of care for male internees in Belgium: Results after 33 months. *Community Mental Health Journal, 54*(1), 58–65. https://doi.org/10.1007/s10597-017-0153-4

Marshall, W. L., & Marshall, L. E. (2015). Psychological treatment of the paraphilias: A review and an appraisal of effectiveness. *Current Psychiatry Reports, 17*(6), 47. https://doi.org/10.1007/s11920-015-0580-2

McCrone, P., Killaspy, H., Bebbington, P., Johnson, S., Nolan, F., Pilling, S., & King, M. (2009). The REACT study: Cost-effectiveness analysis of assertive community treatment in north London. *Psychiatric Services, 60*(7), 908–913. https://doi.org/10.1176/ps.2009.60.7.908

McGrew, J. H., Wilson, R. G., & Bond, G. R. (1996). Client perspectives on helpful ingredients of assertive community treatment. *Psychiatric Rehabilitation Journal, 19*(3), 13–21. https://doi.org/10.1037/h0101291

McGrew, J. H., Wilson, R. G., & Bond, G. R. (2002). An exploratory study of what clients like least about assertive community treatment. *Psychiatric Services, 53*(6), 761–763. https://doi.org/10.1176/appi.ps.53.6.761

Messina, N., Burdon, W., Hagopian, G., & Prendergast, M. (2004). One year return to custody rates among co-disordered offenders. *Behavioral Sciences & the Law, 22*(4), 503–518. https://doi.org/10.1002/bsl.600

Monroe-DeVita, M., Teague, G. B., & Moser, L. L. (2011). The TMACT: A new tool for measuring fidelity to assertive community treatment. *Journal of the American Psychiatric Nurses Association, 17*(1), 17–29. https://doi.org/10.1177/1078390310394658

Morrissey, J. P. (2013). *Forensic assertive community treatment: Updating the evidence*. Rockville, MD: SAMHSA's GAINS Center for Behavioral Health and Justice Transformation. Retrieved from https://www.ncjrs.gov/App/Publications/abstract.aspx?ID=269465

Mueser, K. T., Bond, G. R., Drake, R. E., & Resnick, S. G. (1998). Models of community care for severe mental illness: A review of research on case management. *Schizophrenia Bulletin, 24*(1), 37–74. https://doi.org/10.1093/oxfordjournals.schbul.a033314

Nelson, G., Aubry, T., & Lafrance, A. (2007). A review of the literature on the effectiveness of housing and support, assertive community treatment, and intensive case management interventions for persons with mental illness who have been homeless. *American Journal of Orthopsychiatry, 77*(3), 350–361. https://doi.org/10.1037/0002-9432.77.3.350

O'Connell, M., Tondora, J., Croog, G., Evans, A., & Davidson, L. (2005). From rhetoric to routine: Assessing perceptions of recovery-oriented practices in a state mental health and addiction system. *Psychiatric Rehabilitation Journal, 28*(4), 378–386. https://doi.org/10.2975/28.2005.378.386

Peterson, J., Skeem, J., Kennealy, P., Bray, B., & Zvonkovic, A. (2014). How often and how consistently do symptoms directly precede criminal behavior among offenders with mental illness? *Law and Human Behavior, 38*(5), 439–449. https://doi.org/10.1037/lhb0000075

Prins, S. J. (2014). Prevalence of mental illnesses in U.S. state prisons: A systematic review. *Psychiatric Services, 65*(7), 862–872. https://doi.org/10.1176/appi.ps.201300166

Salyers, M. P., & Tsemberis, S. (2007). ACT and recovery: Integrating evidence-based practice and recovery orientation on assertive community treatment teams. *Community Mental Health Journal, 43*(6), 619–641. https://doi.org/10.1007/s10597-007-9088-5

Skeem, J. L., Steadman, H. J., & Manchak, S. M. (2015). Applicability of the risk-need responsivity model to persons with mental illness involved in the criminal justice system. *Psychiatric Services, 66*(9), 916–922. https://doi.org/10.1176/appi.ps.201400448

Skeem, J. L., Winter, E., Kennealy, P. J., Louden, J. E., & Tatar, J. R. I. I. (2014). Offenders with mental illness have criminogenic needs, too: Toward recidivism reduction. *Law and Human Behavior, 38*(3), 212–224. https://doi.org/10.1037/lhb0000054

Solomon, P., Draine, J., & Marcus, S. C. (2002). Predicting incarceration of clients of a psychiatric probation and parole service. *Psychiatric Services, 53*(1), 50–56. https://doi.org/10.1176/appi.ps.53.1.50

Steadman, H. J., Osher, F. C., Clark Robbins, P., Case, B., & Samuels, S. (2009). Prevalence of serious mental illness among jail inmates. *Psychiatric Services, 60*(6), 761–765. https://doi.org/10.1176/ps.2009.60.6.761

Stein, L. I., & Test, M. A. (1985). The evolution of the training in community living model. *New Directions for Mental Health Services, 1985*(26), 7–16. https://doi.org/10.1002/yd.23319852603

Substance Abuse and Mental Health Services Administration. (2010). *Mental health, United States, 2008. HHS publication no. (SMA) 10–4590*. Rockville, MD: Center for Mental Health Services, Substance Abuse and Mental Health Services Administration. Retrieved from https://www.samhsa.gov/

Swartz, M. S., & Swanson, J. W. (2004). Involuntary outpatient commitment, community treatment orders, and assisted outpatient treatment: What's in the data? *The Canadian Journal of Psychiatry, 49*(9), 585–591. https://doi.org/10.1177/070674370404900903

Talbott, J. A. (2004). Deinstitutionalization: Avoiding the disasters of the past. *Psychiatric Services, 55*(10), 1112–1115. https://doi.org/10.1176/appi.ps.55.10.1112

Teague, G. B., Bond, G. R., & Drake, R. E. (1998). Program fidelity in assertive community treatment: Development and use of a measure. *American Journal of Orthopsychiatry, 68*(2), 216–232. https://doi.org/10.1037/h0080331

Thompson, K. S., Griffith, E. E. H., & Leaf, P. J. (1990). A historical review of the Madison model of community care. *Psychiatric Services, 41*(6), 625–634. https://doi.org/10.1176/ps.41.6.625

Torrey, E. F. (2012). *The insanity defense: How America's failure to treat the seriously mentally ill endangers its citizens*. New York, NY: W. W. Norton & Company.

Tsemberis, S., Gulcur, L., & Nakae, M. (2004). Housing first, consumer choice, and harm reduction for homeless individuals with a dual diagnosis. *American Journal of Public Health, 94*(4), 651–656. https://doi.org/10.2105/AJPH.94.4.651

West, M. L., Yanos, P. T., & Mulay, A. L. (2014). Triple stigma of forensic psychiatric patients: Mental illness, race, and criminal history. *International Journal of Forensic Mental Health, 13*(1), 75–90. https://doi.org/10.1080/14999013.2014.885471

Yang, J., Law, S., Chow, W., Andermann, L., Steinberg, R., & Sadavoy, J. (2005). Best practices: Assertive community treatment for persons with severe and persistent mental illness in ethnic minority groups. *Psychiatric Services, 56*(9), 1053–1055. https://doi.org/10.1176/appi.ps.56.9.1053

Yanos, P. T., Knight, E. L., Vayshenker, B., Gonzales, L., & DeLuca, J. S. (2017). Community protection versus individual healing: Two traditions in community mental health. *Behavioral Sciences & the Law, 35*(4), 288–302. https://doi.org/10.1002/bsl.2297

Ziguras, S. J., & Stuart, G. W. (2000). A meta-analysis of the effectiveness of mental health case management over 20 years. *Psychiatric Services, 51*(11), 1410–1421. https://doi.org/10.1176/appi.ps.51.11.1410

Chapter 13
Multisystemic Therapy for Serious Juvenile Offenders: From Development to Dissemination

Charles M. Borduin, Cynthia E. Brown, and Kaitlin M. Sheerin

13.1 Introduction

Violent criminal acts and other serious crimes committed by youths present significant problems at several levels of analysis, and these problems argue for the development of effective treatment approaches. On a personal level, youths who commit serious crimes experience numerous psychosocial problems as well as reduced educational and occupational opportunities (Lyons, Baerger, Quigley, Erlich, & Griffin, 2001; Odgers et al., 2008). Moreover, serious criminal activity perpetrated by youths has extremely detrimental emotional, physical, and economic consequences for victims, their families, and society at large (Britt, 2001; Kilpatrick & Acierno, 2003; Miller, Fisher, & Cohen, 2001; Robinson & Keithley, 2000). Therefore, effective treatment may not only benefit the youth and his or her family but may also save many persons from victimization.

On an epidemiological level, youths under the age of 18 account for nearly 12% of all index offenses in the United States, including 19% of robberies and 16% of rapes (Federal Bureau of Investigation, 2016), and such offenses greatly underestimate the actual prevalence of youth criminal activity (Farrington et al., 2003). In addition, even though only about 25% of youths arrested for delinquent acts could be characterized as serious offenders, serious juvenile offenders account for nearly half of the total volume of youth crime in a community (Farrington et al., 2003; Loeber & Farrington, 2012). Thus, if one purpose of treating juvenile offenders is to decrease crime, then serious juvenile offenders are a logical target for treatment.

On a social service level, serious juvenile offenders consume a disproportionate amount of resources across multiple service systems (e.g., child mental health, juvenile justice, special education) and are overrepresented in the most intensive

C. M. Borduin (✉) · C. E. Brown · K. M. Sheerin
Department of Psychological Sciences, University of Missouri, Columbia, MO, USA
e-mail: borduinc@missouri.edu; cebm9c@mail.missouri.edu; ksgfd@mail.missouri.edu

E. L. Jeglic, C. Calkins (eds.), *New Frontiers in Offender Treatment*,
https://doi.org/10.1007/978-3-030-01030-0_13

(i.e., "deep end") interventions provided by these systems (Shufelt & Cocozza, 2006). Moreover, serious criminal behavior committed by juveniles has other financial consequences for society, including costs pertaining to law enforcement, the maintenance and expansion of the correctional system, and victimization (McCollister, French, & Fang, 2010; Miller et al., 2001). In addition, youths who engage in serious criminal behaviors often continue to require mental health and criminal justice interventions well into adulthood (Farrington, Ttofi, & Coid, 2009; Odgers et al., 2008). Therefore, the development of effective treatments for serious juvenile offending may help to free resources to address other important problems of children and their families.

Unfortunately, as numerous reviewers have concluded (e.g., Howell, 2009; McCart & Sheidow, 2016), the development and dissemination of effective interventions for criminality in youths have been challenging. Indeed, until the 1990s, the conclusion that "nothing works" (e.g., Lipton, Martinson, & Wilks, 1975) in treating the behavior of serious juvenile offenders was generally accurate. In fact, it is still the case that most (approximately 95%) of serious juvenile offenders do not receive evidence-based interventions (Greenwood, 2008; Henggeler & Schoenwald, 2011). Moreover, a number of juvenile justice interventions (e.g., shock incarceration, residential placement) that are intended to reduce the criminal activity of offenders have had the unintended consequence of increasing youth antisocial behavior (see Drake, Aos, & Miller, 2009; Howell, 2009, for reviews). Furthermore, the most common interventions (e.g., individual therapy, residential treatment) do not address well-established risk factors for serious juvenile offending (e.g., poor parenting skills, involvement with antisocial peers) and are delivered in settings (e.g., training school, group home) that bear little relation to the problems being addressed. It seems clear that there is a pressing need for effective alternatives to the narrowly focused and restrictive practices that currently dominate mental health interventions for serious juvenile offenders.

Multisystemic therapy (MST; Henggeler & Borduin, 1990; Henggeler, Schoenwald, Borduin, Rowland, & Cunningham, 2009) is an intensive family- and community-based treatment that has demonstrated significant effects on the serious and violent criminal activities of juvenile offenders. MST was originally developed in the late 1970s to address major limitations of existing mental health services for serious juvenile offenders (see Henggeler & Schoenwald, 2011) and is now viewed as an effective treatment for criminality in youths (e.g., Blueprints for Healthy Youth Development, 2018; Dopp, Borduin, White, & Kuppens, 2017; McCart & Sheidow, 2016). Indeed, McCart and Sheidow (2016) concluded that MST was one of only two treatment models that met the most rigorous criteria of research support (i.e., "well-established") for juvenile offenders. The present chapter will describe how MST interventions address serious and violent criminal behaviors in juvenile offenders. More specifically, we provide a discussion of the theoretical, empirical, and clinical foundations of MST; a review of findings from controlled evaluations that demonstrate the clinical and economic benefits of MST; and a description of ongoing efforts to disseminate MST into community settings.

13.2 Theoretical Foundations

Family systems theory (Bateson, 1972; Hoffman, 1981; Minuchin, 1985) and the theory of social ecology (Bronfenbrenner, 1979) are consistent with research findings on the correlates and causes of criminality in youths and serve as a basis for case conceptualization and treatment planning in MST. Family systems theory views the family as a rule-governed system that possesses qualities beyond the characteristics of individual family members. Although there are differences in how various approaches to family therapy interpret systems theory, most attempt to understand how symptoms and problem behaviors "fit" within the context of an individual's family relations and emphasize the reciprocal and circular nature of such relations. In the context of youth criminality, a family systems therapist might consider how caregiver discipline strategies influence youth violent behaviors, how the violent behaviors of the youth shape and guide the behaviors of the caregiver, and what function each of these behaviors serve in the family's daily functioning, all within a unified conceptual framework.

The theory of social ecology (Bronfenbrenner, 1979) shares some of the basic concepts of family systems theory but encompasses broader and more numerous contextual influences on a youth's functioning. The individual youth is seen as being nested within a complex of interconnected systems that include the youth's family, peers, school, neighborhood, and community (see Fig. 13.1). The youth's behavior is viewed as being largely determined by the interactions between the youth and these systems as well as by the reciprocal interplay between the systems (e.g., contacts between caregivers and school personnel). It is assumed, then, that youth antisocial behaviors can be maintained by problematic transactions between the youth and a given system or between various combinations of pertinent systems. The theory of social ecology also emphasizes the importance of "ecological validity" in understanding human behavior, that is, the assumption that behavior should be considered within its naturally occurring contexts.

The MST theory of change (see Fig. 13.2) makes two assumptions that are consistent with family systems theory and the theory of social ecology (Henggeler, Schoenwald, et al., 2009). First, the MST theory of change assumes that youth criminality is driven by the interactions of risk factors at various levels of the youth's social ecology (e.g., individual, family, peer, school, and neighborhood). Thus, effective interventions have the capacity to address a comprehensive and individualized (i.e., specific to a particular youth and family) set of risk factors while simultaneously promoting protective factors. Second, the MST theory of change assumes that caregivers are the most proximal influence on reductions in youth antisocial behavior and improvements in youth functioning. Consequently, MST interventions focus on empowering caregivers with the resources and skills necessary for effective parenting (e.g., ability to guide and nurture the youth). The MST therapist collaborates with the caregivers, using family strengths (e.g., supportive caregiver-youth relations, positive and age-appropriate goals for the youth) to overcome barriers to caregiver effectiveness (e.g., high levels of family

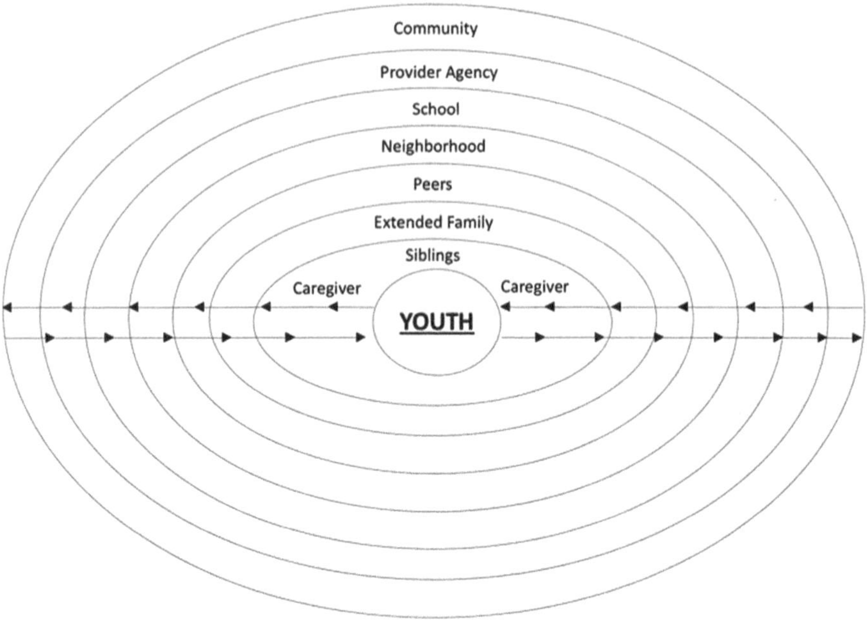

Fig 13.1 Social-ecological environment. The youth and family are embedded in multiple systems with dynamic and reciprocal influences (represented by arrows) on the behavior of family members. Youth offending can be maintained by problematic transactions within and/or between any one or combination of these systems

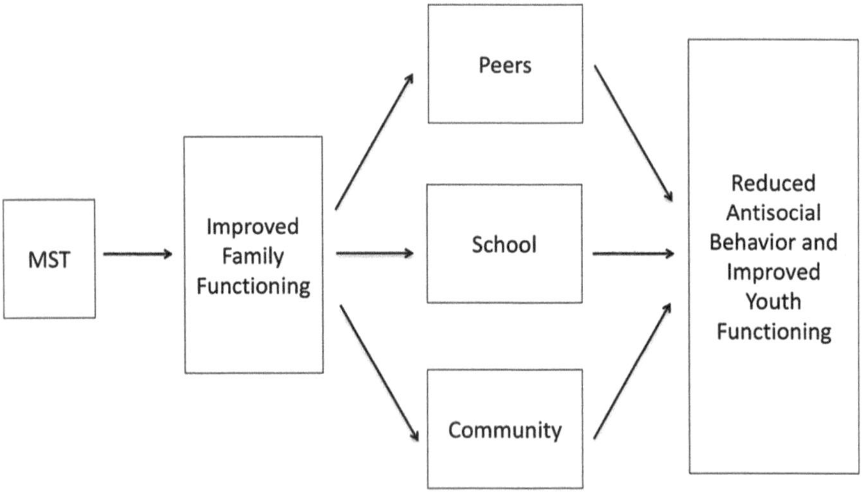

Fig 13.2 The multisystemic therapy (MST) theory of change

disorganization, caregiver substance abuse or mental health difficulties). As parenting skills improve, the therapist and caregivers collaborate to create strategies to, for example, disengage their teenager from deviant peers and enhance school performance. Therefore, a well-functioning family unit is viewed as critical to achieving and sustaining decreased youth criminality and improved youth functioning across multiple contexts. In summary, the MST theory of change emphasizes the importance of creating an endogenous social network for the youth's family that supports prosocial behavior (e.g., involved and effective caregivers, prosocial friends, supportive school figures, social support for caregivers) rather than antisocial behavior.

13.3 Empirical Foundations

Numerous studies have identified correlates of violence and other serious antisocial behaviors in youths. In general, these correlates are characteristics of the individual youth and of the social-ecological systems (family, peers, school, neighborhood) in which the youth is embedded (for reviews, see Loeber, Burke, & Pardini, 2009; Voisin, Hong, & King, 2012). Moreover, many research groups have developed multidimensional causal models of serious antisocial behaviors in youths. Specifically, these researchers have used path analysis or structural equation modeling to examine the interrelations among the various social-ecological correlates of youths' serious and violent antisocial behavior. The results of such studies have provided valuable information about the direct and indirect effects of different variables on serious antisocial behavior while controlling for confounds between correlates. Findings across studies (e.g., Loeber et al., 2009; Monahan, Steinberg, & Cauffman, 2009; Witkiewitz et al., 2013) are relatively clear and consistent:

1. Involvement with deviant peers is virtually always a powerful direct predictor of violence and other antisocial behaviors.
2. Family relations predict serious antisocial behaviors either directly (i.e., contributing unique variance) or indirectly by predicting involvement with deviant peers.
3. School difficulties predict involvement with deviant peers.
4. Neighborhood and community support characteristics add small portions of unique variance or indirectly predict serious antisocial behaviors by, for example, affecting family, peer, or school behavior.

Thus, across studies that varied substantially in measurement strategies and analytic methods, investigators have shown that youths' serious antisocial behaviors are linked directly or indirectly with key characteristics of youths and their social systems.

Based on the above findings, treatments that aim to decrease rates of youth violence and other serious antisocial behaviors should have the capacity to intervene comprehensively at individual, family, peer, school, and possibly even neighborhood levels. Indeed, there is a growing consensus among reviewers that the major limitation of most treatments for serious antisocial behavior is their failure to account for the multidetermined nature of such behavior and that effective treatments must have the ability to flexibly address multidimensional risk factors (Dopp, Borduin, Rothman, & Letourneau, 2017; Henggeler & Schoenwald, 2011; Howell, 2009; Loeber et al., 2009; McCart & Sheidow, 2016). An essential feature of MST is its capacity to address the multiple determinants of youths' serious antisocial behavior in an intensive, comprehensive, and individualized fashion.

13.4 Clinical Foundations

MST interventions are designed to provide intensive support for families of youths with serious antisocial behaviors. Caregivers and other family members are directly involved in therapy and are viewed as valuable resources, even when they have significant and multiple needs (e.g., mental health problems, resistance to treatment). In addition, MST therapists maximize the ecological validity of services by conducting assessments and delivering interventions for juvenile offenders in relevant social contexts, including home, school, and community settings. Delivery of interventions in these natural settings has the added benefit of decreasing barriers to service access, thereby promoting increased session attendance rates and decreased attrition compared to more traditional services (e.g., clinic-based treatment).

MST teams typically consist of two to four master's-level therapists, each with caseloads of four to six families, and a half-time supervisor. The MST therapist is a generalist who directly provides the vast majority of mental health services and coordinates access to other important services (e.g., educational, recreational, financial) to youths and their families during a 3- to 5-month course of treatment. To maximize participation in MST, the therapist schedules treatment sessions at times convenient to the family (e.g., evenings and weekends), with crisis management services available 24 hours a day, 7 days a week. Nevertheless, therapeutic intensity is titrated to clinical need, such that therapists spend more time with families in the initial weeks of therapy (daily, if needed) and gradually taper off as youth and family functioning improves (as infrequently as once a week).

MST is generally used with complex cases that present a variety of clinical needs and strengths, and thus it would not be possible to specify the content of each session or the sequence in which interventions should be delivered. Rather, the MST model includes nine treatment principles that guide therapists' case conceptualizations, prioritization and development of interventions, and implementation of intervention strategies. Briefly, these principles state that multisystemic interventions (1) are based on the fit between identified problems and their broader systemic context; (2) emphasize and leverage family strengths; (3) promote responsible behavior and decrease irresponsible behavior among family members; (4) are present-focused, action-oriented, and problem-specific; (5) target sequences of behavior within and between the multiple systems that maintain problems; (6) are consistent with the developmental needs of the youth; (7) require continuous (i.e., daily or weekly) effort by the youth and family; (8) are evaluated continuously for effectiveness, with providers assuming primary responsibility for intervention success; and (9) promote generalization and long-term maintenance of treatment gains by empowering caregivers to address family members' needs. The MST treatment principles are explained in greater detail in a clinical volume (Henggeler & Borduin, 1990) and a treatment manual (Henggeler, Schoenwald, et al., 2009). As described in more detail later in this chapter, MST teams employ a number of dissemination and quality assurance strategies to promote therapist adherence to the treatment principles.

13.5 Clinical and Economic Benefits

The evaluation of MST outcomes with serious and violent offenders and their families has been a priority since the development of this treatment model four decades ago (see Henggeler & Schoenwald, 2011; Henggeler, Schoenwald, et al., 2009, for reviews). The results of more than a dozen clinical trials demonstrate that MST can produce clinical and economic benefits with two populations of youths that exhibit serious antisocial behaviors: (1) violent and chronic juvenile offenders and (2) juvenile sexual offenders.

13.5.1 MST with Violent and Chronic Juvenile Offenders

The findings of MST efficacy and effectiveness trials have been aggregated in several meta-analytic studies and have consistently demonstrated long-lasting positive outcomes with violent and chronic juvenile offenders (i.e., Curtis, Ronan, & Borduin, 2004; Dopp, Borduin, White, et al., 2017; van der Stouwe, Asscher, Stams, Deković, & van der Laan, 2014). Across studies, findings have shown that:

1. Youths who participate in MST commit fewer crimes relative to youths in comparison conditions (e.g., individual therapy, family court, probation services).
2. MST yields more improvement in secondary outcomes (e.g., family functioning, peer relations) relative to comparison conditions.
3. MST has been shown to be effective for both female and male juvenile offenders of various ages and from diverse backgrounds.
4. MST can be successfully transported to different nations and cultures.

Several long-term follow-up studies have also illustrated the success of MST in reducing recidivism for both target youths and their family members. A 21.9-year follow-up (Sawyer & Borduin, 2011) of the largest randomized clinical trial of MST (N = 176; Borduin et al., 1995) revealed that youths who received MST had a significantly lower rate of recidivism for felony offenses than did youths who received individual therapy (34.8% vs. 54.8%, respectively) and that the frequency of misdemeanor offending was five times lower for MST participants. Furthermore, MST participants were half as likely to be involved in family-related civil suits (i.e., divorce, paternity, and/or child support suits). In a subsequent follow-up of siblings from the same clinical trial, Wagner, Borduin, Sawyer, and Dopp (2014) found that siblings of youths who received MST were about 30% less likely to have been arrested 25 years later than were siblings of youths who received individual therapy. In addition, siblings of youths in the MST condition were three times less likely to be convicted of a felony and two times less likely to be sentenced to probation or incarceration. More recently, Johnides, Borduin, Wagner, and Dopp (2017) found that caregivers of youths who participated in MST 20 years earlier in the Borduin et al. (1995) trial had 94% fewer felonies and 70% fewer misdemeanors than did caregivers of youths who participated in individual treatment. Caregivers in the MST condition were also sentenced to 92% fewer days of incarceration and had 50% fewer family-related civil suits.

In addition to research conducted by MST developers, several groups of independent investigators have examined the effectiveness of MST. The first of these replications (Ogden & Hagen, 2006; Ogden & Halliday-Boykins, 2004), which was conducted in Norway, found that antisocial youths who participated in MST had fewer internalizing problems, externalizing problems, and out-of-home placements up to 2 years postreferral than did youths who received usual child welfare services. In a second study conducted in the United States, Timmons-Mitchell, Bender, Kishna, and Mitchell (2006) found that MST participants had fewer rearrests at a 2-year follow-up than did participants who received usual services. More recently, a study in the United Kingdom (Butler, Baruch, Hickey, & Fonagy, 2011) found that relative to usual services, MST was associated with greater reductions in youths' behavior problems and psychopathy at posttreatment as well as a lower rate of rearrest for nonviolent crimes at an 18-month follow-up. Finally, in a clinical trial in the Netherlands, Asscher, Deković, Manders, van der Laan, and Prins (2013) found that MST was more effective than treatment-as-usual in decreasing youths' externalizing behaviors and property offenses as well as in improving parenting skills and prosocial peer relationships at posttreatment. Taken together, the results of these independent studies suggest that individuals other than the treatment developers can effectively implement MST with violent and chronic juvenile offenders.

Recent studies have also examined the economic impact of MST. Dopp, Borduin, Wagner, and Sawyer (2014) found that reductions in criminality for youths and their siblings who participated in MST 25 years earlier were linked with lasting benefits to both crime victims and taxpayers, with cumulative benefits of MST estimated at $35,582 per juvenile offender and $7,798 per sibling. Furthermore, every dollar spent on MST recovered $5.04 in savings to crime victims and taxpayers. Similarly, in a more recent study, Dopp, Coen, et al. (2017) demonstrated that implementation of MST in New Mexico over a 7-year period yielded a savings of $4,643 per youth in prevented behavioral health claims and $15,019 per youth through reductions in juvenile crime. In sum, these results indicate that MST can yield long-term economic benefits.

13.5.2 MST with Juvenile Sexual Offenders

MST for Problem Sexual Behaviors (MST-PSB; Borduin & Munschy, 2014) is an adaptation of standard MST that has been developed with juvenile sexual offenders. The MST-PSB model is guided by the same theoretical, empirical, and clinical foundations as in standard MST but focuses on aspects of the youth's social ecology that are functionally related to problem sexual behavior (e.g., caregiver and youth denial about sexual offenses), relapse prevention, and victim safety. To date, three outcome studies of MST-PSB with juvenile sexual offenders are the only randomized clinical trials that have been conducted with this challenging clinical population (see Dopp, Borduin, & Brown, 2015; Dopp, Borduin, Rothman, & Letourneau, 2017).

In the first clinical trial (Borduin, Henggeler, Blaske, & Stein, 1990) with a small sample of juvenile sexual offenders (N = 16), results from a 3-year follow-up demonstrated that MST-PSB was more effective than outpatient individual therapy in reducing rates of rearrests for sexual crimes (12.5% vs. 75.0%); the mean frequency of rearrests for sexual crimes (0.12 vs. 1.62) and nonsexual crimes (0.62 vs. 2.25) was also considerably lower for MST-PSB. These favorable effects of MST-PSB supported the viability of conducting a second, larger evaluation with juvenile sexual offenders. The second trial (Borduin, Schaeffer, & Heiblum, 2009; N = 48), which compared MST-PSB with cognitive-behavioral group and individual treatment, showed that MST-PSB participants had (a) greater reductions in behavior problems and psychiatric symptoms as well as greater improvements in family, peer, and school functioning at posttreatment; (b) lower rearrest rates for sexual (8% vs. 46%) or nonsexual (29% vs. 58%) offenses at an 8.9-year follow-up; and (c) fewer days incarcerated at follow-up. In the third trial (N = 127), Letourneau et al. (2009) demonstrated that MST-PSB produced greater reductions in deviant sexual interest/risk behaviors, delinquency, externalizing symptoms, and out-of-home placements at a 12-month follow-up than did cognitive-behavioral group therapy. More recently, Letourneau et al. (2013) found that the favorable 12-month outcomes among MST-PSB participants in the third trial were sustained through a second year of follow-up.

Consistent with the literature on standard MST, MST-PSB has also been found to be highly cost-effective. Indeed, Borduin and Dopp (2015) estimated that MST-PSB yielded a total benefit of $343,455 per participant when compared to usual community services (i.e., cognitive-behavioral group and individual treatment). Stated differently, every dollar spent on MST-PSB recovered $48.81 in savings to taxpayers and crime victims over an 8.9-year follow-up period. These cost benefits are even greater than those provided by standard MST (see Dopp et al., 2014) and further demonstrate the effectiveness of the MST-PSB model.

13.6 Dissemination and Treatment Fidelity

13.6.1 Implementation

MST programs now exist in 34 states and 14 countries outside the United States and together have served more than 200,000 families since their inception (MST Services, 2018). These programs are usually implemented by public (i.e., juvenile justice, mental health, social welfare) or private service providers. These providers contract with MST purveyor organizations (MST Services for standard MST, MST Associates for MST-PSB) to receive orientation and booster training as well as ongoing quality assurance. Prior to entering a contract with an MST purveyor organization, the service provider (including key administrators, supervisors, and therapists) must be committed to the philosophical and empirical framework of the MST approach. This includes an understanding of the role of each member of the treatment team and of the infrastructure for maintaining accountability for clinical outcomes. Indeed, the service provider should have dedicated staff for its MST program (i.e., 100%-time MST therapists) and a supervisor who has credible authority regarding clinical decisions and training in the model. Significant changes in policies and staff members' work routines are often necessary to successfully implement the clinical approach of MST, and logistical support must be evident from the administration of the service provider (e.g., scheduling supervision and consultation times, providing highly competitive salaries and incentives, enacting flex time and comp time policies for staff).

Before an MST program can begin, the MST purveyor organization must support the service provider as it evaluates the environment in which the program services will be delivered, plans for actual program implementation, and establishes written and locally defined program goals and guidelines. During the initial stages of the planning and assessment process, collaborative dialogues are initiated with key stakeholders from funding agencies, child protection agencies, local school systems, court systems, probation and parole departments, and victim advocacy and mental health agencies. Agreement among stakeholders is sought around several critical issues, including which youths can be treated safely in a community setting, what roles will be assumed by various agencies involved with the youths, and how program success will be defined and measured. The two primary purposes of coordinating MST program activities with other agencies are (a) to ensure that the program is likely to attain a sufficient referral base as well as consistent funding and (b) to integrate services that will lead to favorable clinical outcomes.

13.6.2 *Quality Assurance*

The successful transport of MST (or MST-PSB) to a community provider organization is possible only when there are specific mechanisms in place to ensure treatment fidelity. Adherence to treatment practices, parameters, and evaluation protocols is essential if a provider expects to achieve outcomes similar to those obtained in the clinical trials of the treatment model.

The MST purveyor organization employs a number of quality assurance mechanisms that increase fidelity to the treatment model. First, all MST teams participate in an ongoing, comprehensive training program, beginning with a 5-day orientation training in the general MST model (two additional days of training are provided for teams that specialize in MST-PSB). This training is followed by quarterly on-site "booster" trainings that are tailored to meet the unique needs of each team. Second, treatment fidelity is maintained by 2-hour weekly group supervision meetings involving a clinical supervisor and two to four therapists. During supervision, the treatment team (i.e., supervisor, therapists, and other consultants as needed) reviews the goals and progress of each case to ensure the multisystemic focus of therapists' intervention strategies and to identify barriers to success. Third, each treatment team participates in a weekly clinical consultation from an MST/MST-PSB expert to further ensure fidelity, skill building, and positive outcomes. Consultations typically follow group supervision meetings and build upon the quality assurance process initiated by the supervisor. Lastly, treatment fidelity is managed and monitored continuously at multiple levels. More specifically, empirically validated measures are regularly used to examine *therapist adherence* to treatment practices and principles as well as *supervisor adherence* to established program-level practices (e.g., duration of treatment, therapist caseload size). *Clinical outcomes* (e.g., percentage of youths living at home or with no new arrests at the time of therapy closure) are monitored frequently by the MST/MST-PSB expert to promote continuous quality improvement. Research has demonstrated that ongoing training, supervision, consultation, and monitoring of treatment adherence and outcomes are essential for the success of an MST team (e.g., Henggeler, Melton, Brondino, Scherer, & Hanley, 1997; Smith-Boydston, Holtzman, & Roberts, 2014).

13.7 Future Directions in Treatment with Serious Juvenile Offenders

This chapter provided an overview of MST, a family- and community-based treatment approach that directly addresses multiple risk factors for serious and violent juvenile offending. Research studies have demonstrated that MST can successfully reduce criminality in youths and that treatment gains continue well into adulthood. Of course, given the many problems that serious juvenile offenders present for their communities as well as the significant costs of providing these youths with interventions that do not produce durable changes, the continued development and refinement of effective intervention programs such as MST should be a priority for scientists and policymakers alike. Thus, we close this chapter by discussing several key research challenges and by offering pertinent recommendations.

First, understanding the mechanisms of change that underlie the MST intervention model is necessary for the continued refinement of the model and may ultimately help to improve outcomes. To date, several studies have demonstrated that the favorable effects of MST (Deković, Asscher, Manders, Prins, & van der Laan, 2012; Huey, Henggeler, Brondino, & Pickrel, 2000) and MST-PSB (Henggeler, Letourneau, et al., 2009) on youths' antisocial behavior are mediated by changes in caregivers' discipline practices and youth's association with deviant peers. Moreover, there is also evidence that the relative efficacy of MST in reducing criminality and civil suits among caregivers of serious juvenile offenders is mediated by improved caregiver-youth relations during treatment (Johnides et al., 2017). Given the consistency of results across these studies, the most important goal of future research in this area should be to identify the specific components of MST (e.g., protocols, in-session behaviors) that lead to improved caregiver competence and disengagement of youths from deviant peers.

Second, clinical trials that have evaluated treatments for youths' mental health problems, including juvenile offending and other antisocial behaviors, have typically included short (i.e., less than 1–2 years) follow-ups of participant outcomes (see Weisz et al., 2017, for a review). Therefore, our understanding of the sustainability of favorable outcomes achieved in most evidence-based treatments for youths is surprisingly limited. Although Sawyer and Borduin (2011) provided the longest (i.e., 21.9 years) follow-up to date of an evidence-based intervention (i.e., MST) for serious juvenile offenders, additional studies of long-term treatment outcomes with this population are needed. Information on the lasting benefits of empirically supported treatments could greatly assist program administrators and policymakers in selecting and implementing mental health programs for serious juvenile offenders. However, if treatment effects similar to those observed at shorter follow-ups were not sustained over a longer period of time, then such findings could suggest a need for refining treatment, such as providing posttreatment booster sessions or support services in early adulthood.

Finally, the economic costs and benefits of MST should continue to be evaluated, given that treatments that are clinically effective with serious juvenile offenders are also likely to be cost effective. Although methodologies for performing economic analyses of mental health interventions have been well defined (e.g., French, Salome, Sindelar, & McLellan, 2002; Singh, Hawthorne, & Vos, 2001), such work has clearly lagged behind tests of clinical effectiveness of these interventions. Indeed, only a handful of studies have examined the costs and benefits of intervention programs designed for juvenile offenders, and most of those studies have relatively severe methodological limitations (for a review, see Byford, McCrone, & Barrett, 2003). Nonetheless, notable exceptions (e.g., Borduin & Dopp, 2015; Dopp et al., 2014; Dopp, Coen, et al., 2017) have demonstrated that both MST and MST-PSB produce substantial and lasting (i.e., across decades) cost savings to taxpayers and crime victims. Although encouraging, these findings were based on estimates of treatment costs and benefits from only a few provider sites and should be replicated by other service providers. Furthermore, future studies should expand the scope of costs and benefits beyond the criminal justice system to explore the possibility of cost shifting to other service sectors (e.g., primary care, mental health) and of additional benefits (e.g., income tax revenue resulting from increased employment, reduced use of social welfare services) during treatment or follow-up.

In conclusion, a growing body of research indicates that MST can successfully reduce serious and violent offending in juvenile offenders and that these reductions in offending are sustained in adulthood. The favorable results of MST have been linked with considerable cost savings for taxpayers and crime victims and likely correspond to improved life outcomes for youths and families who participate in this treatment. Moreover, the effectiveness of MST bodes well for other evidence-based treatments for serious juvenile offenders (e.g., Treatment Foster Care Oregon; Chamberlain, 2003), given similar clinical emphases (i.e., focus on key risk factors related to juvenile offending, ecologically valid service delivery). As evidence-based treatments are disseminated on a broader scale, our findings should be considered by service providers and policymakers in the selection of interventions for serious juvenile offenders. Of course, even the most successful treatment models require additional replication and validation. Nevertheless, given the many problems that youths who engage in serious and violent criminal acts present for our society, as well as the significant costs and questionable ethics of providing these youths with treatments that do not produce durable changes or that even have deleterious effects, we believe that future evaluation and dissemination efforts should prioritize well-validated treatment models such as MST.

References

Asscher, J. J., Deković, M., Manders, W. A., van der Laan, P. H., & Prins, P. J. M. (2013). A randomized controlled trial of the effectiveness of multisystemic therapy in the Netherlands: Post-treatment changes and moderator effects. *Journal of Experimental Criminology, 9*, 169–187. https://doi.org/10.1007/s11292-012-9165-9

Bateson, G. (1972). *Steps to an ecology of the mind*. San Francisco, CA: Chandler Publishing Company.

Blueprints for Healthy Youth Development. (2018). *Blueprints programs*. Retrieved from http://www.blueprintsprograms.com/allPrograms.php

Borduin, C. M., & Dopp, A. R. (2015). Economic impact of multisystemic therapy with juvenile sexual offenders. *Journal of Family Psychology, 29*, 687–696. https://doi.org/10.1037/fam0000113

Borduin, C. M., Henggeler, S. W., Blaske, D. M., & Stein, R. J. (1990). Multisystemic treatment of adolescent sexual offenders. *International Journal of Offender Therapy and Comparative Criminology, 34*, 105–113. https://doi.org/10.1177/0306624X9003400204

Borduin, C. M., Mann, B. J., Cone, L. T., Henggeler, S. W., Fucci, B. R., Blaske, D. M., & Williams, R. A. (1995). Multisystemic treatment of serious juvenile offenders: Long-term prevention of criminality and violence. *Journal of Consulting and Clinical Psychology, 63*, 569–578. https://doi.org/10.1037/0022-006X.63.4.569

Borduin, C. M., & Munschy, R. M. (2014). *Multisystemic therapy for youths with problem sexual behaviors*. Unpublished manuscript, Department of Psychological Sciences, University of Missouri, Columbia, United States.

Borduin, C. M., Schaeffer, C. M., & Heiblum, N. (2009). A randomized clinical trial of multisystemic therapy with juvenile sexual offenders: Effects on youth social ecology and criminal activity. *Journal of Consulting and Clinical Psychology, 77*, 26–37. https://doi.org/10.1037/a0013035

Britt, C. L. (2001). Health consequences of criminal victimization. *International Review of Victimology, 8*, 63–73. https://doi.org/10.1177/026975800100800104

Bronfenbrenner, U. (1979). *The ecology of human development: Experiments by nature and design*. Cambridge, MA: Harvard University Press.

Butler, S., Baruch, G., Hickey, N., & Fonagy, P. (2011). A randomized controlled trial of multisystemic therapy and a statutory therapeutic intervention for young offenders. *Journal of the American Academy of Child and Adolescent Psychiatry, 50*, 1220–1235. https://doi.org/10.1016/j.jaac.2011.09.017

Byford, S., McCrone, P., & Barrett, B. (2003). Developments in the quantity and quality of economic evaluations in mental health. *Current Opinion in Psychiatry, 16*, 703–707. https://doi.org/10.1097/00001504-200311000-00017

Chamberlain, P. (2003). The Oregon multidimensional treatment foster care model: Features, outcomes, and progress in dissemination. *Cognitive and Behavioral Practice, 10*, 303–312. https://doi.org/10.1016/S1077-7229(03)80048-2

Curtis, N. M., Ronan, K. R., & Borduin, C. M. (2004). Multisystemic treatment: A meta-analysis of outcome studies. *Journal of Family Psychology, 18*, 411–419. https://doi.org/10.1037/0893-3200.18.3.411

Deković, M., Asscher, J. J., Manders, W. A., Prins, P. J. M., & van der Laan, P. (2012). Within-intervention change: Mediators of intervention effects during multisystemic therapy. *Journal of Consulting and Clinical Psychology, 80*, 574–587. https://doi.org/10.1037/a0028482

Dopp, A. R., Borduin, C. M., & Brown, C. E. (2015). Evidence-based treatments for youths with problem sexual behaviors: Review and recommendations. *Journal of Aggression, Conflict, and Peace Research, 7*, 223–236. https://doi.org/10.1108/JACPR-01-2015-0155

Dopp, A. R., Borduin, C. M., Rothman, D. B., & Letourneau, E. J. (2017). Evidence-based treatments for youths who engage in illegal sexual behaviors. *Journal of Clinical Child and Adolescent Psychology, 46*, 631–645. https://doi.org/10.1080/15374416.2016.1261714

Dopp, A. R., Borduin, C. M., Wagner, D. V., & Sawyer, A. M. (2014). Economic impact of multisystemic therapy through midlife: A cost-benefit analysis with serious juvenile offenders and their siblings. *Journal of Consulting and Clinical Psychology, 82*, 694–705. https://doi.org/10.1037/a0036415

Dopp, A. R., Borduin, C. M., White, M. H., II, & Kuppens, S. (2017). Family-based treatments for serious juvenile offenders: A multilevel meta-analysis. *Journal of Consulting and Clinical Psychology, 85*, 335–354. https://doi.org/10.1037/ccp0000183

Dopp, A. R., Coen, A. S., Smith, A. B., Reno, J., Bernstein, D. H., Kerns, S. E., & Altschul, D. (2017). Economic impact of the statewide implementation of an evidence-based treatment: Multisystemic therapy in New Mexico. *Behavior Therapy, 49*, 551–566. https://doi.org/10.1016/j.beth.2017.12.003

Drake, E. K., Aos, S., & Miller, M. G. (2009). Evidence-based public policy options to reduce crime and criminal justice costs: Implications in Washington state. *Victims and Offenders, 4*, 170–196. https://doi.org/10.1080/15564880802612615

Farrington, D. P., Jolliffe, D., Hawkins, J. D., Catalano, R. F., Hill, K. G., & Kosterman, R. (2003). Comparing delinquency careers in court records and self-reports. *Criminology, 41*, 933–958. https://doi.org/10.1111/j.1745-9125.2003.tb01009.x

Farrington, D. P., Ttofi, M. M., & Coid, J. W. (2009). Development of adolescence-limited, late onset, and persistent offenders from age 8 to age 48. *Aggressive Behavior, 35*, 150–163. https://doi.org/10.1002/ab.20296

Federal Bureau of Investigation. (2016). *Crime in the United States, 2015*. Washington, DC: U.S. Department of Justice. Retrieved from https://ucr.fbi.gov/crime-in-the-u.s/2015/crime-in-the-u.s.-2015

French, M. T., Salome, H. J., Sindelar, J. L., & McLellan, A. T. (2002). Benefit-cost analysis of addiction treatment: Methodological guidelines and empirical application using the DATCAP and ASI. *Health Services Research, 37*, 433–455. https://doi.org/10.1111/1475-6773.031

Greenwood, P. (2008). Prevention and intervention programs for juvenile offenders: The benefits of evidence-based practice. *The Future of Children, 18*, 11–36. https://doi.org/10.1353/foc.0.0018

Henggeler, S. W., & Borduin, C. M. (1990). *Family therapy and beyond: A multisystemic approach to treating the behavior problems of children and adolescents*. Pacific Grove, CA: Brooks/Cole.

Henggeler, S. W., Letourneau, E. J., Chapman, J. E., Borduin, C. M., Schewe, P. A., & McCart, M. R. (2009). Mediators of change for multisystemic therapy with juvenile sexual offenders. *Journal of Consulting and Clinical Psychology, 77*, 451–462. https://doi.org/10.1037/a0013971

Henggeler, S. W., Melton, G. B., Brondino, M. J., Scherer, D. G., & Hanley, J. H. (1997). Multisystemic therapy with violent and chronic juvenile offenders and their families: The role of treatment fidelity in successful dissemination. *Journal of Consulting and Clinical Psychology, 65*, 821–833. https://doi.org/10.1037/0022-006X.65.5.821

Henggeler, S. W., & Schoenwald, S. K. (2011). Evidence-based interventions for juvenile offenders and juvenile justice policies that support them: *Society for Research in Child Development: Social Policy Report, 25*, 1–20. Retrieved from https://eric.ed.gov/?id=ED519241

Henggeler, S. W., Schoenwald, S. K., Borduin, C. M., Rowland, M. D., & Cunningham, P. B. (2009). *Multisystemic therapy for antisocial behavior in children and adolescents* (2nd ed.). New York, NY: Guilford Press.

Hoffman, L. (1981). *Foundations of family therapy*. New York, NY: Basic Books.

Howell, J. C. (2009). *Preventing and reducing juvenile delinquency: A comprehensive framework* (2nd ed.). Thousand Oaks, CA: Sage.

Huey, S. J., Henggeler, S. W., Brondino, M. J., & Pickrel, S. G. (2000). Mechanisms of change in multisystemic therapy: Reducing delinquent behavior through therapist adherence and improved family and peer functioning. *Journal of Consulting and Clinical Psychology, 68*, 451–467. https://doi.org/10.1037//0022-006X.68.3.451

Johnides, B. D., Borduin, C. M., Wagner, D. V., & Dopp, A. R. (2017). Effects of multisystemic therapy on caregivers of serious juvenile offenders: A 20-year follow-up to a randomized clinical trial. *Journal of Consulting and Clinical Psychology, 85*, 323–334. https://doi.org/10.1037/ccp0000199

Kilpatrick, D. G., & Acierno, A. (2003). Mental health needs of crime victims: Epidemiology and outcomes. *Journal of Traumatic Stress, 16*, 119–132. https://doi.org/10.1023/A:1022891005388

Letourneau, E. J., Henggeler, S. W., Borduin, C. M., Schewe, P. A., McCart, M. R., Chapman, J. E., & Saldana, L. (2009). Multisystemic therapy for juvenile sexual offenders: 1-year results from a randomized effectiveness trial. *Journal of Family Psychology, 23*, 89–102. https://doi.org/10.1037/a0014352

Letourneau, E. J., Henggeler, S. W., McCart, M. R., Borduin, C. M., Schewe, P. A., & Armstrong, K. S. (2013). Two-year follow-up of a randomized effectiveness trial evaluating MST for juveniles who sexually offend. *Journal of Family Psychology, 27*, 978–985. https://doi.org/10.1037/a0034710

Lipton, D., Martinson, R., & Wilks, J. (1975). *The effectiveness of correctional treatment: A survey of treatment evaluation studies*. New York, NY: Praeger.

Loeber, R., Burke, J. D., & Pardini, D. A. (2009). Development and etiology of disruptive and delinquent behavior. *Annual Review of Clinical Psychology, 5*, 291–310. https://doi.org/10.1146/annurev.clinpsy.032408.153631

Loeber, R., & Farrington, D. P. (Eds.). (2012). *From juvenile delinquency to adult crime: Criminal careers, justice policy and prevention*. New York, NY: Oxford University Press.

Lyons, J. S., Baerger, D. R., Quigley, P., Erlich, J., & Griffin, E. (2001). Mental health service needs of juvenile offenders: A comparison of detention, incarceration, and treatment settings. *Children's Services: Social Policy, Research, and Practice, 4*, 69–85. https://doi.org/10.1207/S15326918CS0402_2

McCart, M. R., & Sheidow, A. J. (2016). Evidence-based psychosocial treatments for adolescents with disruptive behavior. *Journal of Clinical Child and Adolescent Psychology, 45*, 529–563. https://doi.org/10.1080/15374416.2016.1146990

McCollister, K. E., French, M. T., & Fang, H. (2010). The cost of crime to society: New crime specific estimates for policy and program evaluation. *Drug and Alcohol Dependence, 108*, 98–109. https://doi.org/10.1016/j.drugalcdep.2009.12.002

Miller, T. R., Fisher, D. A., & Cohen, M. A. (2001). Costs of juvenile violence: Policy implications. *Pediatrics, 107*, e3. https://doi.org/10.1542/peds.107.1.e3

Minuchin, P. P. (1985). Families and individual development: Provocations from the field of family therapy. *Child Development, 56*, 289–302. https://doi.org/10.2307/1129720

Monahan, K. C., Steinberg, L., & Cauffman, E. (2009). Affiliation with antisocial peers, susceptibility to peer influence, and antisocial behavior during the transition to adulthood. *Developmental Psychology, 45*, 1520–1530. https://doi.org/10.1037/a0017417

MST Services. (2018). *MST services*. Retrieved from http://www.mstservices.com

Odgers, C. L., Moffitt, T. E., Broadbent, J. M., Dickson, N., Hancox, R. J., Harrington, H., … Caspi, A. (2008). Female and male antisocial trajectories: From childhood origins to adult outcomes. *Development and Psychopathology, 20*, 673–716. https://doi.org/10.1017/S0954579408000333

Ogden, T., & Hagen, K. A. (2006). Multisystemic therapy of serious behaviour problems in youth: Sustainability of therapy effectiveness two years after intake. *Child and Adolescent Mental Health, 11*, 142–149. https://doi.org/10.1111/j.1475-3588.2006.00396.x

Ogden, T., & Halliday-Boykins, C. A. (2004). Multisystemic treatment of antisocial adolescents in Norway: Replication of clinical outcomes outside of the US. *Child and Adolescent Mental Health, 9*, 77–83. https://doi.org/10.1111/j.1475-3588.2004.00085.x

Robinson, F., & Keithley, J. (2000). The impacts of crime on health and health services: A literature review. *Health, Risk and Society, 2*, 253–266. https://doi.org/10.1080/713670168

Sawyer, A. M., & Borduin, C. M. (2011). Effects of multisystemic therapy through midlife: A 21.9-year follow-up to a randomized clinical trial with serious and violent juvenile offenders. *Journal of Consulting and Clinical Psychology, 79*, 643–652. https://doi.org/10.1037/a0024862

Shufelt, J. S., & Cocozza, J. C. (2006). *Youth with mental health disorders in the juvenile justice system: Results from a multi-state, multi-system prevalence study*. Delmar, NY: National Center for Mental Health and Juvenile Justice. Retrieved from https://www.ncmhjj.com/resources/youth-mental-health-disorders-juvenile-justice-system-results-multi-state-prevalence-study/

Singh, B., Hawthorne, G., & Vos, T. (2001). The role of economic evaluation in mental health care. *Australian and New Zealand Journal of Psychiatry, 35*, 104–117. https://doi.org/10.1046/j.1440-1614.2001.00845.x

Smith-Boydston, J. M., Holtzman, R. J., & Roberts, M. C. (2014). Transportability of multisystemic therapy to community settings: Can a program sustain outcomes without MST services oversight? *Child and Youth Care Forum, 43*, 593–605. https://doi.org/10.1007/s10566-014-9255-0

Timmons-Mitchell, J., Bender, M. B., Kishna, M. A., & Mitchell, C. C. (2006). An independent effectiveness trial of multisystemic therapy with juvenile justice youth. *Journal of Clinical Child and Adolescent Psychology, 35*, 227–236. https://doi.org/10.1207/s15374424jccp3502_6

van der Stouwe, T., Asscher, J. J., Stams, G. J. J. M., Deković, M., & van der Laan, P. H. (2014). The effectiveness of multisystemic therapy (MST): A meta-analysis. *Clinical Psychology Review, 34*, 468–481. https://doi.org/10.1016/j.cpr.2014.06.006

Voisin, D. R., Hong, J. S., & King, K. (2012). Ecological factors associated with sexual risk behaviors among detained adolescents: A systematic review. *Children and Youth Services Review, 34*, 1983–1991. https://doi.org/10.1016/j.childyouth.2012.07.003

Wagner, D. V., Borduin, C. M., Sawyer, A. M., & Dopp, A. R. (2014). Long-term prevention of criminality in siblings of serious and violent juvenile offenders: A 25-year follow-up to a randomized clinical trial of multisystemic therapy. *Journal of Consulting and Clinical Psychology, 82*, 492–499. https://doi.org/10.1037/a0035624

Weisz, J. R., Kuppens, S., Ng, M. Y., Eckshtain, D., Ugueto, A. M., Vaughn-Coaxum, R., ... Forwood, S. R. (2017). What five decades of research tells us about the effects of youth psychological therapy: A multilevel meta-analysis and implications for science and practice. *American Psychologist, 72*, 79–117. https://doi.org/10.1037/a0040360

Witkiewitz, K., King, K., McMahon, R. J., Wu, J., Luk, J., Bierman, K. L., ... Conduct Problems Prevention Research Group. (2013). Evidence for a multi-dimensional latent structural model of externalizing disorders. *Journal of Abnormal Child Psychology, 41*, 223–237. https://doi.org/10.1007/s10802-012-9674-z

Chapter 14
Treatments that Work for Intimate Partner Violence: Beyond the Duluth Model

Alexandra L. Snead, Victoria E. Bennett, and Julia C. Babcock

14.1 Introduction

Intimate partner violence (IPV) is a serious public health problem that impacts millions of individuals around the world. IPV is defined as physical, sexual, or psychological harm perpetrated by a current or former romantic partner (Saltzman, Fanslow, McMahon, & Shelley, 2002). Physical violence is the intentional use of physical force that has potential to cause death, injury, or harm (Breiding, Basile, Smith, Black, & Mahendra, 2015). Sexual violence consists of rape or penetration (the victim was made to penetrate someone else), nonphysically pressured unwanted penetration, unwanted sexual contact, and noncontact unwanted sexual experience (Breiding et al., 2015). Psychological aggression is the use of verbal or nonverbal communication with the intent to harm another person mentally or emotionally (Breiding et al., 2015). Stalking is characterized by a pattern of repeated, unwanted attention and contact that causes fear or concern for one's safety (Breiding et al., 2015). Mental and physical health consequences of IPV include chronic pain, difficulty sleeping, activity limitations, depression, anxiety, PTSD, and low self-esteem (Black et al., 2011). IPV has been found to cost the United States $5.8 billion each year, with direct medical and mental health care services accounting for $4.1 billion (National Center for Injury Prevention and Control, 2003).

In the United States, nearly one in four women (22.3%) and one in seven men (14%) have been victims of severe physical violence (Breiding et al., 2014). Further, more than one in three women (35.6%) and more than one in four men (28.5%) have been the victims of rape, physical violence, and/or stalking by a romantic partner in their lifetimes (Black et al., 2011). Current research has found that IPV perpetrated

A. L. Snead (✉) · V. E. Bennett · J. C. Babcock
University of Houston, Houston, TX, USA
e-mail: asnead@uh.edu; vebennet@central.uh.edu; jbabcock@uh.edu

E. L. Jeglic, C. Calkins (eds.), *New Frontiers in Offender Treatment*,
https://doi.org/10.1007/978-3-030-01030-0_14

by women is equal to or higher than IPV perpetrated by men (Straus, 2008; Whitaker, Haileyesus, Swahn, & Saltzman, 2007). In a review of 31 studies (Williams, Ghandour, & Kub, 2008) examining the prevalence rates of female perpetrated IPV in adult populations, estimates for physical IPV perpetrated in the last year ranged from 13% to 68%. It is important to note that the study with the highest estimate (68%) included a sample of women seeking alcohol treatment, which may have increased prevalence rates, as alcohol is a risk factor for IPV perpetration and victimization (Chase, O'Farrell, Murphy, Fals-Stewart, & Murphy, 2003). Mutual violence was reported among 45–95% of couples who reported physical violence (Caetano, Ramisetty-Mikler, & Field, 2005; Straus, 2008).

Same-sex partner violence, including prevalence rates and treatment options, has not been studied as comprehensively as heterosexual partner violence. In a review of 19 same-sex and heterosexual partner violence comparison studies, Burke and Follingstad (1999) found IPV to be equally prevalent in same-sex and heterosexual relationships. While studying a large, ethnically diverse community sample of gay men, Turell (2000) found that 44% experienced physical violence, 83% experienced emotional abuse, and 13% experienced sexual abuse. Other researchers have found that IPV ranges from 25% to 50% among lesbian relationships (Alexander, 2002; Brand & Kidd, 1986; Lockhart, White, Causby, & Isaac, 1994).

Historically, intimate partner violence was seen as a gender-based phenomenon in which men batter women as a way to maintain their authority in our patriarchal society. Violent men were classified into different types of batterers (Holtzworth-Munroe & Stuart, 1994; Waltz, Babcock, Jacobson, & Gottman, 2000). However, research shows that a significant number of women (Williams et al., 2008), transgender individuals (Yerke & DeFeo, 2016), and same-sex couples (Messinger, 2011) also perpetrate intimate partner violence. Rather than classifying types of male batterers, researchers have moved toward typifying types of violence. In order to more broadly capture types of IPV, some of which may not constitute battering, researchers have found merit in categorizing IPV into two major types: situational and characterological (Johnson & Ferraro, 2000). Situational violence is mutual, low-level violence (i.e., slapping, grabbing, and pushing) that is perpetrated by both partners normally as a means of conflict management (Johnson & Ferraro, 2000). Characterological violence occurs when the perpetrator uses severe violence as a means of inducing fear and to control the victim (Johnson & Ferraro, 2000). Characterologically violent perpetrators are more likely to endorse violence-supporting attitudes (Leone, Johnson, & Cohan, 2007) and exhibit borderline and antisocial personality features (Kelly & Johnson, 2008) than situationally violent perpetrators. Among a community sample, situational violence accounted for 89% of IPV, while characterological violence accounted for 11% (Johnson, 2006). Additionally, situationally violent couples report lower levels of relationship violence than couples experiencing characterological violence (Friend, Bradley, Thatcher, & Gottman, 2011).

14.2 Treatments

Current interventions for IPV perpetrators are normally court-ordered as a part of criminal adjudication for domestic abuse charges (Babcock & Steiner, 1999), as IPV perpetrators often do not seek treatment on their own (Healey, Smith, & O'Sullivan, 1998). There are two common types of treatment for IPV, which are often called batterers intervention programs (BIPs): the Duluth model and cognitive behavioral therapy (CBT). The most current BIPs are provided in a weekly group format and last between 8 and 52 weeks (Eckhardt et al., 2013). Although group interventions are more cost-effective, others are developing modalities for treating IPV, including individual (Murphy & Eckhardt, 2005) and conjoint treatments (Bradley & Gottman, 2012).

14.2.1 Duluth Model

The Duluth model, named after its originating US city, is the most predominant BIP in the United States. It was not created by therapists but by paraprofessionals through information gathered from interviewing IPV victims in shelters and using principles from feminist and sociological frameworks (Pence & Paymar, 1993). The feminist theoretical model views IPV as a male phenomenon and proposes that IPV is used as a way for men to show power and establish control over their female partners (Pence & Paymar, 1993). Based on interviews of battered women describing their abuse, the creators of the Duluth model developed the "power and control wheel," which theorizes that IPV serves to preserve male privilege (Pence & Paymar, 1993). The main goal in this model is for the male perpetrator to abandon authoritarian relationships and achieve effective types of behavior that fall on the "equality wheel," which fosters a more egalitarian attitude regarding relationships. The goal is not to provide male IPV perpetrators with therapy, but rather to reeducate men on their beliefs regarding IPV, women, and gender stereotypes (Pence & Paymar, 1993).

Some criticize the Duluth model for eliminating the psychology of violence from treatment and replacing it with gender politics (Dutton & Corvo, 2006). According to the model, men in our patriarchal society are likely to be violent in order to maintain control, but there is no research that has found that males with more sexist attitudes are more likely to be violent (Holtzworth-Munroe, Bates, Smutzler, & Sandin, 1997). Additionally, the psychoeducational model focuses mainly on cognition rather than emotion, even though IPV is highly emotionally driven (Babcock, Canady, Graham, & Schart, 2007). Moreover, the Duluth model views the "client" of therapy as the victim rather than the male perpetrator (Pence & Paymar, 1993), and the psychoeducational groups do not consider any of the perpetrators' personal histories during treatment (Dutton & Corvo, 2006), which can make the treatment less engaging. The Duluth model ignores the reality that women can also be perpetrators of IPV (Babcock, Miller, & Siard, 2003). With the Duluth model targeting men's perceived control over women, this method cannot be utilized for same-sex couples or female perpetrated IPV.

There have been few studies that have utilized true experimental designs to examine the efficacy of the Duluth model. One study examined the effects of a psychoeducational-feminist intervention that was similar to the Duluth model; the study contained 404 batterers who were randomly assigned to a 26-week Duluth-type intervention group or a no-treatment control group (Feder & Dugan, 2002). Findings indicated that there was no significant difference between the two groups in terms of recidivism rates posttreatment, according to both victim reports and police records, though, for men that did complete all 26 weeks (40%), treatment produced a minimal but significant effect (Babcock, Green, & Robie, 2004; Feder & Dugan, 2002). There have been several quasi-experimental studies supporting the efficacy of Duluth-type interventions (Babcock & Steiner, 1999; Gondolf, 2004, 2007); however, these have failed to determine causality for IPV reduction.

Gender-Based Cognitive Behavioral Interventions An alternative model developed by psychologists and other social scientists is cognitive behavioral therapy (CBT). Violence is treated as a learned behavior and thus must in turn be replaced by a learned nonviolent behavior. The functionality of the violent behavior is explored along with the pros and cons of using violence to solve problems, and alternative solutions for dealing with antecedents of violence are discussed during CBT sessions (Babcock et al., 2007; Eckhardt, 2007; Wexler, 2013). Strategies used during CBT sessions include cognitive restructuring of negative attributions, anger management techniques, and resocialization (Sonkin, Martin, & Walker, 1985).

Dunford (2000) examined CBT as a battering intervention among domestically violent male US Navy personnel. Men were assigned to one of four groups, a 36-week CBT intervention, a 26-week couples treatment, 12 months of rigorous monitoring, or a no-treatment control group. Based on partner and police report, there were no significant differences in recidivism rates between the CBT group and the no-treatment control group. Morrel, Elliot, Murphy, and Taft (2003) compared the effects of CBT and supportive group therapy among male IPV perpetrators. Both conditions showed significant decreases in IPV when compared to participants who discontinued treatment. However, this study lacked randomization and a control group.

14.2.2 Conjoint Treatments

The use of conjoint or couples-based treatments for IPV is controversial, as some argue that couples therapy for IPV places the victim at a greater risk for abuse. Research has demonstrated that conjoint level treatments are safe for couples in which there is situational couple violence (O'Leary, 1996; O'Leary, Heyman, & Neidig, 1999) and in which the violence typically arises when an argument escalates and the violence is low-level. Most IPV researchers agree that conjoint treatments would be unethical for couples in which there is characterological violence, as therapy would place the victim at greater risk for abuse (Armenti, Iyican, Sommer, & Babcock, 2017; LaTaillade, Epstein, & Werlinich, 2006). Although research has demonstrated that conjoint treatments would be safe (O'Leary et al., 1999), a recent meta-analysis indicated that a limited number of studies ($n = 6$) have explored the efficacy of conjoint treatments (Karakurt, Whiting, van Esch, Bolen, & Calabrese, 2016). They found that across the six studies, couples therapy demonstrated greater reductions in IPV when compared to a control group or standard IPV treatment. One of the new programs explored in the meta-analysis was the Creating Healthy Relationships Program (CHRP), which is described below.

CHRP: Creating Healthy Relationships Program Researchers have recently begun to examine the effectiveness of conjoint intervention for IPV perpetration. Creating Healthy Relationships Program (CHRP) was created from over 30 years of research conducted by Gottman and colleagues (Gottman, 1994; Gottman & Silver, 2000; Jacobson & Gottman, 1998; Shapiro & Gottman, 2005) to strengthen couples' relationships and decrease low levels of mutual violence. CHRP was designed to be effective within low-income, situationally violent couples.

CHRP is comprised of 22 weekly 2-h sessions, attended by 6–8 couples; each session is focused on a different topic. CHRP sessions are generally focused on constructive conflict management related to different topics; five areas are covered: managing stress, establishing emotional connections in the family with partners and children, maintaining intimacy, creating shared meaning, and managing conflict. Each session begins with a video depicting couples participating in a mock talk show that is focused on the session topic. Couples then voice their own opinion on the topic, and then group facilitators present an educational component including research-based information. A skill-building segment is also combined in each session, where couples participate in exercises that allow them to practice relationship skills.

Bradley, Friend, and Gottman (2011) conducted a study testing the efficacy of CHRP when compared to a control group in a sample of 155 couples experiencing situational violence. Results indicated that female participants receiving CHRP were more satisfied with their relationships when compared to the control group after the program, while there was a trend toward significance for male participants (Bradley et al., 2011). Men in the CHRP group reported less conflict after the program compared to the control group (Bradley et al., 2011). Additionally, involvement in CHRP led to greater use of healthy relationship skills (Bradley et al., 2011) and less use of physical and/or psychological aggression while trying to resolve their conflicts (Bradley, Drummey, Gottman, & Gottman, 2014). Research examining the mechanisms of change in CHRP found that the reduction in psychological abuse was induced through the therapeutic principles involved in CHRP, which include conflict management skills, sex/romance/passion, friendship, and shared meaning within the relationship (Bradley & Gottman, 2012). While the differences in couples' IPV perpetration between the control group and the CHRP group were not significantly different, those in the CHRP group reported fewer instances of IPV following the intervention than those in the control group (Bradley et al., 2014). The lack of significance could be attributed to the low rates of IPV in the situationally violent couples at baseline—a floor effect due to screening in only low-level violent couples. Nonetheless, the results do suggest that couples who experience situational violence, in which domination, control, and fear are not the driving forces, can improve their relationship in a safe manner (Bradley et al., 2011).

Attempts to replicate and extend CHRP with court-mandated couples have been logistically challenging (Babcock, Armenti, & Warford, 2017). Many states mandate against couples interventions in cases of IPV. Existing community-coordinated response systems are geared toward one perpetrator and an identified victim. Efforts to recruit situationally violent couples from the courts in Yamhill County, Oregon, have been stymied by low referral rates and political roadblocks (Babcock et al., 2017). Thus, it is questionable if couples interventions are feasible in statewide court-mandated samples in the current political climate.

14.2.3 Military Interventions

The literature has shown that military populations have a three times higher frequency of IPV than community samples, as trauma exposure and PTSD place veterans at greater risk for IPV perpetration (Marshall, Panuzio, & Taft, 2005). A new intervention targets IPV among active-duty and military veterans, called Strength at Home (SAH; Taft et al., 2013). SAH utilizes the social processing model of IPV, which suggests that individuals who have experienced trauma, such as military populations, may be more likely to interpret daily social cues as threatening and subsequently react aggressively (Taft, Walling, Howard, & Monson, 2011). SAH uses a trauma-focused cognitive behavioral group therapy format with four stages. These stages as described by Love et al. (2015, p. 2353) are "psychoeducation, conflict management skills, coping strategies, and communication skills."

Strength at Home for Men There is strong evidence for Strength at Home as a men-focused intervention (SAH-M; Taft, Macdonald, Creech, Monson, & Murphy, 2016) and a couples-prevention program (SAH-C; Taft et al., 2016). In a randomized controlled trial, Taft, Macdonald, et al. (2016) recruited a sample of 135 male servicemen and veterans who had engaged in at least 1 act of male-to-female IPV within the past 6 months and 111 of their female partners for corroborating reports of IPV. Male participants were excluded if they met criteria for a current substance abuse disorder or had an untreated bipolar or psychotic disorder. Participants were randomly assigned to the Strength at Home-Men (SAH-M) or a treatment as usual (TAU) condition with referrals to external therapy sources. After 12 weeks of treatment, participants in the SAH-M group had larger clinically significant decreases (e.g., large effect sizes) in physical and psychological IPV at posttreatment than individuals in the TAU condition.

Strength at Home for Couples Strength at Home-Couples (SAH-C) targets distressed couples who are at increased risk for situational IPV. The core modules of SAH-C are psychoeducation surrounding trauma, relationships, and IPV; establishing healthy conflict management skills; enhancing communication skills; developing assertiveness skills; and listening skills. Taft, Creech, et al. (2016) tested the efficacy of SAH-C as a prevention program for physical and psychological IPV using a randomized controlled trial. Sixty-nine couples were randomly assigned to the SAH-C or the supportive prevention group. Couples randomized to SAH-C participated in a 10-week trauma-focused cognitive behavioral couples group therapy program, and couples randomized to the supportive prevention program (SP) followed a group therapy format that emphasized relationship conflicts and how they relate to IPV. Exclusionary criteria were the presence of a substance use disorder not in remission, female partners engaging in severe physical IPV (e.g., using a weapon or causing injury), as well as any male-to-female physical IPV. Couples in SAH-C reported less IPV and had lower rates of both partners engaging in physical IPV across all time points compared to those in the SP program. Similar results were found with psychological IPV, such that SAH-C resulted in lower rates of both men and women's psychological abuse perpetration.

Strength at Home is the first efficacious military-focused IPV intervention program with men and prevention program with couples. While these programs were greatly needed due to the rates of IPV in military populations, there are some limitations to them. Strength at Home excludes participants in which the service member is female, there is co-occurring substance abuse and IPV, as well as couples in which there is predominantly female-to-male partner violence. IPV in community samples is commonly bidirectional, and women are as frequently as violent as men (Schumacher & Leonard, 2005; Straus, 2004), yet those couples were excluded from the SAH-C clinical trial. This is likely to be true among military samples as well. Service members with co-occurring substance use disorders were also excluded from participating in either SAH-M or SAH-C. Given the wealth of research providing evidence for the link between substance use and IPV (Foran & O'Leary, 2008), research into the efficacy of SAH among those populations is warranted. Finally, SAH's samples have been largely conducted with Caucasian participants, and research examining the efficacy of SAH-M and SAH-C using a diverse sample is needed.

14.2.4 Achieving Change Through Values-Based Behavior Program

One of the most exciting new interventions being tested for IPV reduction is Achieving Change Through Values-Based Behavior (ACTV; Lawrence, Langer Zarling, & Orengo-Aguayo, 2014). ACTV is based on acceptance and commitment therapy (ACT) principles (ACT; Hayes, Strosahl, & Wilson, 1999). ACT emphasizes the importance of psychological flexibility (Hayes et al., 1999). Within an ACT framework, clients are encouraged to master skills, including recognizing and labeling both positive and negative emotions, diminishing attachment to thoughts, present awareness, and perspective-taking, and are taught effective strategies for controlling their emotional reactions (Hayes et al., 1999). One's personal values, defined as activities that give life meaning, are used as motivating factors for behavior change in the ACTV model, and training occurs to help make the valued behavior possible. ACTV has an emphasis on equalizing the relationship between program facilitators and participants by creating a nonjudgmental and collaborative environment.

ACTV was designed as a 24-week program for men or women who are court-mandated to complete a BIP after receiving a domestic violence conviction. The ACTV program centers on experiential learning and altering one's relationship with their thoughts and emotions and does not include challenging one's thoughts (Lawrence et al., 2014). Therefore, a major difference between Duluth/CBT and ACTV is that ACTV focuses on the idea that a participant's behavior can change without targeting distorted beliefs (Zarling, Bannon, & Berta, 2017). In addition, whereas the Duluth model believes that violence occurs because of sexist beliefs and the desire of men to have power and control over women, there are no inferred reasons as to the cause of one's violent behavior in ACTV (Zarling et al., 2017). Each participant is encouraged to identify their own antecedents and consequences to their behavior (Zarling et al., 2017), thus making it a gender-neutral intervention and appropriate for all individuals who perpetrate IPV.

ACTV consists of five modules including big picture/core skills, emotion regulation skills, cognitive skills, behavioral skills, and barriers to change (Zarling et al., 2017). Research has found promising results for ACTV. In a study comparing Duluth/CBT to ACTV in men ($N = 3474$) who were arrested for domestic violence and court-ordered to attend treatment, participants in the ACTV program acquired fewer new charges, domestic assault charges, or violent charges than participants in the Duluth/CBT program during the intervention period (Zarling et al., 2017). Additionally, participants in the ACTV program had on average fewer charges in the year after the treatment than participants in the Duluth/CBT program (Zarling et al., 2017). Treatment improvements were mediated by experiential avoidance and emotion dysregulation, which are both treatment targets in ACTV. It should be noted that participants were not randomized, and an RCT investigating ACTV in court-mandated male batterers is currently ongoing (Zarling, 2018). While the ACTV program seems superior to Duluth/CBT interventions, including the ability of trained correctional officers to administer the program, the dropout rates were significantly higher when compared to Duluth/CBT. This high dropout rate may be explained by the early implementation phase and the fact that this was the first time ACTV had been implemented (Zarling et al., 2017).

These findings have not been without criticism, as some IPV researchers believe that Zarling et al. (2017) overinterpreted their findings, thus prematurely prompting policy changes (Gondolf, Bennett, & Mankowski, 2018). However, Zarling and colleagues indicated that their findings were preliminary and it was the Iowa Department of Corrections (2012) that chose to implement and test ACTV at a statewide level based on their own internal review concluding that the existing Duluth/CBT models were "a waste of taxpayer dollars" (Iowa Department of Corrections, 2012, p. 4). Gondolf et al. (2018) state that "ACTV appears to have links to factions promoting a more gender-neutral theory and programming of domestic violence, in contrast to the gender-based perspective represented in the Duluth program" (p. 6), as if gender neutrality is antithetical to proper IPV intervention. Zarling and colleagues' study demonstrates the feasibility of implementing ACTV within the structure of the existing coordinated community response to IPV.

14.2.5 Alcohol-Based Interventions

Within the IPV literature, there is a well-established link between alcohol and intimate partner violence (Foran & O'Leary, 2008). Despite this relationship, the majority of BIPs do not incorporate alcohol treatment into their programs (Easton et al., 2007), perhaps because alcohol can be used as an excuse for violent behavior and could theoretically decrease perpetrators' accountability. Studies that have integrated alcohol treatment into their programs have found that programs that also target substance abuse demonstrate decreased IPV reoccurrence. Several interventions have been developed that combine substance use and IPV treatments in order to decrease the number of IPV incidents that occur while one or both partners are intoxicated.

Brief Alcohol Interventions Stuart et al. (2013) conducted a RCT in which men arrested for domestic violence and were enrolled in a BIP were randomly assigned to receive a brief (90-min) alcohol intervention prior to beginning IPV treatment or treatment as usual (e.g., BIP alone). The authors examined the impact of the enhanced treatment on alcohol use (e.g., number of drinks per drinking day and percentage of days abstinent) and frequency of IPV. Data was collected at baseline, 3-, 6-, and 12-month follow-up. At 3-month follow-up, participants receiving the enhanced treatment reported less severe physical IPV compared to the treatment as usual participants. Although these initial findings were promising, they did not hold up over time. Specifically, there were no differences between the TAU and the enhanced groups at 6- and 12-month follow-up.

More recently, Stuart, McGreary, Shorey, and Knopik (2016) examined the role of cumulative genetic score (CGS) as a moderator of alcohol use and IPV in a subset of the original sample used by Stuart et al. (2013). Results demonstrated that those at a higher genetic risk (i.e., high scores on CGS) who received the enhanced treatment reported lower physical IPV and partner injuries. These findings provide preliminary evidence for the utility of tailoring treatment for the individual on the basis of biologic factors. More research is needed to examine the utility of CGS specifically when tailoring treatments.

Intensive Substance Abuse Treatments The most robust evidence comes from an integrated treatment, substance abuse-domestic violence (SADV; Easton et al., 2007; Easton, Crane, & Mandel, 2017). SADV is a 12-week intervention that is taught in a group or individually and focuses on psychoeducation surrounding IPV and alcohol, recognizing situations in which they are likely to occur, teaching problem solving, coping, and communication skills, as well as emotion regulation strategies. SADV has been tested in two studies, one of which compared SADV to a treatment program specifically targeting alcohol abuse (Easton et al., 2007), while the other compared SADV to a combined substance and alcohol use treatment program (Easton et al., 2017). Participants were men voluntarily seeking services (Study 1) or court-mandated to substance abuse treatment (Study 2) at an outpatient treatment clinic. Easton et al. (2007) argued that addressing IPV through substance abuse programs reaches a larger audience than BIPs, as the vast majority of BIP attendees are court-mandated to treatment.

In Study 1, participants in the SADV treatment demonstrated a 32% reduction in physical violence compared to 15% reduction in the control group. Despite these promising results, there was no significant difference between the two groups at 6-month follow-up for physical violence (Easton et al., 2007). In Study 2, SADV was individualized for each participant rather than following the standard same-sex group format, as participants had the option of replacing four sessions with couples-focused sessions (Easton et al., 2017). Results demonstrated that physical violence was 1.85 times more likely to occur in the control group compared to those in the SADV group. Furthermore, at the 3-month follow-up, the average number of violent days was less for those receiving the SADV intervention than those only receiving substance use treatment. SADV is a promising treatment for comorbid substance use and IPV; however, it would be important to examine its efficacy in longer-term studies as well as in community samples.

Pharmacological Treatments One RCT by George et al. (2011) examined the effect of incorporating an SSRI into an alcohol abuse treatment on reducing anger and physical IPV among a sample of IPV perpetrators receiving a combined CBT and alcohol abuse treatment. The authors chose to examine the effect of an SSRI because the biological model of IPV (George, Phillips, Doty, Umhau, & Rawlings, 2006) posits that IPV perpetrators are excessively responsive to variables within their environments. Serotonin directly impacts the neuronal processing of one's environment and therefore may help to desensitize IPV perpetrators. In this study, 60 treatment-seeking IPV perpetrators who abused alcohol were randomized to take the SSRI or a placebo pill for 12 weeks. Results indicated that those who received the SSRI had lower self-reported anger and physical IPV scores than those in the placebo-control condition. This study provided preliminary evidence that SSRI could be an effective treatment for reducing violence among alcoholic IPV perpetrators. Despite this preliminary evidence, this study had high rates of treatment dropout, leading to a small sample size at analysis. Therefore, more studies need to be conducted before we can shut down BIPs and replace them with SSRIs.

Regardless of the mechanism of treatment (i.e., pharmacologic, brief, or long-term alcohol interventions), the results reported by George et al. (2011), Stuart et al. (2013), and Easton et al. (2017) underscore the importance of combining alcohol and IPV treatment for populations at risk. Easton and colleagues' two studies provide evidence for a longer-term (i.e., 12 weeks) psychotherapeutic treatment for alcohol, rather than a brief intervention (e.g., Stuart et al., 2013). However, there is also preliminary evidence that biologic treatments, such as medication or tailoring treatment based on genetic risk, may be beneficial in the treatment of co-occurring IPV and alcohol abuse. It would be important for future research to compare a psychotherapeutic intervention, like SADV, to a pharmacologic treatment, like an SSRI, to determine which treatments are the most efficacious and cost-effective for IPV perpetrators.

14.3 Conclusions

IPV is a serious public health problem that results in physical (Black et al., 2011), emotional (Black et al., 2011; Breiding et al., 2014), and economic (Jones, 2000) consequences. The current review explored the efficacy of various IPV interventions, including the Duluth model, CBT, conjoint treatments, military-specific interventions, substance abuse treatments, psychopharmacological, and acceptance- and mindfulness-based interventions. Even the most ardent supporters of the Duluth and CBT models can only assert that they demonstrate modest success rates (Gondolf, 2007). New interventions aim at boosting the efficacy of reducing IPV and tailoring treatments to specific groups (Babcock et al., 2004; Dutton & Corvo, 2006; Eckhardt & Schram, 2009; Labriola, Rempel, & Davis, 2008).

With the field's improved knowledge of the factors contributing to IPV perpetration, researchers are moving toward evidence-based treatments. Recently, there has been success with conjoint treatments (Karakurt et al., 2016), suggesting that couples therapy is efficacious for couples experiencing situational couple violence who want to remain together. However, only a limited number of studies have been conducted, in part for the commonly accepted and politically entrenched structure of same-sex group format for BIPs. The new-wave treatment, ACTV, has demonstrated promising results for court-ordered men (Zarling et al., 2017) and a community sample of men and women (Zarling, Lawrence, & Marchman, 2015). These findings are preliminary, as the first RCT examining ACTV's efficacy when compared to BIPs is currently underway. Some limitations of ACTV include high rates of treatment dropouts and non-randomization of BIP participants, which may have impacted results. However, the principles of addressing relationship communication problems and emotional regulation appear to be promising new additions to battering intervention curricula.

Additional evidence argues for targeting treatments for populations at a greater risk for IPV (i.e., military and substance abusing populations). Strength at Home (SAH) provides the first efficacious treatment for male veterans with co-occurring

PTSD and IPV perpetration. Though a limited number of studies have been conducted, the VA has adopted SAH across the United States. More large-scale studies of SAH are forthcoming. As with many IPV treatments, SAH targets male veterans without co-occurring PTSD and substance use. Given the high comorbidity of IPV and substance use among veterans, logical next steps would be to examine SAH's appropriateness for treating substance abuse-related IPV as well as its efficacy with female veterans. Another promising approach to IPV treatment utilizes an integrated substance abuse and IPV treatment (e.g., SADV), as the two are likely to co-occur. A limited number of studies have tested its efficacy at reducing both substance use and partner violence, but preliminary results have demonstrated long-term effects (Easton et al., 2007, 2017).

Considering high dropout rates of Duluth, CBT (Bennett, Stoops, Call, & Flett, 2007; Buttell & Carney, 2002; Daly & Pelowski, 2000), and ACTV (Zarling et al., 2017), even when perpetrators are court-mandated to attend, more research is needed to address factors that contribute to high dropout rates as well as methods to motivate individuals to complete treatment. Additionally, there appear to be gaps in the literature regarding mechanisms of change in relation to treatments for IPV. Future research may benefit from examining the mechanisms of change in order to create more effective and efficient treatments. Furthermore, research examining what types of treatment is most effective for different types of partner violence (e.g., situational, characterological) may prove beneficial, as individuals use violence for different reasons, thus potentially impacting treatment outcomes (Cantos & O'Leary, 2014). Overall, recent, novel battering intervention programs have demonstrated preliminary efficacy in reducing intimate partner violence. Although these programs are greatly needed, more research is required to address the gaps in the current interventions including uncovering mechanisms of change and how to reduce dropout rates, adapt curriculum for female perpetrators, ensure generalizability to ethnic and racially diverse populations, and maintain cessation or reduction of violence over the long term.

Due to most states mandating the use of a Duluth model type of curriculum for battering intervention programs, researchers experience hurdles when attempting to test different interventions, especially those that do not adhere to the same-sex group format. Without continued legislative changes, the development of novel interventions will continue to be hindered. Our goal is not to undermine coordinated community responses to domestic violence or upend the battering intervention industry. Rather, our goal is to find and disseminate interventions or therapeutic techniques that are empirically shown to decrease or stop intimate partner violence. Our previous meta-analysis found existing battering interventions to have only a small effect at stopping intimate partner assaults (Babcock et al., 2004), but in the past we could offer little advice as to what to do instead. We speculated that just as general field of clinical psychology moved away from dogma and toward evidence-based practice, more novel treatments would emerge that work to reduce or stop partner violence (Babcock et al., 2007). The recent push toward evidence-based practice is slowly revealing new directions for alternative treatment modalities, techniques, and curricula that include formerly taboo ideas of couples-based approaches, alcohol as a causal or facilitating factor in violence, and emotion-focused work. The path to developing empirically supported treatments for domestic violence appears to require thinking outside the state-mandated box of men-only, feminist psychoeducational group interventions and tailoring the treatment to the individuals and couples devastated by domestic abuse.

References

Alexander, C. J. (2002). Violence in gay and lesbian relationships. *Journal of Gay & Lesbian Social Services, 14*(1), 95–98. https://doi.org/10.1300/J041v14n01_06

Armenti, N. A., Iyican, S., Sommer, J. M., & Babcock, J. C. (2017). Treatment of batterers: What works? In P. Sturmey (Ed.), *The Wiley handbook of violence and aggression*. New York, NY: Wiley.

Babcock, J. C., Armenti, N. A., & Warford, P. (2017). The trials and tribulations of testing couples-based interventions for intimate partner violence. *Partner Abuse, 8*(1), 110–122. https://doi.org/10.1891/1946-6560.8.1.110

Babcock, J. C., Canady, B., Graham, K. H., & Schart, L. (2007). The evolution of battering interventions: From the dark ages into the scientific age. In J. Hamel & T. Nicholls (Eds.), *Family therapy for domestic violence: A practitioner's guide to gender-inclusive research and treatment* (pp. 215–244). New York, NY: Springer Publishing Company.

Babcock, J. C., Green, C. E., & Robie, C. (2004). Does batterers' treatment work? A meta-analytic review of domestic violence treatment. *Clinical Psychology Review, 23*(8), 1023–1053. https://doi.org/10.1016/j.cpr.2002.07.001

Babcock, J. C., Miller, S. A., & Siard, C. (2003). Toward a typology of abusive women: Differences between partner-only and generally violent women in the use of violence. *Psychology of Women Quarterly, 27*(2), 153–161. https://doi.org/10.1111/1471-6402.00095

Babcock, J. C., & Steiner, R. (1999). The relationship between treatment, incarceration, and recidivism of battering: A program evaluation of Seattle's coordinated community response to domestic violence. *Journal of Family Psychology, 13*(1), 46–59. https://doi.org/10.1037/0893-3200.13.1.46

Bennett, L. W., Stoops, C., Call, C., & Flett, H. (2007). Program completion and re-arrest in a batterer intervention system. *Research on Social Work Practice, 17*(1), 42–54. https://doi.org/10.1177/1049731506293729

Black M. C., Basile, K. C., Breiding, M. J., Smith S. G., Walters M. L., Merrick M. T., … & Stevens, M. R. (2011). *The national intimate partner and sexual violence survey (NISVS): 2010 summary report*. Atlanta, GA: National Center for Injury Prevention and Control, Centers for Disease Control and Prevention. Retrieved from https://www.cdc.gov/violenceprevention/nisvs/summaryreports.html

Bradley, R. P. C., Drummey, K., Gottman, J. M., & Gottman, J. S. (2014). Treating couples who mutually exhibit violence or aggression: Reducing behaviors that show a susceptibility for violence. *Journal of Family Violence, 29*(5), 549–558. https://doi.org/10.1007/s10896-014-9615-4

Bradley, R. P. C., & Gottman, J. M. (2012). Reducing situational violence in low-income couples by fostering healthy relationships. *Journal of Marital and Family Therapy, 38*(s1), 187–198. https://doi.org/10.1111/j.1752–0606.2012.00288.x

Bradley, R. P. C., Friend, D. J., & Gottman, J. M. (2011). Supporting healthy relationships in low-income, violent couples: Reducing conflict and strengthening relationship skills and satisfaction. *Journal of Couple & Relationship Therapy, 10*(2), 97–116. https://doi.org/10.1080/15332691.2011.562808

Brand, P. A., & Kidd, A. H. (1986). Frequency of physical aggression in heterosexual and female homosexual dyads. *Psychological Reports, 59*(3), 1307–1313. https://doi.org/10.2466/pr0.1986.59.3.1307

Breiding, M. J., Basile, K. C., Smith, S. G., Black, M. C., & Mahendra, R. R. (2015). *Intimate partner violence surveillance: Uniform definitions and recommended data elements, version 2.0*. Atlanta, GA: National Center for Injury Prevention and Control, Centers for Disease Control and Prevention. Retrieved from https://www.cdc.gov/violenceprevention/intimatepartnerviolence/definitions.html

Breiding, M. J., Smith, S. G., Basile, K. C., Walters, M. L., Chen, J., & Merrick, M. T. (2014). Prevalence and characteristics of sexual violence, stalking, and intimate partner violence victimization—National Intimate Partner and Sexual Violence Survey, United States, 2011. *Morbidity and Mortality Weekly Report (MMWR), Surveillance Summaries, 63*(SS08), 1–18. Retrieved from https://www.cdc.gov/mmwr/preview/mmwrhtml/ss6308a1.html

Burke, L. K., & Follingstad, D. R. (1999). Violence in lesbian and gay relationships: Theory, prevalence, and correlational factors. *Clinical Psychology Review, 19*(5), 487–512. https://doi.org/10.1016/S0272-7358(98)00054-3

Buttell, F. P., & Carney, M. M. (2002). Psychological and demographic predictors of attrition among batterers court ordered into treatment. *Social Work Research, 26*(1), 31–41. https://doi.org/10.1093/swr/26.1.31

Caetano, R., Ramisetty-Mikler, S., & Field, C. A. (2005). Unidirectional and bidirectional intimate partner violence among White, Black, and Hispanic couples in the United States. *Violence and Victims, 20*(4), 393–406. https://doi.org/10.1891/088667005780927584

Cantos, A. L., & O'Leary, D. K. (2014). One size does not fit all in treatment of intimate partner violence. *Partner Abuse, 5*(2), 204–236. https://doi.org/10.1891/1946-6560.5.2.204

Chase, K. A., O'Farrell, T. J., Murphy, C. M., Fals-Stewart, W., & Murphy, M. (2003). Factors associated with partner violence among female alcoholic patients and their male partners. *Journal of Studies on Alcohol, 64*(1), 137–149. https://doi.org/10.15288/jsa.2003.64.137

Daly, J. E., & Pelowski, S. (2000). Predictors of dropout among men who batter: A review of with implications for research and practice. *Violence and Victims, 15*(2), 137–160. Retrieved from http://psycnet.apa.org/record/2000-16729-002

Dunford, F. W. (2000). The San Diego navy experiment: An assessment of interventions for men who assault their wives. *Journal of Consulting and Clinical Psychology, 68*(3), 468–476. https://doi.org/10.1037/0022-006x.68.3.468

Dutton, D. G., & Corvo, K. (2006). Transforming a flawed policy: A call to revive psychology and science in domestic violence research and practice. *Aggression and Violent Behavior, 11*(5), 457–483. https://doi.org/10.1016/j.avb.2006.01.007

Easton, C. J., Crane, C. A., & Mandel, D. (2017). A randomized controlled trial assessing the efficacy of cognitive behavioral therapy for substance-dependent domestic violence offenders: An integrated substance abuse-domestic violence treatment approach (SADV). *Journal of Marital and Family Therapy, 44*, 483. https://doi.org/10.1111/jmft.12260

Easton, C. J., Mandel, D. L., Hunkele, K. A., Nich, C., Rounsaville, B. J., & Carroll, K. M. (2007). A cognitive behavioral therapy for alcohol-dependent domestic violence offenders: An integrated substance abuse-domestic violence treatment approach (SADV). *The American Journal on Addictions, 16*(1), 24–31. https://doi.org/10.1080/10550490601077809

Eckhardt, C. I. (2007). Effects of alcohol intoxication on anger experience and expression among assaultive men. *Journal of Consulting and Clinical Psychology, 75*(1), 61–71. https://doi.org/10.1037/0022-006X.75.1.61

Eckhardt, C. I., Murphy, C. M., Whitaker, D. J., Sprunger, J., Dykstra, R., & Woodard, K. (2013). The effectiveness of intervention programs for perpetrators and victims of intimate partner violence. *Partner Abuse, 4*(2), 196–231. https://doi.org/10.1891/1946-6560.4.2.196

Eckhardt, C. I., & Schram, J. (2009). Cognitive behavioral interventions for partner abusive men. In P. Lehmann & C. A. Simmons (Eds.), *Strengths-based batterer intervention: A new paradigm in ending family violence* (pp. 137–188). New York, NY: Springer Publishing Company.

Feder, L., & Dugan, L. (2002). A test of the efficacy of court-mandated counseling for domestic violence offenders: The Broward experiment. *Justice Quarterly, 19*(2), 343–375. https://doi.org/10.1080/07418820200095271

Friend, D. J., Bradley, R. P. C., Thatcher, R., & Gottman, J. M. (2011). Typologies of intimate partner violence: Evaluation of a screening instrument for differentiation. *Journal of Family Violence, 26*, 551–563. https://doi.org/10.1007/s10896-011-9392-2

Foran, H. M., & O'Leary, K. D. (2008). Alcohol and intimate partner violence: A meta-analytic review. *Clinical Psychology Review, 28*(7), 1222–1234. https://doi.org/10.1016/j.cpr.2008.05.001

George, D. T., Phillips, M. J., Doty, L., Umhau, J. C., & Rawlings, R. R. (2006). A model linking biology, behavior, and psychiatric diagnoses in perpetrators of domestic violence. *Medical Hypotheses, 67*(2), 345–353. https://doi.org/10.1016/j.mehy.2006.01.049

George, D. T., Phillips, M. J., Lifshitz, M., Lionetti, T. A., Spero, D. E., Ghassemzedeh, N., … Rawlings, R. R. (2011). Fluoxetine treatment of alcoholic perpetrators of domestic violence: A 12-week, double-blind, randomized, placebo-controlled intervention study. *Journal of Clinical Psychiatry, 72*(1), 60–65. https://doi.org/10.4088/JCP.09m05256gry

Gondolf, E. W. (2004). Evaluating batterer counseling programs: A difficult task showing some effects and implications. *Aggression and Violent Behavior, 9*(6), 605–631. https://doi.org/10.1016/j.avb.2003.06.001

Gondolf, E. W. (2007). Theoretical and research support for the Duluth model: A reply to Dutton and Corvo. *Aggression and Violent Behavior, 12*(6), 644–657. https://doi.org/10.1016/j.avb.2007.03.001

Gondolf, E., Bennett, L., & Mankowski, E. (2018). Lessons in program evaluation: The ACTV batterer program study and its claims. *Violence Against Women*. https://doi.org/10.1177/1077801217741994

Gottman, J. M. (1994). *What predicts divorce? The relationship between marital processes and marital outcomes*. Hillsdale, NJ: Lawrence Erlbaum Associates.

Gottman, J., & Silver, N. (2000). *The seven principles for making marriage work: A practical guide from the country's foremost relationship expert*. New York, NY: Three Rivers Press.

Hayes, S. C., Strosahl, K. D., & Wilson, K. G. (1999). *Acceptance and commitment therapy: An experiential approach to behavior change*. New York, NY: The Guilford Press.

Healey, K., Smith, C., & O'Sullivan, C. (1998). *Batterer intervention: Program approaches and criminal justice strategies*. Rockville, MD: National Institute of Justice. Retrieved from https://www.ncjrs.gov/App/Publications/abstract.aspx?ID=168638

Holtzworth-Munroe, A., Bates, L., Smutzler, N., & Sandin, E. (1997). A brief review of the research on husband violence: Part I: Maritally violent versus nonviolent men. *Aggression and Violent Behavior, 2*(1), 65–99. https://doi.org/10.1016/S1359-1789(96)00015-8

Holtzworth-Munroe, A., & Stuart, G. L. (1994). Typologies of male batterers: Three subtypes and the differences among them. *Psychological Bulletin, 116*(3), 476–497. https://doi.org/10.1037/0033-2909.116.3.476

Iowa Department of Corrections. (2012). *Return on investment: Evidence based options to improve outcomes*. Retrieved from http://publications.iowa.gov/13320/

Jacobson, N., & Gottman, J. (1998). *When men batter women: New insights into ending abusive relationships*. New York, NY: Simon & Schuster.

Johnson, M. P. (2006). Conflict and control: Gender symmetry and asymmetry in domestic violence. *Violence Against Women, 12*(11), 1003–1018. https://doi.org/10.1177/1077801206293328

Johnson, M. P., & Ferraro, K. (2000). Research on domestic violence in the 1990's: Making distinctions. *Journal of Marriage and Family, 62*(4), 948–963. https://doi.org/10.1111/j.1741-3737.2000.00948.x

Jones, A. S. (2000). The cost of batterer intervention programs: How much and who pays. *Journal of Interpersonal Violence, 15*(6), 566–586. https://doi.org/10.1177/088626000015006002

Karakurt, G., Whiting, K., van Esch, C., Bolen, S. D., & Calabrese, J. R. (2016). Couples therapy for intimate partner violence: A systematic review and meta-analysis. *Journal of Marital & Family Therapy, 42*(4), 567–583. https://doi.org/10.1111/jmft.12178

Kelly, J. B., & Johnson, M. P. (2008). Differentiation among types of intimate partner violence: Research update and implications for interventions. *Family Court Review, 46*(3), 476–499. https://doi.org/10.1111/j.1744-1617.2008.00215.x

Labriola, M., Rempel, M., & Davis, R. C. (2008). Do batterer programs reduce recidivism? Results from a randomized trial in the Bronx. *Justice Quarterly, 25*(2), 252–282. https://doi.org/10.1080/07418820802024945

LaTaillade, J. J., Epstein, N. B., & Werlinich, C. A. (2006). Conjoint treatment of IPV: A cognitive behavioral approach. *Journal of Cognitive Psychotherapy, 20*(4), 393–410. https://doi.org/10.1891/jcpiq-v20i4a005

Lawrence, E., Langer Zarling, A., & Orengo-Aguayo, R. (2014). *Achieving change through value-based behavior (ACTV)*. Iowa City, IA: University of Iowa Foundation.

Leone, J. M., Johnson, M. P., & Cohan, C. L. (2007). Victim help seeking: Differences between intimate terrorism and situational couple violence. *Family Relations, 56*(5), 427–439. https://doi.org/10.1111/j.1741-3729.2007.00471.x

Lockhart, L. L., White, B. W., Causby, V., & Isaac, A. (1994). Letting out the secret: Violence in lesbian relationships. *Journal of Interpersonal Violence, 9*(4), 469–492. https://doi.org/10.1177/088626094009004003

Love, A. R., Morland, L. A., Menez, U., Taft, C., Macdonald, A., & Mackintosh, M.-A. (2015). "Strength at Home" intervention for male veterans perpetrating intimate partner aggression: Perceived needs survey of therapists and pilot effectiveness study. *Journal of Interpersonal Violence, 30*(13), 2344–2362. https://doi.org/10.1177/0886260514552445

Marshall, A. D., Panuzio, J., & Taft, C. T. (2005). Intimate partner violence among military veterans and active duty servicemen. *Clinical Psychology Review, 25*(7), 862–876. https://doi.org/10.1016/j.cpr.2005.05.009

Messinger, A. M. (2011). Invisible victims: Same-sex IPV in the national violence against women survey. *Journal of Interpersonal Violence, 26*(11), 2228–2243. https://doi.org/10.1177/0886260510383023

Morrel, T. M., Elliot, J. D., Murphy, C. M., & Taft, C. T. (2003). Cognitive behavioral and supportive group treatments for partner-violent men. *Behavior Therapy, 34*(1), 77–95. https://doi.org/10.1016/s0005-7894(03)80023-0

Murphy, C. M., & Eckhardt, C. I. (2005). *Treating the abusive partner: An individualized cognitive-behavioral approach*. New York, NY: The Guilford Press.

National Center for Injury Prevention and Control. (2003). *Costs of intimate partner violence against women in the United States*. Atlanta, GA: Centers for Disease Control and Prevention. Retrieved from https://www.cdc.gov/violenceprevention/pub/IPV_cost.html

O'Leary, K. D. (1996). Physical aggression in intimate relationships can be treated within a marital context under certain circumstances. *Journal of Interpersonal Violence, 11*(3), 450–452. https://doi.org/10.1177/088626096011003011

O'Leary, K. D., Heyman, R. E., & Neidig, P. H. (1999). Treatment of wife abuse: A comparison of gender-specific and conjoint approaches. *Behavior Therapy, 30*(3), 475–505. https://doi.org/10.1016/S0005-7894(99)80021-5

Pence, E., & Paymar, M. (1993). *Education group for men who batter: The Duluth model*. New York, NY: Springer Publishing Company.

Saltzman, L. E., Fanslow, J. L., McMahon, P. M., & Shelley, G. A. (2002). *Intimate partner violence surveillance: Uniform definitions and recommended data elements, version 1.0*. Atlanta, GA: National Center for Injury Prevention and Control, Centers for Disease Control and Prevention. Retrieved from https://www.cdc.gov/violenceprevention/pdf/ipv/intimate-partner-violence.pdf

Schumacher, J. A., & Leonard, K. E. (2005). Husbands' and wives' marital adjustment, verbal aggression, and physical aggression as longitudinal predictors of physical aggression in early marriage. *Journal of Consulting and Clinical Psychology, 73*(1), 28–37. https://doi.org/10.1037/0022-006X.73.1.28

Shapiro, A. F., & Gottman, J. M. (2005). Effects on marriage of a psycho-communicative-educational intervention with couples undergoing the transition to parenthood. *Journal of Family Communication, 5*(1), 1–24. https://doi.org/10.1207/s15327698jfc0501_1

Sonkin, D. J., Martin, D., & Walker, L. E. A. (1985). *The male batterer: A treatment approach*. New York, NY: Springer Publishing Company.

Straus, M. A. (2004). Prevalence of violence against dating partners by male and female university students worldwide. *Violence Against Women, 10*(7), 790–811. https://doi.org/10.1177/1077801204265552

Straus, M. A. (2008). Dominance and symmetry in partner violence by male and female university students in 32 nations. *Children and Youth Services Review, 30*(3), 252–275. https://doi.org/10.1016/j.childyouth.2007.10.004

Stuart, G. L., McGreary, J., Shorey, R. C., & Knopik, V. S. (2016). Genetics moderate alcohol and intimate partner violence treatment outcomes in a randomized controlled trial of hazardous drinking men in batterer intervention programs: A preliminary investigation. *Journal of Consulting and Clinical Psychology, 84*(7), 592–598. https://doi.org/10.1037/a0040219

Stuart, G. L., Shorey, R. C., Moore, T. M., Ramsey, S. E., Kahler, C. W., O'Farrell, T. J., … Monti, P. M. (2013). Randomized clinical trial examining the incremental efficacy of a 90-minute motivational alcohol intervention as an adjunct to standard batterer intervention for men. *Addiction, 108*(8), 1376–1384. https://doi.org/10.1111/add.12142

Taft, C. T., Creech, S. K., Gallagher, M. W., Macdonald, A., Murphy, C. M., & Monson, C. M. (2016). Strength at Home Couples program to prevent military partner violence: A randomized controlled trial. *Journal of Consulting and Clinical Psychology, 84*(11), 935–945. https://doi.org/10.1037/ccp0000129

Taft, C. T., Macdonald, A., Creech, S. K., Monson, C. M., & Murphy, C. M. (2016). A randomized controlled clinical trial of the Strength at Home Men's program for partner violence in military veterans. *Journal of Clinical Psychiatry, 77*(9), 1168–1175. https://doi.org/10.4088/JCP.15m10020

Taft, C. T., Macdonald, A., Monson, C. M., Walling, S. M., Resick, P. A., & Murphy, C. M. (2013). "Strength at Home" group intervention for military populations engaging in intimate partner violence: Pilot findings. *Journal of Family Violence, 28*(3), 225–231. https://doi.org/10.1007/s10896-013-9496-y

Taft, C. T., Walling, S. M., Howard, J. M., & Monson, C. (2011). Trauma, PTSD, and partner violence in military families. In S. M. Wadsworth & D. Riggs (Eds.), *Risk and resilience in U.S. military families* (pp. 195–212). New York, NY: Springer Science + Business Media, LLC.

Turell, S. C. (2000). A diverse analysis of same-sex relationship violence for a diverse sample. *Journal of Family Violence, 15*(3), 281–293. https://doi.org/10.1023/A:1007505619577

Waltz, J., Babcock, J. C., Jacobson, N. S., & Gottman, J. M. (2000). Testing a typology of batterers. *Journal of Consulting and Clinical Psychology, 68*(4), 658–669. https://doi.org/10.1037/0022-006X.68.4.658

Wexler, D. B. (2013). *The STOP domestic violence program: Group leader's manual*. New York, NY: W. W. Norton & Company.

Whitaker, D. J., Haileyesus, T., Swahn, M., & Saltzman, L. S. (2007). Differences in frequency of violence and reported injury between relationships with reciprocal and nonreciprocal intimate partner violence. *American Journal of Public Health, 97*(5), 941–947. https://doi.org/10.2105/AJPH.2005.079020

Williams, J. R., Ghandour, R. M., & Kub, J. E. (2008). Female perpetration of violence in heterosexual intimate relationships: Adolescence through adulthood. *Trauma, Violence & Abuse, 9*(4), 227–249. https://doi.org/10.1177/1524838008324418

Yerke, A. F., & DeFeo, J. (2016). Redefining intimate partner violence beyond the binary to include transgender people. *Journal of Family Violence, 31*(8), 975–979. https://doi.org/10.1007/s10896-016-9887-y

Zarling, A. (2018). Reply to lessons in program evaluation: The ACTV batterer program study and its claims. *Violence Against Women*, 1077801218794301. https://doi.org/10.1177/1077801218794301

Zarling, A., Bannon, S., & Berta, M. (2017). Evaluation of acceptance and commitment therapy for domestic violence offenders. *Psychology of Violence*. https://doi.org/10.1037/vio0000097

Zarling, A., Lawrence, E., & Marchman, J. (2015). A randomized controlled trial of acceptance and commitment therapy for aggressive behavior. *Journal of Consulting and Clinical Psychology, 83*(1), 199–212. https://doi.org/10.1037/a0037946

Chapter 15
Can Psychopathy Be Treated? What the Research Tells Us

Mark E. Olver

15.1 Introduction

Psychopathy is a serious personality disorder marked by a constellation of interpersonal, affective, and behavioral characteristics. Interpersonally psychopathic persons are superficially charming, grandiose, deceitful, and manipulative. Affectively, they tend to be without a conscience, lack empathy and remorse for wrongdoing, and are impaired in the capacity to form stable affective bonds. And behaviorally, psychopathic individuals lead an impulsive, irresponsible, unstable lifestyle, frequently characterized by a persistent pattern of versatile, rule-defying behavior. High scores on the tool most frequently used to assess psychopathy, the Hare Psychopathy Checklist-Revised (PCL-R; Hare, 1991, 2003) or its derivatives, are associated with a host of antisocial behavioral outcomes including violence and other forms of criminal recidivism (Leistico, Salekin, DeCoster, & Rogers, 2008), institutional behavior problems (Guy, Edens, Anthony, & Douglas, 2005), failure on conditional release (Hart, Kropp, & Hare, 1988), and lengthier criminal careers (Olver & Wong, 2015). The base rates of psychopathy are approximately 15–25% in most adult male offender settings yet only approximately 1% in the general population (Hare, 1996).

This chapter provides an overview of the psychopathy treatment literature. It begins with a review of the challenges associated with working with psychopathic clientele, followed by a review of key findings from meta-analytic reviews in terms of what has been attempted, what has been shown not to work, and what approaches have promise. Specifically, characteristics of ineffective approaches and concordant research are reviewed, followed by a proposed treatment framework for promising approaches with recent findings. Although psychopathic offenders present as a high-risk–high-need group often resistant to change, the central premise of this

M. E. Olver (✉)
Department of Psychology, University of Saskatchewan, Saskatoon, SK, Canada
e-mail: mark.olver@usask.ca

E. L. Jeglic, C. Calkins (eds.), *New Frontiers in Offender Treatment*,
https://doi.org/10.1007/978-3-030-01030-0_15

chapter is that there is little reason to believe that they are not also capable of making substantive treatment changes and reducing their risk for criminal recidivism.

15.2 An Overview of PCL-R-Measured Psychopathy

For the purposes of this chapter, psychopathy will be operationalized by the PCL-R. Briefly, the PCL-R is a 20-item symptom construct rating scale designed to assess and diagnose psychopathic personality disorder. With each item rated on a 0 (characteristic absent), 1 (maybe/possible present), and 2 (characteristic present), possible scores range from 0 to 40 and represent the extent to which the individual rated has the characteristics of prototypical psychopathy. Results from confirmatory factor analyses demonstrate that the PCL-R items can be arranged into four first-order factors or facets (Neumann, Hare, & Newman, 2007) termed interpersonal (superficial, grandiose, deceitful, manipulative), affective (lack of remorse, callousness, shallow emotions, doesn't accept responsibility), lifestyle (need for stimulation, parasitic, lacks goals, impulsivity, irresponsibility), and antisocial (poor behavior controls, early behavior problems, juvenile delinquency, release failure, criminal versatility). Two items tend not to load on the factors (sexual promiscuity, multiple short-term marital relationships). Two second-order factors subsume the four facets; Factor 1 subsumes the interpersonal and affective facets, while Factor 2 subsumes the lifestyle and antisocial facets.

Typically rated on the basis of a comprehensive semi-structured interview and file review, PCL-R total scores of 30 have frequently been used to characterize psychopathy, although lower scores (e.g., 27) have been employed given the standard error of measurement, or for research-based archival ratings (e.g., 25), given that some of the interpersonal and affective traits may be underrated without the interview (Wong, 1988). The base rates of psychopathy previously referenced are generated from 25- to 30-point range of cut scores. An important distinction can also be made between psychopathy and antisocial personality disorder or ASPD; the latter is recognized as a formal entry within the fifth edition of *Diagnostic and Statistical Manual of Mental Disorders* (DSM-5; American Psychiatric Association, 2013) as well as previous editions of DSM, while the former is not. In essence, ASPD is a persistent pattern of rule-defying behavior captured most prominently in the lifestyle and antisocial features (i.e., Factor 2) but lacking most of the interpersonal and affective features as reflected in the DSM-5 symptom criteria for the disorder. Historically, the distinction between ASPD and psychopathy has been a source of some diagnostic confusion, but they are not one and the same (Hare, 1996).

In sum, psychopathy is a serious personality disorder marked by a constellation of stable and problematic traits. Although psychopathy is associated with high rates of criminal recidivism post-release and the PCL-R is a strong predictor of recidivism, not all psychopathic offenders inexorably reoffend violently or otherwise (Burt, Olver, & Wong, 2016).

15.3 Psychopathy and Therapeutic Pessimism

It may seem unsurprising that psychopathy has also been associated with therapeutic pessimism (Salekin, 2002), with such doubts about the rehabilitative potential of this client group dating back to the early works of Cleckley (1941), whose 16 criteria informed the development of the PCL-R. Indeed, research demonstrates high psychopathy persons to have high rates of treatment attrition from correctional programs, to struggle with motivation, and often showing limited improvement (Ogloff, Wong, & Greenwood, 1990). A meta-analysis of offender treatment attrition found PCL-R score and diagnosis of psychopathy to be among the strongest predictors of program noncompletion (Olver, Stockdale, & Wormith, 2011). Empirical examination at the PCL-R factor and facet level among offender populations has demonstrated Factor 1 to be associated with treatment-interfering behaviors (Hobson, Shine, & Roberts, 2000) and for scores on the affective facet specifically to be associated with increased treatment dropout (Daly, 2017; Olver & Wong, 2011), decreased therapeutic progress (Olver, Lewis, & Wong, 2013; Sewall & Olver, in press), and weaker working alliances, particularly the emotional bond between client and therapist (DeSorcy, Olver, & Wormith, 2017).

15.3.1 Challenges in Working with Psychopathic Offenders

Although it may seem self-explanatory, why are psychopathic offenders so challenging to treat and what accounts for these negative therapeutic correlates? Psychopathic offenders are more likely to display a series of treatment-interfering behaviors that can make them an administrative burden to institutions and a threat to the welfare of staff and rehabilitative progress of co-patients. For instance, psychopathic offenders can often be disruptive and attention seeking in group; they can monopolize or derail discussion, bully group mates, or deflect personal responsibility. They can be deceitful and manipulative, lying about a number of things both big and small, diminishing their credibility and potentially placing staff on guard. Psychopathic patients can also be adept at spotting vulnerable staff or patients, setting up alliances, and in some instances pitting one staff member against another. Most concerning, psychopathic offenders may attempt to manipulate staff or patients to provide special favors or break institutional rules (e.g., bringing in contraband), violate boundaries, or even develop personal or sexualized relationships. Psychopathic patients can be interpersonally abrasive and grandiose, antagonizing staff and patients, contributing to an uncomfortable and anti-therapeutic milieu. They can be overpowering in their interpersonal presentation, aggressive, argumentative, verbally abusive, and intimidating, keeping people at a distance and walking on eggshells so as not to provoke them. Accordingly, in such instances, psychopathic men are not challenged, they are not confronted on negative behaviors, they do not develop new prosocial behavior skills, and they do not benefit from treatment interventions.

As a result, staff can feel victimized by lies and deceit, they may feel preyed upon, or they may feel helpless and hopeless in their capacity to effect positive change. The failure of these men to develop and display authentic guilt, remorse, and empathy for their offenses may contribute to further feelings of failure. By contrast, staff may lash out angrily and retaliate, resort to their own verbal or emotional abuse, or conduct themselves in unprofessional ways not befitting a treatment service provider. Or, as alluded to above, staff may develop personal, romantic, or sexual feelings and commit serious boundary violations in a misguided effort to help the individual. In all, the consequences are an erosion of treatment integrity equating to increased attrition, reduced progress, and deteriorated alliances.

15.4 Meta-analytic Reviews of Treatment Outcome

Although therapeutic pessimism in the treatment of psychopathic persons is nothing new, neither are efforts to treat the syndrome of psychopathy. Salekin (2002) conducted one of the first meta-analyses of the treatment of psychopathy in an aggregate review of 42 studies that spanned 60 years of clinical research. Several themes were evident. First, there were a startling array of interventions employed that, among the most common, included psychoanalytic, therapeutic communities (TCs), and cognitive behavioral treatment (CBT) approaches, followed by less frequent interventions such as electroconvulsive shock therapy, pharmacotherapy, psychodrama, personal construct therapy, rational emotive therapy, and other unspecified interventions. Second, there was a range of indicators of treatment progress, such as personal and emotional developments that would seem to equate to changes in psychopathic personality (e.g., increased feelings of guilt, anxiety, and depression), prosocial changes in social and relationship realms (e.g., improved work ethic, strengthened relationships), or reductions in antisocial behavioral outcomes (e.g., decreased institutional infractions, reduced aggression, decreased criminal charges and convictions). Third, few of the studies involved controlled evaluations and several were case studies. Fourth, few investigations employed a validated operationalization of psychopathy, given that many predated the existence of such a measure (e.g., PCL-R), and it was unclear if a given client was necessarily psychopathic and thus what the nature was of the population being treated. Finally, few of the studies employed a structured assessment of offender risk and need (per the risk principle), which could inform treatment intensity and prioritize target areas for intervention (per the need principle).

These issues notwithstanding, in all, Salekin (2002) found that approximately 60% of the studies reported some improvement in their clientele, leading him to conclude “that there is little scientific basis for the belief that psychopathy is an untreatable disorder” (p. 79). Interestingly, the largest proportion of the studies employed psychoanalytic therapy, 59% of which reported success across 17 studies and 88 cases. CBT programs reported a 62% success rate, which was not meaningfully different from psychoanalytic approaches, based on 5 studies and 246 psychopathic cases. TCs were among the least effective with only a 25% success rate on the basis of 8 studies and 372 psychopathic clients.

Salekin, Worley, and Grimes (2010) conducted an updated review on a select sampling of more methodologically rigorous evaluations that redressed a number of shortcomings of studies from the previous review. In total, 13 studies were reviewed (k = 8 for adult, k = 5 for youth) that examined treatment outcomes of high psychopathy clientele. Common to these studies is that they all employed one of the PCL measures to characterize psychopathy and featured either TC- or CBT-based programs. Some programs were relatively brief, while others were high-intensity multimodal violence reduction programs. A number of the studies examined relevant criminal behavior criterion variables, and several (but not all) featured programs built on a foundation of more contemporary interventions aligned with the "what works" literature. In all, only three of the eight adult outcome studies reported a positive effect, in contrast to six out of eight youth studies. The results reaffirmed the challenging nature of this population to treat and indicated particular value in attempting to intervene with younger groups. With regard to the adult treatment outcomes, Salekin, Worley, and Grimes (2010) offer, "Of the two best methodological studies (Olver & Wong, 2009; Skeem, Monahan, & Mulvey, 2002), there is a glimmer of hope that some treatment may be helpful to at least some psychopathic offenders. Two other well-designed studies showed a negative effect (Richards, Casey, & Lucente, 2003; Van Stelle, Bulmer, & Moberg, 2004), and research to sort out what results in positive versus negative effects is needed" (p. 248). Of note, the two studies featuring positive effects were CBT-based programs, while the two studies with negative results were TCs. These studies speaking to characteristics of promising vs. ineffective treatment approaches, including further relevant works, will be reviewed in the remainder of this chapter.

15.5 Ineffective Therapeutic Approaches

15.5.1 The Penetanguishene Therapeutic Community Study

In 1992, Rice, Harris, and Cormier published a treatment report that turned the psychopathy treatment field on its head. This study would ultimately be the basis for the popular notion that "nothing works" in the treatment of psychopathic offenders. The report featured a special type of TC developed by psychiatrist Elliot Barker in the 1960s at Penetanguishene Mental Health Centre in rural Ontario, Canada. The facility primarily housed men who were adjudicated not criminally responsible (or legally insane in other jurisdictions), who suffered serious mental disorder and frequently had a history of serious violent crime, or who were on remand awaiting sentencing. The program was approximately 2 years in duration and was intense, with the men attending treatment 80 h per week, with a small cohort of men locked in a small room in close quarters, forced to confront each other's behaviors, issues, and conflicts. The men were frequently handcuffed to one another, performed all personal activities together, and were subjected to group pressures, sleep deprivation, and occasional fasting. Frequently, heavy sedative or hallucinogenic drugs were prescribed to patients by their own co-patients, and administered by a nurse or physician, to reduce defensiveness and promote cooperation.

Rice, Harris, and Cormier (1992) conducted an archival quasi-experimental evaluation of this program several years after its discontinuation, with the PCL-R rated on the men from institutional file information. In total, 176 men were divided into high (PCL-R 25+) and low (PCL-R < 25) psychopathy groups as well as those who attended the TC and those who did not (i.e., TC vs. no TC, respectively). The men were then followed up in the community post-release to examine rates of recidivism and rehospitalization. Low psychopathy men who attended the TC had significantly lower rates of violent reconviction post-release (20%) compared to the no-TC low psychopathy men (35%). By contrast, 77% of high psychopathy men attending the TC were convicted for a new violent offense post-release, in contrast to 55% of no-TC high psychopathy men; a significant difference! Rice et al. (1992) concluded, "The results strongly suggest that the kind of therapeutic community described in this article is the wrong program for serious psychopathic offenders" (p. 408).

15.5.2 Characteristics of Ineffective Approaches

It is not hard to imagine why such a program was not effective, although the alarming reality was that the findings were taken by many as proof positive that psychopathic offenders not only could not be rehabilitated but that treatment probably made them worse. So why have some studies such as these generated negative findings? To this end, Simourd and Hoge (2000) offer, "At a practical level, the treatment of psychopaths has an interesting history, short on quantity and long on lore … Close examination of the treatment studies of psychopaths shows that most treatment efforts have failed to attend to the principles of effective correctional interventions" (p. 269).

In what many have considered to be the inaugural paper outlining the risk (match treatment intensity to offender risk level), need (target dynamic risk factors, aka criminogenic needs, for treatment), and responsivity (use CBT model of service delivery adapted to the client's unique needs and circumstances) principles of effective correctional intervention (also known as RNR), Andrews et al. (1990) conducted a meta-analysis of 80 correctional program outcome studies. Appropriate interventions (i.e., broadly adhering to RNR) generated the largest (30%) reductions in recidivism followed by unspecified programs (13% reduction); however, criminal justice sanctions (e.g., prison, more probation) alone generated a small increase in recidivism (7%) as did inappropriate programs (6%). Andrews et al. (1990) defined inappropriate programs as nondirective, unstructured general counselling-based approaches or milieu-based approaches that placed an emphasis on within-group communication and consequent failure to target criminogenic need. An updated meta-analysis (Andrews & Bonta, 2010) of 374 studies reaffirmed these findings, with little reduction in recidivism found for programs adhering to only one RNR principle (ES = 0.02) and successively larger reductions in recidivism associated with adherence to two (ES = 0.18) vs. all three (ES = 0.26) principles. By contrast, as with the previous review, inappropriate services (ES = −0.01) and criminal justice sanctions (ES = −0.03) were associated with small increases in recidivism.

In short, the Penetanguishene TC was not therapeutically aligned with the RNR principles; even though it predated formal articulation of RNR, programs existed at the time that did have components consistent with the model. The TC also had a number of features of inappropriate services. First, the program overtreated the men. Even the highest intensity programs are 400–500 h spaced out over several months, amounting to about 15 h of treatment per week (Hanson et al., 2017). In the span of several weeks, the Penetanguishene TC would meet and exceed this dose. Relatedly, men were not screened for recidivism risk, and consequently low- and high-risk offenders could be intermixed (or even shackled together) in the program, creating the potential for iatrogenic effects, manipulation, and victimization of vulnerable men. Third, the programs did not target criminogenic need (e.g., pro-criminal attitudes, criminal peers, substance abuse, family/marital problems) or foster the development of prosocial behavior skills (e.g., problem-solving, vocational skills, assertiveness, anger control) essential to successful community reintegration. Fourth, the programs, rather, often had inappropriate therapeutic foci, such as sharing and expressing feelings, fostering empathy, and instilling guilt, which did little to reduce risk and had the potential to involve the development of skills that could be misused. Fifth, a number of the interventions were frankly inappropriate and actively harmful, such as involuntary administration of drugs or exposure to group and environmental stressors. Finally, there was little staff supervision or input, and hence many missed opportunities for what would later be termed core correctional practices (Dowden & Andrews, 2004), such as prosocial role modeling, a firm but fair attitude, effective use of authority, and effective use of disapproval among others. Rather, the men were left unsupervised to treat each other, at times with devastating consequences.

15.6 Promising Therapeutic Approaches

The Salekin reviews (Salekin, 2002; Salekin et al., 2010) give some room for cautious optimism, particularly with juvenile offenders, but also provide some potential insights as to what approaches may have promise in the treatment of psychopathic offenders. Arguably many criminal justice jurisdictions internationally have routinely been treating and managing psychopathic offenders within their prisons and hospitals, without the condition necessarily being formally diagnosed. Do such programs work? Is a different or specialized treatment approach needed for psychopathic offenders?

15.6.1 A Two-Component Model for the Treatment of Psychopathy: Overview and Rationale

Wong (2015) and colleagues (Wong, Gordon, Gu, Lewis, & Olver, 2012; Wong & Hare, 2005) assert that the treatment of psychopathy should have one primary goal in mind: to reduce violence or the potential for violence through a risk reduction treatment regime. The two-component model is grounded in this objective and the notion that the target of intervention is something that should be changeable and also linked to violence and/or antisocial behavior in general. Thus, should the objective of treatment be to change a psychopathic individual's emotional experience and character structure (i.e., Factor 1), to change their risk for violence and antisocial behavior (i.e., Factor 2), or both? Using the PCL-R as the operational definition of psychopathy, in a large cross-sectional study of PCL-R scores across adult age cohorts of 889 prison inmates, Harpur and Hare (1994) found that Factor 1 scores remained remarkably stable across the lifespan, while Factor 2 scores dropped precipitously, particularly after age 45. Moreover, Yang, Wong, and Coid (2010) conducted a multilevel modeling meta-analysis that examined the comparative predictive accuracy of nine forensic assessment tools for future violence, including the PCL-R and its constituent factors. While different clinical assessment measures generally yielded moderate and respectable predictive accuracy, the exception was the PCL-R factors, in which Factor 2 performed comparably to other stand-alone instruments (area under the receiver operating curve; AUC = 0.67) while Factor 1 did not (AUC = 0.56). Although other meta-analyses have found Factor 1 to predict recidivism outcomes, its predictive accuracy has consistently been substantially lower than that of Factor 2 (e.g., Guy et al., 2005; Leistico et al., 2008).

As such, there is little evidence that Factor 1 changes appreciably or that it is a particularly strong predictor of violence or other forms of recidivism. However, as noted at the outset of this chapter, evidence abounds that Factor 1, particularly the affective facet, embodies treatment-interfering characteristics and has linkages to negative treatment outcomes. As such, Wong (2015) and colleagues suggest that Factor 1 primarily constitutes a set of responsivity issues to be managed in order to retain psychopathic men in treatment. By contrast, evidence does exist that Factor 2 can change and, reflecting one's propensity for criminal behavior, is a stronger predictor of all recidivism outcomes. In addition, research has demonstrated that Factor 2 and its constituent facets have high correlations with dynamic risk assessment tools, that is, measures of criminogenic need (Douglas, Yeomans, & Boer, 2005; Olver & Wong, 2009; Simourd & Hoge, 2000; Wong & Gordon, 2006), underscoring its risk relevance. Accordingly, Wong (2015) and colleagues (Wong et al., 2012; Wong & Hare, 2005) assert that the Factor 2 domains and concordant criminogenic needs should be targeted for risk reduction services per the risk and need principles. In sum, this model emphasizes the correctional or forensic treatment of violence risk as the primary objective in the treatment of psychopathy, rather than attempting to fundamentally alter their personality traits. It is possible that some emotional or characterological changes can happen, which may be a side benefit, but this is not the mainstay of intervention.

15.6.2 Implementing Component 1

Managing Factor 1 as a set of responsivity issues is a challenging process, but it is critical to maintaining treatment integrity, promoting staff and patient safety, and retaining challenging clientele in treatment. Some guidelines are offered here.

Staff Training, Selection, and Support

Knowledge is power, and a key element of working with psychopathic offenders is for service providers to understand the construct and to be savvy about the population they are working with, especially their penchant for manipulation, tendency to push boundaries, and to develop a healthy expectation of the challenges that lie ahead. Moral and educational support is equally important in this line of work, as is selecting and training people for the job who may be a good fit (e.g., rehabilitative orientation, ability to maintain boundaries, conscientiousness, etc.).

Open Lines of Communication

Related to the above is the need for staff to maintain clear lines of communication and for the patients to be aware that staff do speak to one another. Staff should not be keeping secrets about patients from other staff. Even awareness of this reality can serve as a deterrent for some patients to attempt to curry favor with some staff and attempt to form alliances. This would extend to routine written documentation of all patient contacts in the patient's chart notes regular consultation and ward rounds to review patient progress.

Maintaining Boundaries and Managing Countertransference

Part of staff training is maintaining good boundaries with their clientele, which includes refraining from sharing much in the way of personal information; being able to recognize attempts at manipulation, to document and process these behaviors, and to not partake; and maintaining a warm but professional relationship. Part of this is awareness of, and management of, one's emotional reactions to the clients they work with (i.e., countertransference) to prevent unhelpful or unprofessional interactions.

Motivating the Unmotivated

The principles of Miller and Rollnick's (2002) seminal motivational interviewing (MI) work are essential for working constructively with challenging clients and briefly include the following: express empathy (i.e., providing validation, even though psychopathic individuals likely will not reciprocate), develop discrepancy (i.e., point out how self-defeating behaviors are sabotaging their best interests), roll with resistance (i.e., responding nondefensively to a client's opposition or reluctance to change), support self-efficacy (i.e., strengthen and support the client's belief in their ability to change), and avoid argumentation (i.e., adopt a nondefensive posture and refrain from a tug of war battle).

Core Correctional Practices (CCPs)

CCPs (see Dowden & Andrews, 2004) have much in common with MI but, briefly, reflect a collection of attitudes and interpersonal behaviors that shape positive interactions with offenders and help them learn to behave more prosocially. In brief, they include effective use of authority (i.e., fair but firm attitude), prosocial role modeling (i.e., role modeling the very behaviors they wish for their clients to exhibit), problem-solving (i.e., problem identification and resolution), effective use of community resources (e.g., application of skills to release contexts), and interpersonal relationships (i.e., a warm, empathic, and humane interpersonal style, consistent with general responsivity).

Managing the Working Alliance

As noted previously, some research has demonstrated that psychopathic offenders tend to struggle the most with the emotional bond with their therapists, as measured by the Working Alliance Inventory (Horvath & Greenberg, 1989). Given the affective deficits possessed by psychopathic offenders, greater progress may be engendered by focusing on other elements of the working alliance, such as common goals (e.g., violence reduction and community reintegration) and mutually agreed upon therapeutic tasks (e.g., cognitive restructuring, role-playing assertiveness, practicing time outs).

15.6.3 Implementing Component 2

Targeting Criminogenic Need

Psychopathic offenders have the same treatment targets as non-psychopathic offenders and are candidates for the same types and range of services. Psychopathic offenders, however, frequently score as high risk for a range of recidivism outcomes and have a larger number and density of criminogenic needs. Simourd and Hoge (2000), for instance, found, in a sample of 321 male federal inmates, that high PCL-R scoring men had more pronounced concerns on all of the central eight criminogenic needs including education/employment deficits, family/marital concerns, pro-criminal attitudes, substance abuse problems, criminal peers, poor use of leisure recreation, as well as more serious criminal histories. Consistent with the risk principle, psychopathic offenders are usually candidates for high-intensity risk reduction services, should be placed with other moderate- to high-risk offenders, and stand to benefit from a comprehensive multimodal program. Such programs are typically group oriented, with the opportunity for individual therapy, and target a number of criminogenic needs, consistent with the need principle. Some foci may differ, however, depending on whether the individual has committed a sexual offense and requires a sexual offender treatment program, or if they are a general violent offender with a history of nonsexually motivated violence, or if they have no history of violence, etc.

Assessing and Evaluating Risk

To link assessment and treatment per Component 2, a dynamic risk assessment would be conducted at the point of intake to assess risk to inform service intensity and to identify criminogenic needs to inform the prioritization of services. A dynamic tool such as the HCR-20 Version 3 (HCR-20-V3; Douglas, Hart, Webster, & Belfrage, 2011), Violence Risk Scale (VRS; Wong & Gordon, 1999–2003) or its Sexual Offense version (VRS-SO; Wong, Olver, Nicholaichuk, & Gordon, 2003–2017), a variant of the Level of Service Inventory (e.g., LSI-R; Andrews & Bonta, 1995), or other tools could be used to assess baseline risk and inform treatment planning. Repeated administration of a dynamic tool, at mid or end points, can be used to document treatment change and risk reduction, to identify outstanding treatment needs and inform potential follow-up services, release decisions, community supervision conditions or restrictions, and so forth.

Monitoring and Treating OABs and ORBs

Gordon and Wong (2010) use the term offense analogue behaviors (OABs) to refer to offense-linked proxy behaviors that can emerge in an institutional or secure custodial environment. The presence of OABs alerts the presence of criminogenic needs, such as pro-criminal attitudes, patterns of interpersonal aggression, antisocial peers, or impulsivity, that are manifested in an environment where supervision is tighter and structures and supports are available which may decrease opportunities for criminal behavior. For instance, aggressive and intimidating behavior toward staff and patients would be an indication that problems with pro-violence attitudes and aggressive interpersonal tendencies are prevalent and need to be managed. Similar inferences could be made about the presence or use of homemade weapons (an OAB for weapon use), adherence to the con code (OAB for criminal attitudes/orientation), accumulating institutional infractions (OAB for impulsivity), associating with "heavies" on the unit (OAB for criminal peers), and so on. By contrast, offense replacement behaviors (ORBs) refer to positive prosocial behaviors that are essentially opposite to OABs. For instance, assertive and nonaggressive interactions (an ORB for interpersonal aggression), taking a time out to de-escalate conflict (ORB for poor emotional control), avoiding high-status inmates (ORB for criminal peers), challenging and checking distorted perceptions (ORB for criminal attitudes), or learning a vocational trade and maintaining an institutional job (ORB for poor work ethic and unemployment) would all be illustrations of ORBs. In principle, progress, per Component 2, would be indicated by a decrease in OABs and concordant increase in ORBs.

An Illustrative Example: The Violence Reduction Program

As one illustration, the Violence Reduction Program (VRP; Wong & Gordon, 2013; Wong, Gordon, & Gu, 2007) is a high-intensity, RNR/CBT-based, risk reduction program for violent nonsexual offenders divided into three phases. In Phase 1, the VRS is administered at intake to assess risk level, identify treatment targets, and to assess readiness for change on the individual's dynamic risk factors. Individuals develop an understanding of their risk factors and causes of violence, and motivational interviewing strategies are used to help move the individual along the continuum of change. Phase 2 involves the acquisition of skills and strategies to reduce violence risk, such as anger management, restructuring cognitions and attitudes supportive of violence, developing problem-solving skills, strengthening communication skills, and developing alternatives to aggression. Targeting and managing OABs would be part of the treatment regime, particularly as articulated in Phase 2, but has relevance throughout a risk reduction program per Component 2. Phase 3 involves consolidation and transfer of these skills and the formulation of a relapse prevention plan to mitigate risk for future violence. The VRS would also be readministered posttreatment to assess risk reduction and treatment change and to inform possible further services, release decisions, and community release planning.

15.6.4 Promising Therapeutic Approaches: A Literature Recap and Update

Salekin (Salekin, 2002; Salekin et al., 2010) reviews have identified some programs and outcome studies that may lend some optimism for the treatability of psychopathic offenders. This section will review some of the promising programs and outcome studies, building on Salekin reviews, and commencing with the VRP.

Outcome Studies with Violent Offenders

The VRP has been implemented in different jurisdictions and was modeled off the aggressive behavior control (or ABC) program, which was a 6-month high-intensity violence reduction CBT program operated at a maximum security mental health correctional facility in Saskatchewan, Canada. Two outcome studies subsequent to Salekin et al. (2010) have been conducted via the VRP/ABC Program examining treatment responses of violent psychopathic offenders. First, Olver et al. (2013) examined treatment response in 152 men convicted for violent nonsexual offenses admitted to the program in the 1990s and followed up in the community an average of 5 years post-release. This was an exceptionally high-risk sample, with an average PCL-R score of 26 and an average VRS score of 61, the latter of which is approximately 1.5 SD above the normative mean for Canadian Prairie Region violent federal offenders (see Wong & Gordon, 2006). The VRS was scored pre- and posttreatment on the basis of comprehensive institutional file information, and associations were examined between changes in violence risk, as captured by the VRS pre-post change score, with postprogram violent recidivism in the community. VRS change scores were significantly associated with reductions in violent recidivism after controlling for PCL-R scores and, alternatively, Factors 1 or 2 through Cox regression survival analysis. The hazard ratio magnitudes ($e^B = 0.90–0.92$) indicated an 8–10% reduction in the hazard of violent recidivism for every one-point increase in change score, controlling for individual differences in psychopathy. In other words, men who had lowered their violence risk considerably, even those with substantial psychopathic traits, demonstrated lower rates of violent recidivism following the program and upon release to the community. As a further indication of this, high PCL-R men who demonstrated little changes in risk, assessed via the PCL-R, had significantly higher rates of violent recidivism over time than high PCL-R men who fared well in treatment; in turn, even psychopathic men who had lowered their risk had rates of violent recidivism that were not significantly different than other violent men who scored lower by comparison on the PCL-R.

Second, Wong et al. (2012) conducted a quasi-experimental examination of 32 psychopathic men (mean PCL-R 28.6) who had completed the ABC Program to a sample of 32 untreated psychopathic men (mean PCL-R 28), matched on a series of static and dynamic risk, criminal history, sentencing, and demographic variables. Upon follow-up, the two groups were not significantly different in frequency or number of new violent, nonviolent, or general convictions; however, the treated men had significantly shorter sum totals of aggregate sentences for new offenses compared to the untreated men. As sentence length can be taken as an indication of the severity of a criminal offense, treated psychopathic offenders were being convicted for less severe new crimes than the untreated psychopathic men, whose sum total of new aggregate offenses was more than double. Wong et al. (2012) argued this to be an illustration of harm reduction, in which case the treatment regime did not eradicate recidivism outright per se but may have decreased the severity of recidivism. To this effect, Wong and Hare (2005) write:

> … it would be a mistake to believe that … individuals with a history of predatory behavior will become model citizens. *Saul will not become Paul*, to use a biblical analogy. About the best we can hope for is that psychopaths who have gone through the [program] will be significantly (in a practical as well as statistical sense) less prone to engage in violent behavior than they were before the program. Still, even modest reductions in the use of aggression and violence by psychopaths would be of enormous benefit to society. (p. 9)

Finally, Salekin et al. (2010) noted the Skeem et al. (2002) investigation as providing promise for the treatment of psychopathic individuals. This study examined the association of psychopathy and treatment dosage to violent recidivism in a sample of 871 civil psychiatric patients from the MacArthur Violence Risk Assessment Study. Although the study did not feature violent offenders per se, violent recidivism was the primary outcome variable of interest. The study featured short-term verbal treatment plus medication as appropriate (0–10 weekly sessions) followed up over 5–10 week intervals in the community. Whether patients were classified as psychopathic or potentially psychopathic on the basis of their Psychopathy Checklist: Screening Version (PCL: SV; Hart, Cox, & Hare, 1995) scores, individuals receiving 0–6 sessions of treatment had higher rates of violence at a given follow-up than similarly psychopathic patients who received seven or more sessions. Of further interest, Skeem et al. (2002) found that treatment involvement was significantly associated with decreased violence (OR = 2.7) after controlling for several risk-relevant covariates, including PCL: SV score.

Outcome Studies with Sexual Offenders

Salekin et al. (2010) review briefly discussed Olver and Wong (2009), which examined treatment responses of a sample of 156 sexual offenders who had attended a high-intensity, CBT-based, sexual violence reduction program, the Clearwater Program, operated out of the same facility as the ABC Program. The men were rated on the VRS-SO (recall, the sexual violence risk assessment counterpart of the VRS) at pre- and posttreatment as well as the PCL-R from comprehensive institutional file information and followed up an average 10 years post-release. First, although as anticipated, high PCL-R scoring men had higher rates of treatment completion (26.7%) compared to non-psychopathic men (10.0%), importantly, nearly three quarters (73.3%) of the high psychopathy men managed to successfully complete the program; this simply illustrates that psychopathic offenders can be retained in treatment. High PCL-R successful treatment completers also had significantly lower rates of new violent charges and convictions (60.6%) than similarly psychopathic non-completers (91.7%). Changes in sexual violence risk, assessed via the VRS-SO change score, were also significantly associated with reductions in sexual and violent recidivism after controlling for baseline static risk and PCL-R total score. That is, substantive changes in sexual violence risk from pre- to posttreatment were associated with reductions in future sexual violence and any new violence, even for high psychopathy offenders.

Sewall and Olver (in press) extended this line of research, doubling the sample of Clearwater patients ($N = 302$), updating the recidivism data, and increasing the follow-up time to 18 years post-release. The men had previously been rated on the VRS-SO pre- and posttreatment, and new cases were subsequently rated on the PCL-R via file review. The study also served as a direct examination of the two-component model. Consistent with earlier findings, although psychopathic men were more likely to drop out of sexual offender treatment (29.9%), again, most high PCL-R scoring men (70.1%) successfully completed the Clearwater Program. Consistent with Component 1 of the two-component model, Factor 1, and specifically, the affective facet, was significantly and uniquely associated with treatment noncompletion and decreased therapeutic change. In contrast to Olver and Wong (2009), however, there were no significant differences in rates of sexual and violent reconviction over the follow-up between high psychopathy sexual offenders who did or did not successfully complete the program. Sewall and Olver (in press) suggested that treatment completion may be a relatively weaker proxy for risk reduction—that is, not everyone who completes treatment, completes it well—and as such, a measure of treatment-related changes in risk may be a more direct indication of benefit. Of note, the VRS-SO change scores of high PCL-R scoring men were not significantly lower than that of lower PCL-R scoring men. Accordingly, in Cox regression survival analyses, VRS-SO change score was significantly associated with decreases in both sexual and general violent recidivism, after controlling for PCL-R total score and individual differences on static and dynamic risk factors, consistent with Component 2. The magnitude of hazard ratios ($e^B = 0.90–0.91$) indicated an approximate 9–10% reduction in the hazard of future sexual or general violence, for each one-point increase in change score, controlling for psychopathy and baseline pretreatment risk.

Two additional psychopathy sexual offender treatment outcome studies also merit attention that was not captured in Salekin et al. (2010) review. These were also based in Canadian federal institutions (as with Clearwater) and featured moderate- to high-intensity CBT-based programs. Looman, Abracen, Serin, and Marquis (2005) examined treatment responses of a sample of 154 consecutive admissions to the Ontario Regional Treatment Centre's high-intensity sexual offender program. The PCL-R was rated on the sample from institutional file information, and treatment progress was coded in terms of whether the men were evaluated in their treatment reports at program end as (1) having progressed in treatment and (2) having reduced their recidivism risk. There were no differences in rates of violent recidivism among high psychopathy men (PCL-R 25+), who were judged as having improved vs. not improved; however, high psychopathy men who were appraised as having lowered their risk had lower (30%) rates of violent recidivism than similarly psychopathic men who were evaluated as not having lowered their risk (50%) at posttreatment.

A second evaluation featured a program of research conducted out of Warkworth Sexual Behavior Clinic (WSBC), a moderate intensity prison-based sexual offender treatment program in Ontario, Canada. The study featured a large sample of treated adult male federal sexual offenders who were rated on a measure of treatment behavior and the PCL-R. The measure of treatment behavior was dichotomized into high and low scores corresponding to positive vs. negative treatment behavior. The first of a series of evaluations was published by Seto and Barbaree (1999), who found that in a sample of 283 men, those scoring 15 or higher on the PCL-R and who displayed positive treatment behavior actually had significantly higher rates of violent recidivism over a 32-month follow-up than similar PCL-R scoring men in the negative treatment behavior group. In an updated evaluation, Barbaree (2005) extended the follow-up to 5 years post-release with more complete recidivism data obtained from a national database. Barbaree (2005) found that rates of violent recidivism were simply no different among the men scoring 15+ on the PCL-R who demonstrated positive (34%) vs. negative (30%) treatment behavior, concluding there was simply no treatment effect. In the most recent WSBC evaluation, Langton, Barbaree, Harkins, and Peacock (2006) expanded the sample to 418 sexual offenders who had attended the program and followed up 5 years post-release. Both sexual and violent recidivism, captured from national criminal records, were examined, and a PCL-R cut score of 25 was employed to characterize high and low psychopathy groups consistent with the extant literature. Using Cox regression survival analysis, Langton, Barbaree, Harkins, and Peacock (2006) found a significant interaction between psychopathy and treatment behavior, such that high psychopathy men demonstrating negative treatment behavior had significantly higher rates of sexual recidivism than similarly psychopathic men who demonstrated positive treatment behavior. The same trend was observed for general violence, although the interaction was not significant.

Characteristics of Promising Programs

A common thread among promising programs is that these are broadly grounded in the RNR principles and, at least on the surface, would appear to employ practices consistent with the two-component model, such that (1) most high psychopathy men are retained in treatment and successfully complete the program; (2) the programs are broadly CBT-based in their model and method of behavior change; (3) the programs explicitly target criminogenic need; (4) they are of a sufficient and appropriate intensity level for a moderate- to high-risk group of psychopathic violent or sexual offenders; and (5) they have a high level of staff involvement, with staff being explicitly trained in the treatment methods employed and the client population treated, providing coordinated service delivery, with careful supervision and monitoring of patients. When these basic components of programs can be implemented, we concur with the sentiments of Polaschek (2014) that, "Like other high-risk criminals, those with psychopathy can benefit from psychological treatment" (p. 296).

15.7 Conclusions and Future Directions

So, can psychopathy be treated? The answer is: *It depends*. It depends on how one defines treatment success, and it depends on the correctional treatment regime. If treatment success is defined as a reduction in violence or sexual violence and the agent driving the change is a credible, high-intensity, integrated, and evidence-informed change agent (e.g., such a comprehensive CBT program, ancillary programs, and coordinated release planning), then the answer is a qualified *yes*, and there is reason for cautious optimism. And as Polaschek (2014) and others (Salekin, 2002; Salekin et al., 2010; Skeem et al., 2002) contend, there is little reason to believe that psychopathic offenders might not also benefit in the same way as other high-risk high-need offender populations from treatment. And many correctional jurisdictions have been treating and reintegrating men and women with substantial psychopathic traits, who may not have necessarily been formally assessed as such, for years. But as this chapter illustrates, effective correctional treatment and risk management requires resources, teamwork, patience, staff training, as well as managerial, administrative, and organizational support for proper staffing, staff training, and maintenance of treatment integrity. It also requires the coordination of services, if nothing else, to help the transition from the institution to community. Further research will inform future practice. One possible way forward is to routinely assess psychopathy in a correctional treatment context (or to obtain archival ratings from past program evaluations) and examine what evidence exists that people with substantial psychopathic traits benefit any differently from other high-risk offenders with fewer traits and how frequently high psychopathy men do manage to successfully complete a program. As with other offender populations, the question may gradually shift from "if" psychopathic offenders can be treated to "what works" in the treatment of psychopathic offenders. Time and continued evaluations will tell.

References

American Psychiatric Association. (2013). *Diagnostic and statistical manual of mental disorders* (5th ed.). Washington, DC: Author.

Andrews, D. A., & Bonta, J. (1995). *Level of service inventory-revised (LSI-R): An offender assessment system. User's guide*. Toronto, ON: Multi-Health Systems.

Andrews, D. A., & Bonta, J. (2010). Rehabilitating criminal justice policy and practice. *Psychology, Public Policy, and Law, 16*(1), 39–55. https://doi.org/10.1037/a0018362

Andrews, D. A., Zinger, I., Hoge, R. D., Bonta, J., Gendreau, P., & Cullen, F. T. (1990). Does correctional treatment work? A clinically-relevant and psychologically informed meta-analysis. *Criminology, 28*(3), 369–404. https://doi.org/10.1111/j.1745-9125.1990.tb01330.x

Barbaree, H. E. (2005). Psychopathy, treatment behavior, and recidivism: An extended follow-up of Seto and Barbaree. *Journal of Interpersonal Violence, 20*(9), 1115–1131. https://doi.org/10.1177/0886260505278262

Burt, G. N., Olver, M. E., & Wong, S. C. P. (2016). Investigating characteristics of the nonrecidivating psychopathic offender. *Criminal Justice and Behavior, 43*(12), 1741–1760. https://doi.org/10.1177/0093854816661215

Cleckley, H. (1941). *The mask of sanity*. St. Louis, MO: Mosby.
Daly, T. E. (2017). *Why are psychopaths difficult to treat? Testing the two-component model for the treatment of PCL psychopaths* (Unpublished doctoral dissertation). Victoria University of Wellington, Wellington, New Zealand.
DeSorcy, D. R., Olver, M. E., & Wormith, J. S. (2017). Working alliance and psychopathy: Linkages to treatment outcome in a sample of treated sexual offenders. *Journal of Interpersonal Violence*. Advance online publication. https://doi.org/10.1177/0886260517698822
Douglas, K. S., Hart, S. D., Webster, C. D., & Belfrage, H. (2011). *Historical clinical risk management (version 3): Professional guidelines for evaluating risk of violence [draft 2.1]*. Vancouver, BC: Mental Health, Law, and Policy Institute, Simon Fraser University.
Douglas, K. S., Yeomans, M., & Boer, D. P. (2005). Comparative validity analysis of multiple measures of violence risk in a sample of criminal offenders. *Criminal Justice and Behavior, 32*(5), 479–510. https://doi.org/10.1177/0093854805278411
Dowden, C., & Andrews, D. A. (2004). The importance of staff practice in delivering effective correctional treatment: A meta-analytic review of core correctional practice. *International Journal of Offender Therapy and Comparative Criminology, 48*(2), 203–214. https://doi.org/10.1177/0306624X03257765
Gordon, A., & Wong, S. C. P. (2010). Offense analogue behaviours as indicator of criminogenic need and treatment progress in custodial settings. In M. Daffern, L. Jones, & J. Shine (Eds.), *Offence paralleling behaviour: A case formulation approach to offender assessment and intervention* (pp. 171–183). West Sussex, UK: Wiley–Blackwell.
Guy, L. S., Edens, J. F., Anthony, C., & Douglas, K. S. (2005). Does psychopathy predict institutional misconduct among adults? A meta-analytic investigation. *Journal of Consulting and Clinical Psychology, 73*(6), 1056–1064. https://doi.org/10.1037/0022-006X.73.6.1056
Hanson, R. K., Bourgon, G., McGrath, R. J., Kroner, D., D'Amora, D. A., Thomas, S. S., & Tavarez, L. P. (2017). *A five-level risk and needs system: Maximizing assessment results in corrections through the development of a common language*. New York, NY: The Council of State Governments Justice Center. Retrieved from https://csgjusticecenter.org/nrrc/publications/a-five-level-risk-and-needs-system-maximizing-assessment-results-in-corrections-through-the-development-of-a-common-language/
Hare, R. D. (1991). *Manual for the revised psychopathy checklist*. Toronto, ON: Multi-Health Systems.
Hare, R. D. (1996). Psychopathy: A clinical construct whose time has come. *Criminal Justice and Behavior, 23*(1), 25–54. https://doi.org/10.1177/0093854896023001004
Hare, R. D. (2003). *Manual for the revised psychopathy checklist* (2nd ed.). Toronto, ON: Multi-Health Systems.
Harpur, T. J., & Hare, R. D. (1994). Assessment of psychopathy as a function of age. *Journal of Abnormal Psychology, 103*(4), 604–609. https://doi.org/10.1037/0021-843X.103.4.604
Hart, S. D., Cox, D. N., & Hare, R. D. (1995). *The hare psychopathy checklist: Screening version (PCL:SV)*. Toronto, ON: Multi-Health Systems.
Hart, S. D., Kropp, P. R., & Hare, R. D. (1988). Performance of male psychopaths following conditional release from prison. *Journal of Consulting and Clinical Psychology, 56*(2), 227–232. https://doi.org/10.1037/0022-006X.56.2.227
Hobson, J., Shine, J., & Roberts, R. (2000). How do psychopaths behave in a prison therapeutic community? *Psychology, Crime and Law, 6*(2), 139–154. https://doi.org/10.1080/10683160008410838
Horvath, A. O., & Greenberg, L. S. (1989). Development and validation of the working Alliance inventory. *Journal of Counseling Psychology, 36*(2), 223–233. https://doi.org/10.1037/0022-0167.36.2.223
Langton, C. M., Barbaree, H. E., Harkins, L., & Peacock, E. J. (2006). Sex offenders' response to treatment and its association with recidivism as a function of psychopathy. *Sexual Abuse: A Journal of Research and Treatment, 18*(1), 99–120. https://doi.org/10.1007/s11194-006-9004-5

Leistico, A.-M. R., Salekin, R. T., DeCoster, J., & Rogers, R. (2008). A large-scale meta-analysis relating the Hare measures of psychopathy to anti-social conduct. *Law and Human Behavior, 32*(1), 28–45. https://doi.org/10.1007/s10979-007-9096-6

Looman, J., Abracen, J., Serin, R., & Marquis, P. (2005). Psychopathy, treatment change, and recidivism in high-risk, high-need sexual offenders. *Journal of Interpersonal Violence, 20*(5), 549–568. https://doi.org/10.1177/0886260504271583

Miller, W. R., & Rollnick, S. (2002). *Motivational interviewing: Preparing people for change* (2nd ed.). New York, NY: The Guilford Press.

Neumann, C. S., Hare, R. D., & Newman, J. P. (2007). The super-ordinate nature of the psychopathy checklist-revised. *Journal of Personality Disorders, 21*(2), 102–117. https://doi.org/10.1521/pedi.2007.21.2.102

Ogloff, J. D., Wong, S. C. P., & Greenwood, A. (1990). Treating criminal psychopaths in a therapeutic community program. *Behavioral Sciences and the Law, 8*(2), 181–190. https://doi.org/10.1002/bsl.2370080210

Olver, M. E., Lewis, K., & Wong, S. C. P. (2013). Risk reduction treatment of high risk psychopathic offenders: The relationship of psychopathy and treatment change to violent recidivism. *Personality Disorders: Theory, Research, and Treatment, 4*(2), 160–167. https://doi.org/10.1037/a0029769

Olver, M. E., Stockdale, K. C., & Wormith, J. S. (2011). A meta-analysis of predictors of offender treatment attrition and its relationship to recidivism. *Journal of Consulting and Clinical Psychology, 79*(1), 6–21. https://doi.org/10.1037/a0022200

Olver, M. E., & Wong, S. C. P. (2009). Therapeutic responses of psychopathic sexual offenders: Treatment attrition, therapeutic change, and long-term recidivism. *Journal of Consulting and Clinical Psychology, 77*(2), 328–336. https://doi.org/10.1037/a0015001

Olver, M. E., & Wong, S. C. P. (2011). Predictors of sex offender treatment dropout: Psychopathy, sex offender risk, and responsivity implications. *Psychology, Crime, and Law, 17*(5), 457–471. https://doi.org/10.1080/10683160903318876

Olver, M. E., & Wong, S. C. P. (2015). Short and long-term recidivism prediction of the PCL-R and the effects of age: A 24-year follow-up. *Personality Disorders: Theory, Research, and Treatment, 6*(1), 97–105. https://doi.org/10.1037/per0000095

Polaschek, D. L. L. (2014). Adult criminals with psychopathy: Common beliefs about treatability and change have little empirical support. *Current Directions in Psychological Science, 23*(4), 296–301. https://doi.org/10.1177/0963721414535211

Rice, M. E., Harris, G. T., & Cormier, C. A. (1992). An evaluation of a maximum security therapeutic community for psychopaths and other mentally disordered offenders. *Law and Human Behavior, 16*(4), 499–412. https://doi.org/10.1007/BF02352266

Richards, H. J., Casey, J. O., & Lucente, S. W. (2003). Psychopathy and treatment response in incarcerated female substance abusers. *Criminal Justice and Behavior, 30*(2), 251–276. https://doi.org/10.1177/0093854802251010

Salekin, R. T. (2002). Psychopathy and therapeutic pessimism: Clinical lore or clinical reality. *Clinical Psychology Review, 22*(1), 79–112. https://doi.org/10.1016/S0272-7358(01)00083-6

Salekin, R. T., Worley, C., & Grimes, R. D. (2010). Treatment of psychopathy: A review and brief introduction to the mental model approach for psychopathy. *Behavioral Sciences and the Law, 28*(2), 235–266. https://doi.org/10.1002/bsl.928

Seto, M. C., & Barbaree, H. E. (1999). Psychopathy, treatment behavior, and sex offender recidivism. *Journal of Interpersonal Violence, 14*(12), 1235–1248. https://doi.org/10.1177/088626099014012001

Sewall, L. A., & Olver, M. E. (in press). Psychopathy and sexual violence risk: Linkages to therapeutic change, treatment attrition, and recidivism. *Personality Disorders: Theory, Research, and Treatment*. https://doi.org/10.1037/per0000297

Simourd, D. J., & Hoge, R. D. (2000). Criminal psychopathy: A risk-and-need perspective. *Criminal Justice and Behavior, 27*(2), 256–272. https://doi.org/10.1177/0093854800027002007

Skeem, J. L., Monahan, J., & Mulvey, E. P. (2002). Psychopathy, treatment involvement, and subsequent violence among civil psychiatric patients. *Law and Human Behavior, 26*(6), 577–603. https://doi.org/10.1023/A:1020993916404

Van Stelle, K. R., Bulmer, C., & Moberg, D. P. (2004). Treatment retention of dually diagnosed offenders in an institutional therapeutic community. *Behavioral Sciences and the Law, 22*(4), 585–597. https://doi.org/10.1002/bsl.602

Wong, S., & Hare, R. D. (2005). *Guidelines for a psychopathy treatment program.* Toronto, ON: Multi-Health Systems.

Wong, S. C. P. (1988). Is Hare's psychopathy checklist reliable without the interview? *Psychological Reports, 62*(3), 931–934. https://doi.org/10.2466/pr0.1988.62.3.931

Wong, S. C. P. (2015). Treatment of violence prone individuals with psychopathic personality traits. In W. J. Livesley, G. Dimaggio, & J. F. Clarkin (Eds.), *Integrated treatment of personality disorder: A modular approach* (pp. 345–376). New York, NY: The Guildford Press.

Wong, S. C. P., & Gordon, A. (1999–2003). *The violence risk scale.* Saskatoon, SK: Regional Psychiatric Centre and University of Saskatchewan. Retrieved from http://www.psynergy.ca/VRS_VRS-SO.html

Wong, S. C. P., & Gordon, A. (2006). The validity and reliability of the violence risk scale: A treatment-friendly violence risk assessment tool. *Psychology, Public Policy, and Law, 12*(3), 279–309. https://doi.org/10.1037/1076-8971.12.3.279

Wong, S. C. P., & Gordon, A. (2013). The violence reduction programme: A treatment programme for violence-prone forensic clients. *Psychology, Crime & Law, 19*(5–6), 461–475. https://doi.org/10.1080/1068316X.2013.758981

Wong, S. C. P., Gordon, A., & Gu, D. (2007). Assessment and treatment of violence-prone forensic clients: An integrated approach. *British Journal of Psychiatry, 190*(Supplement 49), s66–s74. https://doi.org/10.1192/bjp.190.5.s66

Wong, S. C. P., Gordon, A., Gu, D., Lewis, K., & Olver, M. E. (2012). The effectiveness of violence reduction treatment for psychopathic offenders: Empirical evidence and a treatment model. *International Journal of Forensic Mental Health, 11*(4), 336–349. https://doi.org/10.1080/14999013.2012.746760

Wong, S. C. P., Olver, M. E., Nicholaichuk, T. P., & Gordon, A. (2003–2017). *The violence risk scale: Sexual offense version (VRS-SO).* Saskatoon, SK: Regional Psychiatric Centre and University of Saskatchewan. Retrieved from http://www.psynergy.ca/VRS_VRS-SO.html

Yang, M., Wong, S. C. P., & Coid, J. (2010). The efficacy of violence prediction: A meta-analytic comparison of nine risk assessment tools. *Psychological Bulletin, 136*(5), 740–767. https://doi.org/10.1037/a0020473

Chapter 16
Conclusion: Where Do We Go from Here?

Elizabeth L. Jeglic and Cynthia Calkins

16.1 Introduction

Since Martinson's, 1974 pessimistic conclusion that "nothing works" in correctional treatment, funding and support for rehabilitative efforts in the United States have stagnated. Internationally, however, the rehabilitation movement remained strong, and in the last several decades many of the leading correctional scholars have emerged from Canada, the United Kingdom, Germany, Australia, and New Zealand. It is during this time that Andrews, Bonta, and Hoge (1990) developed the Risk, Needs, Responsivity Model (see Chap. 2), which revolutionized correctional treatment and provided context for why previous researchers, such as Martinson and his colleagues, failed to demonstrate effectiveness. Concurrently, general psychotherapy researchers began conducting meta-analyses of psychotherapy outcome studies demonstrating that those who partook in psychological treatment were better off than 75% of those who did not receive treatment (Smith & Glass, 1977). It was within this backdrop that the evidence-based practice movement emerged and researchers and scholars in the psychotherapy field wanted to develop a means to disseminate effective interventions to those who were working in the field. To bridge the science-practice divide, a task force was established by Division 12 (Clinical Psychology) of the American Psychological Association which results in the development of evidence-based treatments (ESTs) and later to evidence-based practice (EBPs). While the development of ESTs and EBPs has not been without controversy (see Castelnuovo, 2010), they established the precedent for the integration and dissemination of research in the practice of psychology (Chambless & Ollendick, 2001). Simultaneously, with the advent of positive psychology (Seligman & Csikszentmihalyi, 2000), there has been a general movement in the field to move

E. L. Jeglic (✉) · C. Calkins
Department of Psychology, John Jay College of Criminal Justice, City University of New York, New York, NY, USA
e-mail: ejeglic@jjay.cuny.edu; ccalkins@jjay.cuny.edu

E. L. Jeglic, C. Calkins (eds.), *New Frontiers in Offender Treatment*,
https://doi.org/10.1007/978-3-030-01030-0_16

away from emphasizing psychopathology and instead focus on helping individuals live happier and more meaningful lives (Seligman & Csikszentmihalyi, 2000). This positive psychology movement formed the basis for strengths-based approaches in offender rehabilitation, which began to look at human beings more holistically. The positive psychology movement also influenced correctional interventions, as described in Chap. 3. The Good Lives Model (GLM; Ward & Gannon, 2006; Ward & Stewart, 2003) of offender treatment manages risk by helping those who have offended developed "Good Lives Plans" that are incompatible with offending.

From the general therapy literature, we have also learned that process issues cannot be ignored. As described in Chap. 5, regardless of the intervention, the therapeutic alliance is integral for behavior change regardless of whether dealing with general psychotherapy clients or those with a history of offenses. Further, as we learn in Chap. 6, there are characteristics of the therapist that can impact treatment outcome—both positively and negatively. While there is evidence that some of these traits, such as directiveness, can be taught, other characteristics, such as warmth and empathy, may be more innate. We also have to consider how the work itself may impact the therapist and how supervision and self-care practices can help to prevent burnout and vicarious traumatization. One area that has, to date, received little attention in corrections is the how diversity can impact treatment outcomes. While Andrews and Bonta (1998) have emphasized that diversity is encompassed within the responsivity principle of the RNR model, as explained in Chap. 7, we know little about how well therapists attend to issues of diversity and how this impacts treatment outcome within correctional programming.

The last two decades within psychology have marked the advent of numerous new interventions that have deviated from the traditional cognitive behavioral models. Among them, the third wave cognitive behavioral therapies—which include mindfulness and dialectical behavior therapy among others—focus more on the process and relationship to thoughts and emotions as opposed to the content of those thoughts and emotions themselves. These third wave methods have been added to complement many existing treatments based in traditional cognitive behavioral principles (Hayes & Hofmann, 2017). As we learned in Chaps. 8 and 10, practices such as dialectical behavior therapy and mindfulness have also been applied to corrections with some success. However, some of the most exciting work has occurred with populations that have traditionally been more resistant to change. Stinson, in Chap. 11, reveals how motivational interviewing may be uniquely suited for work with court-ordered clients, who are initiating treatment on a voluntary basis and may be resistant to change. As discussed in Chap. 14, these motivational practices may be particularly suited to treating perpetrators of interpersonal violence, as many are court-ordered to attend, and treatment dropout is common. Assertive community treatment approaches for justice-involved persons (i.e., FACT), discussed in Chap. 12, align with the RNR model and utilize the evidence-based ACT approach to build connections to the criminal justice system. Chapter 13, which describes MST interventions for juvenile offenders, demonstrates how a collaborative approach that uses the resources and skills of family caregivers can facilitate youth functioning and decrease criminality, improving the lives of youth as well as their families and others with whom they come into contact. Finally, Olver in Chap. 15 discusses the treatment of psychopathy, traditionally regarded as the clientele most resistant to change. Although early work suggested that treating psychopathic offenders could do more harm than good, more recent reviews give reason for optimism. Modest reductions in recidivism, that themselves have far reaching consequences, give renewed hope for this difficult to treat population.

As can be seen—there are new frontiers in offender treatment. Evidence-based practices from the general psychotherapy literature have begun to be translated for use in correctional settings. While the notion of evidence-based practice is still in its relative naissance within the criminal justice system, we are entering a new and more optimistic era, one where adaptations of "what works" from the general psychotherapy literature are being applied to court-involved clients. However, this does not mean that we can rest on our laurels, as much remains to be done, and the needs of justice-involved clients, as described in these chapters, are many. This volume concludes with the editors' visions and recommendations for the future of evidence-based interventions within the criminal justice system.

16.2 New Directions

16.2.1 Create a Task Force

While research on the effectiveness of correctional interventions has made considerable progress in the last several decades, it still lags behind that of the general psychotherapy literature. Most of what is known about the effectiveness of treatment for those who have offended comes from programs designed to treat sexual offenders, and even that research suffers from methodological limitations (Schmucker & Lösel, 2015; Seto et al., 2008).

While the "gold standard" of psychotherapy research still remains the randomized controlled trial (RCT), the ethics of such designs has been hotly contested by researchers involved in developing programs within the criminal justice field (see the debate between Marshall & Marshall, 2007, 2008 and Seto et al., 2008). Division 12 of the American Psychological Association (Clinical Psychology) has taken the lead in developing, evaluating, and disseminating research-based interventions. However, no corresponding organization exists for those who develop, evaluate, and implement evidence-based practice within the criminal justice system. Division 41 of the American Psychological Association is the American Psychology and Law Society (AP-LS), whose mission is "advancing the science of psychology-law and the translation of psychology-law knowledge into practice and policy" (American Psychology-Law Society, n.d.) has traditionally focused more on experimental rather than clinical aspects of forensic psychology, with issues related to offender rehabilitation generally occupying little interest. The Association for the Advancement of Cognitive and Behavior Therapy (ABCT) has a criminal justice special interest group (SIG); however, the organization is primarily based in the United States and does not have a large membership. Most of the researchers who are developing and evaluating treatment programs belong to the Association for the Treatment of Sexual Abusers (ATSA), though as the name suggests, the focus of this organization is primarily the treatment of those who have committed sexual offenses.

Consequently, we do not have a strong voice advocating broadly for evidence-based treatments within corrections. It is thus suggested that the leaders in the field come together (many of whom have authored chapters in this textbook) and form a forensic evidence-based treatment task force. This can be done through the development of a new organization or simply a working group of key stakeholders. The goal of the task force would be similar to the goals established by the Division 12 Task Force—to develop and disseminate evidence-based interventions. As such, researchers in the field could work together to develop interventions based upon the latest theory and research and establish an agreed upon set of criteria by which these interventions are evaluated. This research and the references to corresponding treatment manuals (where applicable) would be available online for use by clinicians in the field. Additionally, researchers could develop evaluative frameworks that could be shared, and clinicians using the intervention would be encouraged to gather their own program data and share it with a central depository.

16.2.2 Enhance Forensic Training

It is evident from the general psychotherapy literature that the therapist plays the biggest role in the effectiveness of an intervention (see Chaps. 5 and 6 for review), accounting for more variance in treatment outcome than any other treatment-related factor (Webb, DeRubeis, & Barber, 2010). Thus, the quality of the intervention is only as good as the person delivering it. In the general psychotherapy literature, process issues—such as the role of the therapist in treatment outcome—have been well researched. In addition, therapist training and supervision is integrated within most clinically focused doctoral level clinical psychology programs. However, within corrections, there is often no specific forensic training required. While there are some master's and doctoral programs that specialize in forensic psychology, the majority of individuals who work with court-ordered clients do not have any specialized forensic training (Jeglic, Hanson, & Calkins, 2016). As well, a "get tough" approach still predominates, despite knowledge that a challenging but supportive therapeutic alliance can more effectively motivate clients toward change. As such, specialized training for those who work in the field should be required. As reviewed in Chap. 6, there are issues that may be unique to clients who are involved with the criminal justice system, such as mandated treatment, power differentials, a lack of confidentiality in treatment, difficult and aggressive clients, exposure to details of trauma and heinous crimes, a lack of empathy for victims, work environments that are not supportive of rehabilitation, high caseloads, and little access to supervision, that make work with forensic clients particularly challenging. Without proper training and support, these issues can result in burnout and vicarious traumatization. In return, this leads to high job turnover, increased recruitment and training costs, lower client and therapist satisfaction, and poorer treatment outcomes (Greeson, Guo, Barth, Hurley, & Sisson, 2009; Park & Shaw, 2013). Therefore, everyone loses.

In addition, it is integral that those who work in corrections are familiar with the theory and research behind behavior change (Jeglic et al., 2016). As described in Chap. 4, cognitive behavioral interventions have been found to be the most effective for use with those in the criminal justice system. Both the RNR model and the GLM models highlight the need for tailoring the interventions to meet individual client needs—the clinician must be adept at understanding the conceptualization of the criminal behavior and applying appropriate evidence-based interventions to improve quality of life and diminish risk.

The American Psychological Association currently does not accredit forensic clinical doctoral training programs. As a result, there is no core curriculum for those who train to work in the field. While there are several certification programs—none of these is nationally recognized, and they do not focus on evidence-based practice. Hence, specialized training for those working in the criminal justice field must be required and standardized. This can be accomplished in one of two ways. First, a standard curriculum can be established within forensically oriented training programs, where students receive training in areas pertaining to evidence-based practice within corrections, models of correctional interventions, treatment development and evaluation, principles of behavior change, as well as clinical training and supervision on issues specifically related to working with clients in the criminal justice system, including self-care. Another option would be to have nationally accredited post degree certification programs where students with master's and doctoral degrees in psychology, mental health counseling, and social work would take the aforementioned curriculum to become certified as an evidence-based correctional therapist.

16.2.3 Address Diversity

Minority populations have long been overrepresented in the criminal justice system (Rosich, 2007), and as such there is a uniquely pressing need for practitioners and therapists to be more attentive to issues of diversity in justice-related contexts. Diversity not only in terms of race and ethnicity, but also interns of gender, sexual orientation, and religion among others. From the general therapy research, we know that factors related to diversity can impact treatment responsiveness (Meyer & Zane, 2013) and that understanding how someone identifies is integral to being a culturally competent therapist (Sue, Zane, Hall, & Berger, 2009). Further, as treatment providers we cannot ignore the overrepresentation of minorities who are incarcerated and how that may impact their experience within the criminal justice system. In an effort to address the importance of diversity, the APA established a Task Force for Reenvisioning the Multicultural Guidelines for the twenty-first Century which produced a report entitled *Multicultural Guidelines: An Ecological Approach to Context, Identity, and Intersectionality* (APA, 2017). While these guidelines apply broadly to all psychological clients, including those within the criminal justice system, there is no specific mention of factors that may be unique to this population. Further, we know little about how issues of diversity impact correctional treatment. This is particularly salient, as diversity is considered a responsivity factor, and this has been the least studied of the RNR principles. Consequently, we need a call to action for researchers and scholars to systematically evaluate the role of diversity in treatment outcome.

16.2.4 Think Outside the Box

Some of the most exciting and effective treatments in corrections today came about because those involved started to look at the problem differently. That is, they began to think outside of the box when it came to existing treatments. For example, in Chap. 14 the Duluth model of intimate partner violence is reviewed. This has been the dominant model of treatment for perpetrators of IPV in the field. This intervention is based upon the patriarchal model where a man engages in physical violence against a woman based upon patriarchal beliefs of dominance and control (Dobash, 1979). However, the research now shows us that many men do not engage in violence because of patriarchal beliefs and that women and same sex partners are also engaging in IPV, so that the Duluth model will not universally apply. This requires us to re-examine our assumptions and develop new interventions that address the varied root causes of the problem.

Similarly, we used to provide juvenile offenders with individual treatment, but there was little evidence that treating them in isolation of their environments was working. This led to the movement of holding children more accountable for their crimes and giving them longer sentences (Redding, 1997). However, as Hilary Clinton wrote—it takes a village—and that is exactly what the Multisystemic Therapy researchers found. By thinking of the youth as but one part of a larger socioecological model, it was quite obvious that treating the juvenile alone would not solve the problem. As described in Chap. 13, successful treatment of serious juvenile offenders requires working with the youth, their family, their school, and their community.

Some of the most exciting research is coming from the data on the treatment of those with psychopathy. It has long been clinical lore that those with psychopathy was not responsive to treatment and that treatment in fact made them worse. In Chap. 15, this myth is debunked, and we are shown that by training staff to manage the Factor 1 (character structure) and implemented high-intensity intervention to manage the Factor 2 (antisocial) behaviors, those with psychopathy can decrease their risk of recidivating.

16.2.5 Treat Clients Holistically

The principles of behavior change tell us that if we want to make a meaningful and lasting change, we must change our lifestyle (Young, 2014). The same can be said for treatment programs. One of the main criticisms of the RNR model has been its focus on criminogenic needs and risk to the detriment of a more approach-based goals (see Ward, Melser, & Yates, 2007). In other words, the RNR approach emphasizes avoidance of problems over the pursuit of a positive and healthy life. Therefore, holistic models such as the GLM and other strengths-based approaches have been well received in the field, although research on outcome is still lacking.

Further, we need to examine some of the factors that led individuals to become involved in the criminal justice system in the first place. While we do not wish to excuse the offending behavior, it is often the case that those involved in the criminal justice system have suffered significant abuse (e.g., Widom, 1989) which contributed to their delinquency. Thus, as described in Chap. 9, integrating trauma-focused care can complement other evidence-based treatments by helping the individual understand and cope more effectively with the trauma they themselves experienced therein decreasing their offending risk.

We also have to advocate for the reinstatement of university level education behind bars. While education is not a psychological intervention, it is an evidence-based intervention in that educations is one of the more important "hooks for change" among those who have committed a crime. While many prison college programs were disbanded in the 1960s and 1970s as the prison culture change from rehabilitation to punishment, we should not be short sighted. Unequivocally, getting an education decreases recidivism risk and increases the individuals' chances of obtaining meaningful employment, benefiting both the individual and society.

16.3 Conclusion

The promising findings reviewed in this book lead us to believe that the field is ripe for change. That said, while it is clear that we have moved beyond Martinson's "nothing works" conclusion, the field still lacks a clear accounting of and directory for evidence-based interventions. We hope that this text motivates those in the field to continue to adapt current evidence-based practices to the forensic contexts and to test those adaptations for efficacy. We also hope that the field will begin to develop a repository for evidence-based treatments, so that practitioners can readily find and access treatment modalities that have been shown to work. Ultimately, these evidence-based interventions—whether promising or proven to work—have the capacity to change not only the offenders themselves but the lives of all of us, as the treatment of offender populations can help to not only reduce crime but also increase the number of people in our communities living healthy and fulfilling lives.

References

American Psychological Association. (2017). *Multicultural guidelines: An ecological approach to context, identity, and intersectionality*. Retrieved from http://www.apa.org/about/policy/multicultural-guidelines.pdf

American Psychology-Law Society. (n.d.). *AP-LS mission, vision and core values*. Retrieved from http://www.apadivisions.org/division-41/about/mission.aspx

Andrews, D. A., & Bonta, J. (1998). *The psychology of criminal conduct* (2nd ed.). Cincinnati, OH: Anderson.

Andrews, D. A., Bonta, J., & Hoge, R. D. (1990). Classification for effective rehabilitation: Rediscovering psychology. *Criminal Justice and Behavior, 17*(1), 19–52. https://doi.org/10.1177/0093854890017001004

Castelnuovo, G. (2010). Empirically supported treatments in psychotherapy: Towards an evidence-based or evidence-biased psychology in clinical settings? *Frontiers in Psychology, 1*, 27. https://doi.org/10.3389/fpsyg.2010.00027

Chambless, D. L., & Ollendick, T. H. (2001). Empirically supported psychological interventions: Controversies and evidence. *Annual Review of Psychology, 52*, 685–716. https://doi.org/10.1146/annurev.psych.52.1.685

Dobash, R. E. (1979). *Violence against wives: A case against the patriarchy*. New York, NY: Free Press.

Greeson, J. K. P., Guo, S., Barth, R. P., Hurley, S., & Sisson, J. (2009). Contributions of therapist characteristics and stability to intensive in-home therapy youth outcomes. *Research on Social Work Practice, 19*(2), 239–250. https://doi.org/10.1177/1049731508329422

Hayes, S. C., & Hofmann, S. G. (2017). The third wave of cognitive behavioral therapy and the rise of process-based care. *World Psychiatry, 16*(3), 245–246. https://doi.org/10.1002/wps.20442

Jeglic, E. L., Hanson, R. K., & Calkins, C. (2016). Sex offender treatment: The need for cognitive behavioral therapists. *The Behavior Therapist, 39*(5), 162–168. Retrieved from http://www.abct.org/Journals/?m=mJournal&fa=TBT

Marshall, W. L., & Marshall, L. E. (2007). The utility of the random controlled trial for evaluating sexual offender treatment: The gold standard or an inappropriate strategy? *Sexual Abuse, 19*(2), 175–191. https://doi.org/10.1177/107906320701900207

Marshall, W. L., & Marshall, L. E. (2008). Good clinical practice and the evaluation of treatment: A response to Seto et al. *Sexual Abuse, 20*(3), 256–260. https://doi.org/10.1177/1079063208323839

Martinson, R. (1974). What works? Questions and answers about prison reform. *The Public Interest, 35*, 22–54. Retrieved from https://www.nationalaffairs.com/public_interest/issues/spring-1974

Meyer, O. L., & Zane, N. (2013). The influence of race and ethnicity in clients' experiences of mental health treatment. *Journal of Community Psychology, 41*(7), 884–901. https://doi.org/10.1002/jcop.21580

Park, T.-Y., & Shaw, J. D. (2013). Turnover rates and organizational performance: A meta-analysis. *Journal of Applied Psychology, 98*(2), 268–309. https://doi.org/10.1037/a0030723

Redding, R. E. (1997). Juveniles transferred to criminal court: Legal reform proposals based on social science research. *Utah Law Review,1997*(3), 709–763. Retrieved from https://dc.law.utah.edu/ulr/

Rosich, K. J. (2007). *Race, ethnicity, and the criminal justice system*. Washington, DC: American Sociological Association. Retrieved from http://www.asanet.org/sites/default/files/savvy/images/press/docs/pdf/ASARaceCrime.pdf

Schmucker, M., & Lösel, F. (2015). The effects of sexual offender treatment on recidivism: An international meta-analysis of sound quality evaluations. *Journal of Experimental Criminology, 11*(4), 597–630. https://doi.org/10.1007/s11292-015-9241-z

Seligman, M. E. P., & Csikszentmihalyi, M. (Eds.). (2000). Special issue on happiness, excellence, and optimal human functioning. *American Psychologist, 55*(1), 5–183.

Seto, M. C., Marques, J. K., Harris, G. T., Chaffin, M., Lalumière, M. L., Miner, M. H., ... Quinsey, V. L. (2008). Good science and progress in sex offender treatment are intertwined: A response to Marshall and Marshall (2007). *Sexual Abuse, 20*(3), 247–255. https://doi.org/10.1177/1079063208317733

Smith, M. L., & Glass, G. V. (1977). Meta-analysis of psychotherapy outcome studies. *American Psychologist, 32*(9), 752–760. https://doi.org/10.1037/0003-066X.32.9.752

Sue, S., Zane, N., Hall, G. C. N., & Berger, L. K. (2009). The case for cultural competency in psychotherapeutic interventions. *Annual Review of Psychology, 60*, 525–548. https://doi.org/10.1146/annurev.psych.60.110707.163651

Ward, T., & Gannon, T. A. (2006). Rehabilitation, etiology, and self-regulation: The comprehensive good lives model of treatment for sexual offenders. *Aggression and Violent Behavior, 11*(1), 77–94. https://doi.org/10.1016/j.avb.2005.06.001

Ward, T., Melser, J., & Yates, P. M. (2007). Reconstructing the risk-need-responsivity mode: A theoretical elaboration and evaluation. *Aggression and Violent Behavior, 12*(2), 208–228. https://doi.org/10.1016/j.avb.2006.07.001

Ward, T., & Stewart, C. A. (2003). The treatment of sex offenders: Risk management and good lives. *Professional Psychology: Research and Practice, 34*(4), 353–360. https://doi.org/10.1037/0735-7028.34.4.353

Webb, C. A., DeRubeis, R. J., & Barber, J. P. (2010). Therapists' adherence/competence and treatment outcome: A meta-analytic review. *Journal of Consulting and Clinical Psychology, 78*(2), 200–211. https://doi.org/10.1037/a0018912

Widom, C. S. (1989). Child abuse, neglect, and violent criminal behavior. *Criminology, 27*(2), 251–271. https://doi.org/10.1111/j.1745-9125.1989.tb01032.x

Young, S. (2014). Healthy behavior change in practical settings. *The Permenente Journal, 18*(4), 89–92. https://doi.org/10.7812/TPP/14-018

Index

E. L. Jeglic, C. Calkins (eds.), *New Frontiers in Offender Treatment*,
https://doi.org/10.1007/978-3-030-01030-0

N